Pain Medicine
UPDATES
Fast-Track Updates for Pain Clinicians

2025 EDITION

Authors

Guilherme Ferreira Dos Santos, MD, CIPS

Division of Pain Medicine, Department of Anesthesiology, Reanimation, and Pain Medicine, Hospital Clinic de Barcelona, University of Barcelona. Barcelona, Spain

Prof. Admir Hadzic, MD, PhD

NYSORA, New York, USA | Ziekenhuis Oost-Limburg, Genk, Belgium
Northwell health, New York USA

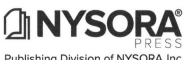

Publishing Division of NYSORA, Inc
2585 Broadway, suite 183, New York, NY10025
info@nysora.com, www.nysora.com

Contributors: NYSORA Educational Board

Introduction

As busy pain clinicians, we face increasing demands on our time - balancing patient care, administrative responsibilities, and the need for continuous professional development. Staying current with the latest research and advancements in pain medicine, pharmacology, and industry developments can be daunting, given the constant flow of new studies, guidelines, and updates from various publications, online platforms, and even social media. Recognizing this, NYSORA created Pain Medicine Updates 2025 with condensed, easy-to-read chapters covering the most significant developments in a format tailored for the busy practitioner.

This book is designed to cut through the noise, offering concise, practical insights that are directly applicable to the clinical practice of pain medicine. Each update has been carefully curated by Dr. Guilherme Ferreira Dos Santos, NYSORA's educational department, and an International Pain Medicine Educational Board, a team of scholars and practicing clinicians who reviewed and condensed essential findings from the past two years. With a unique double-peer-review process - combining internal and external reviews - the result is a distilled collection of the most critical advancements in pain medicine, ensuring accuracy, relevance, and immediate applicability.

The 2025 edition includes a range of relevance-based selected, expertly crafted updates organized into sections for easy navigation. Each topic reflects insights from the latest clinical trials, consensus guidelines, and innovations published in 2023-2024. Space is provided for personal notes, enabling readers to adapt the content to their practice. While references are intentionally limited to key sources, they guide those wishing to explore topics in greater depth.

Whether refreshing your knowledge or seeking the latest clinical insights, Pain Medicine Updates 2025 offers an indispensable resource to help you stay at the forefront of patient care and clinical excellence. It is our hope that this unique book format not only informs but inspires continuous learning and better outcomes for patients.

On behalf of NYSORA's team,
Dr. Guilherme Ferreira Dos Santos, MD, CIPS | Prof. Dr. Admir Hadzic, MD, PhD

Dedication

To the clinicians who strive every day to improve the lives of their patients and to the educators and researchers whose dedication to advancing the field makes this possible-this book is for you.

Your commitment to excellence inspires progress, and it is our privilege to support your journey. May Pain Medicine Updates 2025 serve as a trusted companion in your pursuit of knowledge, growth, and the highest standards of care.

Acknowledgments

We extend our deepest gratitude to the tireless researchers whose dedication and innovation have brought forth the new knowledge presented in this edition of Pain Medicine Updates. Your work is the foundation of progress in our field.

A heartfelt thank you to the NYSORA Fellows, whose meticulous efforts in selecting and curating the most impactful literature have been invaluable. To the ZOL Hospital in Genk, Belgium, your unwavering commitment to patient care and education inspires us daily.

To the exceptional NYSORA team and the NYSORA Pain Medicine Educational Board, your passion and dedication to advancing knowledge and improving outcomes in pain medicine make endeavors like this possible.

This book is a testament to the collective commitment to education, innovation, and excellence in pain medicine. Thank you all for your contributions.

▓ Notice / Disclaimer

The information contained in Pain Medicine Updates 2025 is intended to serve as a guide for practicing clinicians in the field of pain medicine. NYSORA Press and its contributors have made every effort to ensure the accuracy, completeness, and relevance of the content presented. However, medical knowledge is continually evolving, and new research or clinical guidelines may emerge after the publication of this book. NYSORA Press and NYSORA Inc. do not assume any liability or responsibility for any errors, omissions, or potential consequences arising from using the information provided. The clinical recommendations, techniques, and drug dosages presented in this text should be interpreted and applied by qualified healthcare professionals in conjunction with their clinical judgment, institutional protocols, and current best practices. Ultimately, the responsibility for patient care lies with the attending healthcare professional, and any application of the information provided in this text must be tailored to each patient's specific circumstances. NYSORA Press and NYSORA Inc. expressly disclaim any liability for adverse outcomes, including but not limited to injury, illness, or death, that may result from the application or interpretation of the content within Pain Medicine Updates 2025. By utilizing this book, readers acknowledge and accept that the responsibility for safe and effective patient care rests with the clinician's professional judgment and the proper application of current medical standards and practices.

Errata: While every effort has been made to ensure the accuracy and quality of this book, errors or areas for improvement may still exist. If you identify any inaccuracies or have suggestions for enhancing the content or visuals, please send your feedback to info@nysora.com. We value your input and may acknowledge contributions as appropriate. Thank you for supporting our commitment to continuous improvement.

▓ Library of Congress Identification

Authors: Guilherme Ferreira Dos Santos, MD, CIPS | Admir Hadzic, MD, PhD

Title: Pain Medicine Updates
Subtitle: Fast-Track Updates for Pain Clinicians
2025 Edition

Identifiers:
Library of Congress Control Number: 2024926441
ISBN: 979-8-9920578-0-5

Table of Contents

Headache & Orofacial Pain

Profiling migraine patients: Clinical and psychophysical subgroups............................12

Preventive pharmacological treatment of migraine 16

Anti-CGRP monoclonal antibodies for migraine in older adults............................20

Effectiveness of fremanezumab in managing migraine..26

Acute pharmacological treatment of migraine..30

Intranasal ketamine for refractory chronic migraine 34

Greater occipital nerve block with methylprednisolone and lidocaine for episodic cluster headaches 38

OnabotulinumtoxinA injections targeting the sphenopalatine ganglion for refractory headache disorders 42

Epidural blood or fibrin patches for post-dural puncture headache 46

Radiofrequency ablation of the occipital nerves for occipital neuralgia and chronic headaches 50

Cervical stabilization training for headache management 54

Surgical treatments for trigeminal neuralgia 58

DSA-guided ethanol rhizotomy for trigeminal neuralgia 64

Botulinum toxin for temporomandibular dysfunction-related myofascial pain........68

The relationship between insomnia and chronic orofacial pain..............................72

Spinal Pain

Delaying epidural steroid injections: Infection risks and platelet counts 78

Postpartum epidural steroid injections: Lipomatosis and steroid safety....................82

Cervical radicular pain: Diagnosis and management...86

Minimizing risks with cervical epidural injections..90

The safety of cervical transforaminal epidural steroid injections.............................94

Cervical transforaminal epidural steroid injections for cervical radicular pain.........98

Ultrasound-guided medial branch blocks to select patients for cervical facet joint radiofrequency neurotomy 102

Epidural steroid injections in lumbar spinal stenosis...106

The timeline of pain relief after epidural steroid injections 110

Lumbosacral radicular pain: Diagnosis and management 114

Lumbar transforaminal or interlaminar epidural steroid injections.........................118

Pain originating from the lumbar facet joints 122

Osteoarthritis of zygapophysial joints as a cause of back and neck pain................126

Sacroiliac joint pain: Diagnosis and management..130

Persistent spinal pain syndrome type 2: Diagnosis and management 134

Musculoskeletal Pain & Regional Pain Syndromes

Local anesthetic chondrotoxicity and safety in stellate ganglion blocks 140

Oral corticosteroids for complex regional pain syndrome 144

Lumbar sympathetic blocks with thermographic monitoring for complex regional pain syndrome...148

Sympathetic blocks to predict ketamine infusion response in complex
regional pain syndrome 152
Perfusion index for monitoring response to intravenous ketamine in complex
regional pain syndrome 156
Patient outcomes following rehabilitation in early or persistent complex
regional pain syndrome 160
Continuous peripheral nerve blocks for postamputation phantom and residual limb pain ... 164
Radiofrequency thermocoagulation for chronic hip pain 168
Polynucleotide, sodium hyaluronate, or crosslinked sodium hyaluronate for
knee osteoarthritis 172
Genicular nerve radiofrequency ablation for chronic knee pain 176
Genicular nerve ablation for osteoarthritic and post-total knee arthroplasty pain ... 180
Cooled and monopolar radiofrequency ablation for chronic knee pain 184
Cooled or conventional radiofrequency treatment of the genicular nerves for chronic
knee pain 188
Cryoneurolysis for chronic knee pain 192
Shear wave elastography in musculoskeletal injuries 196

Cancer Pain

Predictors and consequences of cancer-related and non-cancer-related
pain in oncology 202
Use of opioids for adults with cancer pain 206
Opioid analgesics for nociceptive cancer pain 210
Neuropathic pain in cancer: Diagnosis and management 214
Predictors of successful opioid response in cancer patients 218
Optimizing opioid dose titration for cancer pain 222
Pain management in cervical cancer 226
Pharmacologic management of cancer-related pain in pregnant patients 230
Cancer pain management in inpatient specialized palliative care settings 234
Multimodal locoregional procedures for cancer pain management 238
Epidural analgesia for intractable cancer pain 242
Intrathecal drug delivery in cancer-related pain 246
Efficacy and safety of intrathecal infusion devices for cancer pain 250
Cancer-related pain management in suitable intrathecal therapy candidates 254
Controversies in intrathecal drug delivery for cancer pain 260

Pharmacology & Transitional Pain

Pharmacodynamic effects of co-administered cannabinoids and opioids in
pain management 266
Opioid tapering in patients with chronic non-cancer pain 272
Long-term postoperative opioid use in orthopedic patients 278
Persistent opioid use following traumatic injury 282
Transitional pain services and postoperative opioid trajectories 286
Low-dose naltrexone for centralized pain conditions 290
Duloxetine for managing central post-stroke pain 294
Soticlestat as adjunctive therapy for complex regional pain syndrome 298

Analgesic properties of anti-osteoporotic drugs...302
Prescribing patterns in older adults with chronic non-cancer pain...........................308

Neuromodulation

A classification and definition framework for neuromodulation for chronic pain 314
Mitigating complications of neurostimulation 318
Long-term outcomes and salvage strategies in spinal cord stimulation.........................322
Factors predicting pain relief after spinal cord stimulation....................................326
Differential target multiplexed spinal cord stimulation for intractable low back pain............330
The duration of carryover effects in spinal cord stimulation...................................334
Impact of prior lumbar spine surgeries on spinal cord stimulation outcomes 338
Outcomes of single-stage spinal cord stimulation..342
Long-term outcomes of closed-loop and open-loop spinal cord stimulation 346
Identifying nonresponders to high-frequency spinal cord stimulation 350
Intrathecal drug delivery for chronic noncancer pain 354
The efficacy of 60-day percutaneous peripheral nerve stimulation after total
knee arthroplasty 360
Pre-implant diagnostic nerve blocks for peripheral nerve stimulation 364
Multifidus dysfunction and restorative neurostimulation 368
Long-term effectiveness of restorative neurostimulation in multifidus
muscle dysfunction..372

Regenerative Medicine

Regenerative medicine treatments for chronic pain 378
Cell transplantation and platelet-rich plasma for disc degeneration-related back and
neck pain...382
Orthobiologic injections for discogenic chronic low back pain 386
Subacromial injection of platelet-rich plasma or corticosteroids for rotator
cuff tendinopathy...390
Platelet-rich plasma therapy for adhesive capsulitis...394
Platelet-rich plasma or corticosteroids for lateral epicondylitis.................................400
Platelet-rich plasma injections for knee osteoarthritis 404
Three doses or one dose of platelet-rich plasma in knee osteoarthritis..........................408
Platelet-rich plasma in foot and ankle pathologies..412
The impact of platelet dose on the efficacy of platelet-rich plasma therapy for
musculoskeletal conditions..416

Psychology, Psychiatry & Neuroscience

Psychologically based interventions for adults with chronic neuropathic pain....................422
Emotion regulation and pain catastrophizing in patients with chronic pain.......................426
The role of chronic pain acceptance in moderating suicidal cognitions..........................430
Predicting quality of life in phantom limb pain using neuropsychiatric drugs and
neurophysiological markers 434
Psychological factors influencing pain medication use in adolescents with
chronic pain 438

Headache & Orofacial Pain

Profiling migraine patients: Clinical and psychophysical subgroups

01

Why this topic is important

Migraine affects approximately 15% of the global population, significantly impacting quality of life and productivity. While advancements in pharmacological treatments such as CGRP inhibitors have shown promise, up to 66% of patients fail to respond to these therapies. Personalized medicine, which tailors treatment based on individual patient profiles, is crucial for improving outcomes.

This study by Di Antonio et al. (2023) uses cluster analysis to classify migraine patients into distinct subgroups based on clinical and psychophysical characteristics. By identifying variations in pain sensitivity, musculoskeletal dysfunctions, and headache-related disability, these findings pave the way for targeted therapies and enhanced care strategies.

Objectives of this update

- Highlight the importance of psychophysical profiling in understanding migraine subgroups.

- Summarize the identified clusters and their clinical implications.

- Discuss how these findings inform personalized and multidisciplinary migraine management.

What is new

This study introduces several advancements in migraine research:

- **Cluster analysis:** Migraine patients were categorized into distinct subgroups during ictal/perictal and interictal phases based on measurable clinical and psychophysical traits.

- **Predictive tools:** Pressure pain thresholds (PPT) and cervical range of motion (AROM) were identified as reliable predictors of subgroup classification.

- **Personalized care:** Insights into how specific subgroups respond differently to pharmacological and physical therapies, fostering precision medicine approaches.

Methodology

- **Design:** Observational, multicenter study involving 198 patients with episodic (EM) or chronic migraine (CM).
- **Phases:** Patients were assessed during ictal/perictal (n=100) or interictal (n=98) phases using AROM measurements, PPT algometry, and standardized disability questionnaires.
- **Analysis:** K-means clustering identified subgroups with shared characteristics.

Results

Ictal/perictal phase

Two clusters were identified:

- **Cluster 1.1 (19%):**
  - Patients showed no psychophysical impairments.
  - A higher percentage of males (32%) and lower headache-related disability scores.
- **Cluster 1.2 (81%):**
  - Patients exhibited widespread pain sensitivity and reduced AROM.
  - Increased headache-related emotional disability and psychological burden (e.g., anxiety and depression).

Interictal phase

Three clusters emerged:

- **Cluster 2.1 (18%):**
  - No psychophysical impairments, mirroring Cluster 1.1.
  - Stable AROM and PPT values.
- **Cluster 2.2 (45%):**
  - Increased pain sensitivity but no cervical musculoskeletal dysfunction.
  - Younger patients with lower headache frequency and disability.

- **Cluster 2.3 (37%):**
  - Combined pain sensitivity and cervical musculoskeletal impairments.
  - Older patients with prolonged disease duration, higher headache frequency, and greater disability.

Implications for clinical practice

This study highlights the heterogeneity of migraine and underscores the importance of psychophysical characteristics in shaping patient care. The distinction between pain sensitivity and musculoskeletal dysfunction provides a foundation for stratifying patients into treatment-specific subgroups.

Predictive tools

1. **PPT assessment:** Lower thresholds over the temporalis, cervical, and distal sites indicate heightened pain sensitivity.
2. **AROM evaluation:** Reduced movement during cervical flexion, extension, and lateral flexion correlates with musculoskeletal dysfunction.

Recommendations for care

- **Subgroup-specific management:**
  - Cluster 1.1/2.1: Pharmacological preventives targeting neural pathways may suffice.
  - Cluster 1.2/2.3: Multidisciplinary approaches incorporating physiotherapy to restore AROM and reduce pain sensitivity are essential.
- **Personalized therapies:**
  - Consider preventive treatments with central nervous system effects for clusters with heightened pain sensitivity.
  - Introduce targeted physical therapies, such as manual techniques, for those with cervical musculoskeletal dysfunctions.

- **Routine assessments:**
  - Integrate PPT and AROM measurements into standard migraine evaluations.
  - Use these metrics to monitor disease progression and therapy response.

Key takeaways

☑ Psychophysical profiling identifies meaningful subgroups among migraine patients, guiding targeted interventions.

☑ Subgroups with combined pain sensitivity and musculoskeletal dysfunction require multidisciplinary management strategies.

☑ Routine use of AROM and PPT tools in clinical settings enhances diagnostic precision and treatment customization.

☑ Ongoing research is needed to refine these findings and develop standardized protocols for personalized care.

Additional recommended reading:

1. Di Antonio S, Arendt-Nielsen L, Castaldo M, et al. Profiling migraine patients according to clinical and psychophysical characteristics: A cluster analysis approach. *Pain Med.* 2023;24(9):1046-1057.

2. Fernández-de-las-Peñas C, Navarro-Santana MJ, et al. Localized and widespread pressure pain hypersensitivity in episodic and chronic migraine. *Cephalalgia.* 2022;42(9):966-980.

3. Pan LLH, Wang YF, Ling YH, et al. Pain sensitivities predict prophylactic treatment outcomes in chronic migraine: A prospective study. *Cephalalgia.* 2022;42(9):899-909.

Preventive pharmacological treatment of migraine

02

Why this topic is important

Migraine is a leading cause of disability worldwide, affecting millions of individuals across all age groups. As a chronic and often debilitating neurological condition, it significantly impacts quality of life, work productivity, and societal costs. Preventive pharmacological treatment is a cornerstone of migraine management, aiming to reduce the frequency, severity, and duration of migraine attacks while minimizing reliance on acute treatments.

Despite the availability of numerous preventive therapies, inconsistent access, lack of standardized approaches, and varying efficacy pose challenges in delivering optimal care. The 2024 IHS global practice recommendations provide a comprehensive, evidence-based framework to guide clinicians in selecting and optimizing preventive treatments for migraine, adapted to diverse healthcare settings worldwide.

Objectives of this update

- Identify candidates for preventive pharmacological treatment based on migraine frequency, disability, and response to acute therapies.

- Highlight evidence-based recommendations for the selection and evaluation of preventive therapies.

- Address practical considerations, including combination therapy, managing comorbidities, and treatment duration.

What is new

The 2024 IHS recommendations integrate key updates:

- **Candidate criteria:** Preventive treatment is recommended for individuals with ≥ 4 monthly migraine days or substantial disability, incorporating shared decision-making.

- **Treatment stratification:** Dual guidance for "Optimal" (full drug availability) and "Essential" (limited availability) scenarios ensures global applicability.

- **Emerging therapies:** Including monoclonal antibodies targeting the calcitonin gene-related peptide (CGRP) pathway and gepants highlights advancements in migraine prevention.

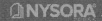

Candidate selection for preventive therapy

Preventive treatment is advised for individuals experiencing:

- **High migraine frequency:** ≥ 4 monthly migraine days.

- **Significant disability:** Impacts personal, professional, or social life.

- **Inadequate response to acute therapies:** Frequent or ineffective acute medication use.

Additional considerations include:

- Presence of hemiplegic migraine or prolonged aura.

- Risk of medication overuse headache.

Recommended preventive therapies

Traditional therapies

- **Beta-blockers** (e.g., propranolol, metoprolol): Effective for episodic migraine, particularly in patients with comorbid hypertension or anxiety.

- **Antiepileptics** (e.g., topiramate, valproate): Effective for episodic and chronic migraines. Topiramate is preferred, but caution is required in women of childbearing potential.

- **Antidepressants** (e.g., amitriptyline): Beneficial for patients with comorbid depression or insomnia.

Emerging therapies

- **CGRP monoclonal antibodies:**

  - Drugs like erenumab, fremanezumab, and galcanezumab target the CGRP pathway, offering efficacy in both episodic and chronic migraine.

  - Advantages include rapid onset, favorable tolerability, and minimal drug-drug interactions.

- **Gepants** (e.g., atogepant, rimegepant): Oral CGRP receptor antagonists with dual utility in acute and preventive settings.

- **OnabotulinumtoxinA:** Approved for chronic migraine, offering sustained benefits in select populations.

Evaluating effectiveness

Timeline for assessment

- **Oral drugs**: Evaluate after 3 months at the target dose.

- **Injectable therapies**: Minimum evaluation period of 3 months for monthly administration and 6 months for quarterly treatments.

Criteria for success

- ≥ 50% reduction in monthly migraine days (30% for chronic migraine).

- Clinically meaningful improvement in patient-reported outcomes (e.g., MIDAS, HIT-6 scores).

Combination therapy

When to consider combinations

Combination therapy is recommended for individuals with:

- Partial response to monotherapy.

- Complex comorbidities requiring treatment overlap.

Evidence and combinations

While formal evidence for combination therapy is limited, common combinations include:

- **Topiramate with propranolol:** Different mechanisms may enhance efficacy.

- **CGRP monoclonal antibodies with onabo-tulinumtoxinA:** Observational studies suggest additive benefits.

Caution is advised to avoid overlapping side effects or drug interactions.

Addressing comorbidities

Preventive therapy selection should consider comorbid conditions to maximize benefits and minimize risks:

- **Hypertension:** Beta-blockers or candesartan.

- **Obesity:** Topiramate.

- **Depression or anxiety:** Amitriptyline or venlafaxine.

- **Epilepsy:** Valproate or topiramate.

Conversely, some medications should be avoided (e.g., beta-blockers in asthma).

Treatment duration and discontinuation

- **Minimum duration:** Continue effective preventive treatment for at least 6 months (oral drugs) or 12 months (injectables).

- **Discontinuation criteria:** Consider tapering after 3 consecutive months of sustained improvement (< 4 monthly migraine days).

- **Monitoring:** Use headache diaries to track symptom recurrence and guide reinitiation if necessary.

Key takeaways

☑ Preventive pharmacological treatment is essential for individuals with frequent or disabling migraines, offering significant reductions in attack burden and improved quality of life.

☑ CGRP-targeting therapies and gepants represent significant advancements, expanding options for refractory cases.

☑ Considering comorbidities and patient preferences, individualized care is crucial for optimizing outcomes.

☑ Consistent monitoring and shared decision-making ensure treatment alignment with patient goals.

Additional recommended reading:

1. Puledda F, Sacco S, Diener HC, et al. International Headache Society global practice recommendations for preventive pharmacological treatment of migraine. *Cephalalgia*. 2024;44(9):1-31.

2. Dodick DW, Silberstein SD. Migraine prevention. *Neurology*. 2018;91(21): e2115-e2125.

3. Lipton RB, Dodick DW, Silberstein SD, et al. Efficacy and safety of fremanezumab for the preventive treatment of chronic migraine. *JAMA*. 2018;319(19): 1999-2008.

Anti-CGRP monoclonal antibodies for migraine in older adults

03

Why this topic is important

Migraine, a prevalent and disabling neurological condition, remains underdiagnosed and undertreated in older adults. Although migraines often diminish in frequency with age, a significant proportion of elderly individuals continue to suffer, often with added challenges of multimorbidity and polypharmacy. The introduction of calcitonin gene-related peptide (CGRP) monoclonal antibodies (mAbs) has transformed migraine prevention. Still, evidence for their use in patients over 65 years old remains limited due to exclusion from clinical trials.

The study by Gonzalez-Martinez et al. (2024) provides critical insights into the real-world effectiveness and safety of anti-CGRP mAbs in older adults, addressing concerns about tolerability and identifying potential predictors of treatment response. This update offers guidance on optimizing migraine care in this underserved population.

Objectives of this update

- Assess the effectiveness of anti-CGRP mAbs in reducing migraine and headache frequency in elderly patients.

- Evaluate the safety profile and tolerability of anti-CGRP mAbs in older adults.

- Identify potential predictors of treatment response to guide clinical decision-making.

What is new

This study highlights significant findings for clinical practice:

- **Effectiveness:** Anti-CGRP mAbs reduced monthly headache days (MHD) and migraine days (MMD) in elderly patients, with comparable results to younger cohorts over time.

- **Safety:** Tolerability in older adults was similar to that in younger patients, with minimal adverse events (AEs) and no treatment discontinuations due to side effects.

- **Predictors of response:** Episodic migraine (EM) diagnosis and lower baseline MHD were associated with better treatment outcomes in elderly patients.

Methods

- **Design:** A multicenter, observational case-control study in nine headache units across Spain.

- **Participants:**

  ○ **Cases:** 114 patients aged ≥ 65 years (mean age 70.1 years).

  ○ **Controls:** 114 sex-matched patients aged < 55 years (mean age 42.9 years).

  ○ **Inclusion criteria:** EM or chronic migraine (CM) diagnosis, failure of ≥ 2 preventive treatments, including onabotulinumtoxinA for CM.

  ○ **Etiology:** 17.5% EM, 82.5% CM.

- **Primary endpoint:** 50% reduction in MHD at 20-24 weeks.

- **Secondary endpoints:** Changes in MHD, MMD, and responder rates (30%, 50%, 75%) at various time points.

Results

Effectiveness

- **Primary endpoint**

  ○ **Elderly patients:** 57.5% achieved a 50% reduction in monthly headache days (MHD) at 20-24 weeks.

  ○ **Younger controls:** 60.8% achieved a 50% reduction in MHD at 20-24 weeks.

- **Responder rates**

  ○ **30% Reduction in Monthly Migraine Days (MMD):**

    • Elderly patients: 68.5% at 20-24 weeks.

    • Younger controls: A higher 30% responder rate at 20-24 weeks compared to elderly patients.

  ○ **50% Reduction in MHD:**

    • Elderly patients: 63.6% by 44-48 weeks.

    • Younger controls: Similar rates were observed by 44-48 weeks.

  ○ **75% Reduction in MMD:**

    • Elderly patients: 21.9% achieved this at 20-24 weeks.

    • Younger controls: Comparable rates to elderly patients at 20-24 weeks.

- **Time to response**

  ○ Elderly patients exhibited **slower initial reductions in MHD** at 8-12 weeks compared to younger controls **(5.0 vs. 8.8 days).**

  ○ These differences diminished by 20-24 weeks, and response rates became more aligned between the two groups.

Safety and tolerability

- **Adverse events:** Reported in 32% of participants across both age groups. Common AEs included:

  ○ Constipation (15.3%)

  ○ Dizziness (8.3%)

  ○ Local injection site reactions (6.6%)

- **Serious adverse events:** None were reported in the elderly group.

- **Tolerability:** No treatment discontinuations occurred due to AEs, and elderly patients tolerated anti-CGRP mAbs comparably to younger individuals.

Predictors of response

- **Positive predictors:**

  ○ Diagnosis of EM (associated with a 50% reduction in MHD at the 20-24 week time point).

  ○ Lower baseline MHD (greater reductions at 20-24 weeks).

- **Initial response as a predictor:** Any degree of reduction MHD reductions at 8-12 weeks strongly correlated with long-term improvements at 20-24 weeks.

Implications for clinical practice

This study supports the inclusion of anti-CGRP mAbs in migraine prevention protocols for elderly patients, addressing the unmet need for effective treatments with minimal systemic risks.

Recommendations

- **Patient selection:**
  - Consider anti-CGRP therapies for patients with EM or CM who have not responded to standard preventive treatments.
  - Evaluate comorbidities, such as vascular risks, to help guide and personalize management plans.

- **Monitoring:**
  - Monitor response during the first 12 weeks to help decide whether to continue treatment.
  - Encourage the use of headache diaries to track changes in MHD and MMD for more accurate assessment.

- **Tolerability considerations:**
  - Discuss potential adverse events (AEs) with patients, highlighting that they are often mild or transient.
  - Schedule regular follow-ups to support early identification and management of side effects if they occur.

Limitations

- **Generalizability:** Findings may not apply to broader populations due to the specific study cohort.
- **Retrospective design:** Potential biases from retrospective data collection.
- **Short-term monitoring:** Limited data on long-term safety and efficacy beyond 48 weeks.
- **Comorbidities:** Impact of untreated vascular risks or other conditions was not fully explored.
- **No placebo control:** Effects may include natural variability or placebo response.
- **Attrition:** Patient dropouts may have influenced long-term results.
- **Predictor analysis:** Limited exploration of complex interactions between response predictors.

Key takeaways

- ☑ Anti-CGRP mAbs reduce headache and migraine frequency in elderly patients, with over 50% achieving a significant reduction in monthly headache days (MHD) by 20-24 weeks.

- ☑ Safety and tolerability profiles are generally favorable, though vascular comorbidities should be monitored closely, especially in older patients.

- ☑ Early reductions in MHD during the first 8-12 weeks can predict long-term response, emphasizing the value of initial treatment evaluations.

- ☑ Anti-CGRP mAbs provide an alternative for older adults with migraine, but further research is needed to confirm long-term safety and effectiveness in this population.

Additional recommended reading:

1. Gonzalez-Martinez A, Sanz-García A, García-Azorín D, et al. Effectiveness, tolerability, and response predictors of preventive anti-CGRP mAbs for migraine in patients over 65 years old: A multicenter real-world case-control study. *Pain Med.* 2024;25(3):194-202.

2. Cetta I, Messina R, Zanandrea L, et al. Comparison of efficacy and safety of erenumab between over and under 65-year-old refractory migraine patients. *Neurol Sci.* 2022;43(9):5769-5771.

3. Nahas SJ, Naegel S, Cohen JM, et al. Efficacy and safety of fremanezumab in clinical trial participants aged ≥60 years with episodic or chronic migraine. *J Headache Pain.* 2022;23(1):57.

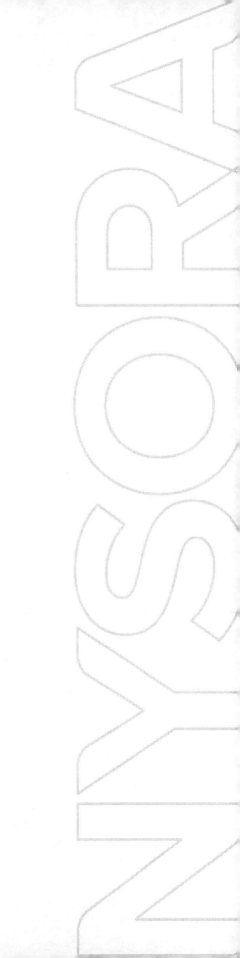

Effectiveness of fremanezumab in managing migraine

04

Why this topic is important

Migraine is a disabling neurological condition with a global prevalence of 14.4%, significantly impacting quality of life and productivity. Chronic migraine (CM) and episodic migraine (EM) pose challenges due to their refractory nature in many patients. The advent of calcitonin gene-related peptide (CGRP) monoclonal antibodies, including fremanezumab, has transformed migraine prevention. However, real-world data are essential to validate clinical trial findings in diverse populations and settings.

The study by Kikui et al. (2024) evaluates fremanezumab's effectiveness and safety in a Japanese cohort, addressing its impact on migraine burden and identifying factors influencing treatment outcomes. This update explores the role of fremanezumab in real-world migraine management, emphasizing the nuanced needs of EM and CM patients.

Objectives of this update

- Assess fremanezumab's effectiveness in reducing migraine and headache days (MMD and MHD) and acute medication days (AMD).

- Highlight differences in response between EM and CM patients.

- Provide insights into safety, tolerability, and factors predicting treatment success or failure.

What is new

This study introduces critical findings for clinical practice:

- **Sustained efficacy:** Fremanezumab significantly reduces MHD, MMD, and AMD across 12 months.

- **Differential response:** EM patients show quicker improvements, while CM patients require longer treatment durations for maximal benefit.

- **Safety profile:** Low adverse event (AE) rates and no treatment discontinuations reinforce fremanezumab's tolerability.

Methods

- **Design**
  - Retrospective real-world study conducted at a Japanese headache center.

- **Participants**
  - The study included 165 patients with migraine (17 males and 148 females; 89.7% female), with an average age of 45.5 ± 16.0 years. Among these patients:
    - 53 had episodic migraine (EM), and 112 had chronic migraine (CM).
    - 67 patients also had medication-overuse headache (MOH).
    - 75.7% (125 patients) were naïve to anti-calcitonin gene-related peptide monoclonal antibodies (anti-CGRP mAbs).

- **Intervention**
  - Fremanezumab administered as 225 mg monthly or 675 mg quarterly based on patient preference for up to one year.

- **Outcome measures**
  - Changes in MMD, MHD, and AMD; responder rates (≥ 50% reduction in MMD); safety and tolerability assessments.

Results

Effectiveness

EM group

- Baseline MHD: 8.1 ± 4.0 days. Reduced to 4.6 ± 3.3 days after 12 months.

- Baseline MMD: 5.9 ± 1.8 days. Reduced to 3.5 ± 2.7 days after 12 months.

- Responder rates (≥ 50% reduction in MMD): Achieved by 57.1% at 12 months.

CM group

- Baseline MHD: 20.9 ± 6.1 days. Reduced to 12.0 ± 9.1 days after 12 months.

- Baseline MMD: 16.8 ± 6.8 days. Reduced to 8.3 ± 7.5 days after 12 months.

- Responder rates: Gradual improvement with 54.2% achieving ≥ 50% reduction in MMD at 12 months.

Safety and tolerability

- **Adverse events:** Reported in 4.8% of patients, including injection site reactions (2.4%), constipation, malaise, rash, and pruritus.

- **Serious adverse events:** None reported.

- **Tolerability in elderly patients:** No AEs were observed in patients aged ≥ 70 years.

Predictors of response

- **Negative predictors:**
  - Medication-overuse headache (MOH): Associated with a 70% reduced likelihood of achieving ≥ 50% reduction in MMD.
  - Long migraine history (> 21 years): 63% reduced likelihood of achieving a ≥ 50% reduction in MMD.
  - Prior failure of ≥ 2 preventive medications: 67% reduced likelihood of achieving a ≥ 50% reduction in MMD.

- **Favorable predictors:**
  - Shorter migraine history and absence of MOH.
  - Earlier response during the first 3 months predicted sustained benefits.

Implications for clinical practice

Fremanezumab has demonstrated effectiveness and safety for both episodic migraine (EM) and chronic migraine (CM), offering sustained benefits over 12 months. While its efficacy may be reduced in patients with multiple negative predictors (e.g., long migraine history, MOH, or failure of multiple prior treatments), it remains an important option for:

- Patients who are unresponsive to traditional oral preventives but have a shorter migraine history or fewer comorbidities such as MOH.
- Individuals with minimal tolerance for side effects or multiple comorbid conditions that limit oral preventive options.

Recommendations for use

- **Patient selection**
  - Consider screening for MOH and other potential negative predictors to help manage treatment expectations effectively.
- **Treatment timeline**
  - For CM: Patients may benefit from continuing treatment for at least 6 months to potentially achieve the full therapeutic effects.
  - For EM: Early improvements may be observed, but sustained treatment may be important for long-term benefits.
- **Monitoring and adjudstments**
  - Encourage the use of headache diaries to document changes in MHD, MMD, and AMD.

  - Periodically assess treatment response and adjust therapy as necessary, particularly for patients who do not show improvement in the early stages of treatment.

Limitations

- **Retrospective design:** Limits causal interpretations and introduces selection bias.
- **Single-center study:** Findings may not generalize to other populations or regions.
- **No placebo control:** Effects of fremanezumab may be confounded by placebo or natural variability.
- **Patient attrition:** Only 60% completed 12 months, potentially biasing outcomes.
- **Heterogeneous population:** Varied treatment histories and comorbidities complicate uniform conclusions.
- **Short-term safety data:** Limited evaluation of rare or long-term adverse effects.
- **Self-reported outcomes:** Potential inaccuracies from headache diaries and patient recall.
- **Concurrent medications:** Use of other treatments may have influenced results.

Key takeaways

☑ Fremanezumab reduces monthly headache and migraine days with sustained benefits over 12 months.

☑ EM patients respond faster, while CM patients may require ≥ 6 months for maximal effects.

☑ Low adverse event rates and high tolerability make it safe for diverse populations, including the elderly.

☑ Predictors like MOH and prior treatment failure highlight the need for tailored treatment strategies.

☑ Study limitations, including retrospective design and patient attrition, should guide interpretation and expectations.

Additional recommended reading:

1. Kikui S, Daisuke D, Miyahara J, et al. Effectiveness of fremanezumab treatment in patients with migraine headache: A real-world study. *Pain Med.* 2024;25:664-670.

2. Goadsby PJ, Silberstein SD, Dodick DW, et al. Long-term efficacy and safety of fremanezumab in migraine prevention. *Neurology.* 2020;95:e2487-e2499.

3. Ferrari MD, Diener HC, Ning X, et al. Fremanezumab for migraine prevention in refractory cases: A phase 3 trial. *Lancet.* 2019;394:1030-1040.

Acute pharmacological treatment of migraine

05

Why this topic is important

Migraine is a complex and disabling neurological condition, ranking among the leading causes of disability worldwide. Acute attacks significantly impair quality of life, productivity, and well-being. While various medications exist for treating migraines, access, efficacy, and tolerability vary widely across populations and settings. Mismanagement of acute attacks can lead to complications like medication overuse headaches (MOH), necessitating a balanced, evidence-based approach to treatment.

The International Headache Society (IHS) developed these global practice recommendations to address the disparities in migraine treatment by categorizing strategies into **optimal** and **essential** levels. This approach ensures applicability in diverse healthcare systems, from resource-rich environments to underserved regions relying on essential medications listed by the World Health Organization (WHO).

Objectives of this update

- Provide evidence-based guidelines for the selection of acute migraine therapies across different resource settings.

- Highlight strategies to minimize risks like medication overuse and optimize patient outcomes.

- Equip clinicians with practical tools for tailoring treatments to individual patient needs.

What is new

This update emphasizes advancements in acute migraine care:

- **Dual-level recommendations:** Differentiating between "optimal" and "essential" strategies ensures broader global applicability.

- **Innovative therapies:** Inclusion of newer drug classes like gepants and lasmiditan, expanding options for patients unresponsive to traditional treatments.

- **Focus on outcomes:** Improved guidelines for timing and combination of medications enhance treatment efficacy and patient satisfaction.

Clinical recommendations

Candidate selection for acute treatment

Acute pharmacological treatment is indicated for individuals with moderate to severe migraine attacks or those experiencing disabling mild migraines. Key factors influencing treatment choice include:

- Attack severity and associated symptoms (e.g., nausea, vomiting, sensitivity to light/sound).

- Comorbidities such as cardiovascular disease or gastrointestinal disorders.

- Accessibility and availability of medications in the patient's healthcare setting.

Recommended medications

- **Analgesics and NSAIDs**

  - **Optimal level:** Ibuprofen (400-600 mg), naproxen (500-1000 mg), or diclofenac (50 mg) are first-line options due to their affordability and efficacy.

  - **Essential level:** Paracetamol (1000 mg) is a viable alternative, especially where NSAIDs are unavailable or contraindicated.

- **Triptans**

  - **Optimal level:** Triptans are highly effective migraine-specific agents. Choices include sumatriptan (50-100 mg), zolmitriptan (2.5 mg), or rizatriptan (5-10 mg), with nasal sprays and subcutaneous forms available for patients with nausea or vomiting.

  - **Essential level:** Sumatriptan remains the most widely available triptan, recommended as a first-line treatment when NSAIDs fail.

- **Gepants and lasmiditan**

  - **Gepants** (e.g., rimegepant, ubrogepant): Suitable for patients who cannot tolerate or do not respond to triptans.

  - **Lasmiditan:** Reserved for patients with cardiovascular contraindications to triptans.

These newer agents are included in the optimal category but are less accessible in resource-limited settings.

- **Ergot derivatives**

  - **Optimal level:** Dihydroergotamine nasal spray or injectable forms may be used when other treatments fail.

  - **Essential level:** Ergotamine tartrate remains an option but is generally less favored due to side effects and limited efficacy than triptans.

- **Anti-nausea medications**

  - Adjunctive antiemetics like metoclopramide (10 mg) or domperidone (10 mg) improve medication absorption and alleviate nausea.

Timing and administration strategies

- **Early intervention:** Medications are most effective when taken at the onset of an attack or during the mild pain phase.

- **Combination therapy:** Combining triptans with NSAIDs (e.g., sumatriptan 85 mg + naproxen 500 mg) enhances efficacy and prevents headache relapse.

- **Non-oral routes:** For patients with nausea or early vomiting, consider subcutaneous, intranasal, or rectal formulations.

Minimizing risks

Excessive use of acute treatments increases the risk of MOH. To prevent this:

- Limit triptan or combination analgesic use to 8 days/month.

- Limit NSAIDs or paracetamol to 10 days/month.

Addressing treatment failure

Patients unresponsive to their initial medication should try alternative options, such as:

- Switching to a different triptan or dose.
- Combining triptans with NSAIDs.
- Exploring newer therapies like gepants.

Special populations

- **Pregnancy and breastfeeding**

    ○ Paracetamol is the preferred first-line therapy during pregnancy.

    ○ Triptans and NSAIDs may be used with caution in select cases, avoiding NSAIDs in the third trimester.

- **Pediatric and geriatric patients**

    ○ Pediatrics: Paracetamol (15 mg/kg) or ibuprofen (10 mg/kg) is recommended for children and adolescents. Rizatriptan is preferred among triptans.

    ○ Geriatrics: Use paracetamol or low-dose NSAIDs cautiously, monitoring for gastrointestinal and cardiovascular risks.

Key takeaways

☑ Acute migraine treatment should be tailored to attack severity, patient preference, and resource availability.

☑ NSAIDs and triptans are first-line therapies, with gepants and lasmiditan offering alternatives for refractory cases.

☑ Early intervention and combination strategies improve efficacy and reduce relapse rates.

☑ Limiting medication use and considering special populations ensures safer, more effective management.

Additional recommended reading:

1. Puledda F, Sacco S, Diener HC, et al. International Headache Society global practice recommendations for the acute pharmacological treatment of migraine. *Cephalalgia*. 2024;44(8):1-45.

2. Tfelt-Hansen P, De Vries P, Saxena PR. Triptans in migraine: A comparative review of pharmacology, pharmacokinetics and efficacy. *Drugs*. 2000;60(6):1259-1287.

3. Lipton RB, Munjal S, Buse DC, et al. Reduction in headache burden with rimegepant: Results from a randomized, double-blind, placebo-controlled trial. *Neurology*. 2019;92(7-e752).

Intranasal ketamine for refractory chronic migraine

06

Why this topic is important

Chronic migraine (CM) is a highly disabling condition, with patients often experiencing 15 or more headache days per month, of which at least 8 are migraine. The refractory subtype, refractory chronic migraine (rCM), poses even greater challenges due to its resistance to standard preventive and acute treatments. This has significant physical, emotional, and economic burdens on affected individuals and healthcare systems.

Ketamine, a dissociative anesthetic with unique mechanisms of action, including N-methyl-D-aspartate (NMDA) receptor antagonism, has shown promise in managing refractory pain conditions. While intravenous (IV) ketamine is well-studied, its use is limited by the need for specialized inpatient settings. Intranasal (IN) ketamine provides a convenient outpatient alternative, but evidence of its safety and efficacy for rCM remains limited. The retrospective study by Yuan et al. (2023) explores real-world outcomes of IN ketamine use in rCM, shedding light on its potential as a rescue therapy for this challenging condition.

Objectives of this update

- Evaluate the effectiveness of IN ketamine in reducing pain intensity and improving quality of life in rCM patients.

- Examine the safety profile and tolerability of IN ketamine in outpatient settings.

- Provide insights into real-world usage patterns and clinical implications for incorporating IN ketamine into migraine management.

What is new

This study contributes novel findings to the literature:

- **Effectiveness:** IN ketamine significantly reduced headache intensity and frequency for many rCM patients.

- **Tolerability:** Despite mild-to-moderate adverse events (AEs), most patients continued using IN ketamine due to its perceived benefits.

- **Practical insights:** Real-world data on dosage, administration, and patient adherence informs clinical protocols.

Methodology

- **Design:** Retrospective chart review and structured telephone interviews conducted at a tertiary headache center.

- **Participants:** 169 rCM patients (79.9% female, median age 44 years) with prior failure of multiple preventive and acute medications.

- **Intervention:** Patients self-administered IN ketamine sprays (10 mg per spray) as needed, with a maximum of 20 sprays per day and 40 sprays per week.

Results

Effectiveness

- **Pain reduction:** Following IN ketamine use, the median pain intensity decreased from 8/10 to 5/10, with a median onset of relief of 27.5 minutes.

- **Consistency of relief:** Over 80% of responders experienced consistent pain relief across multiple uses.

- **Improved quality of life (QoL):**

  ◦ 35.5% of patients reported their QoL as "much better," while 42.6% noted it as "somewhat better."

  ◦ IN ketamine was rated "much better" than other acute treatments by 43.2% of users.

Safety and tolerability

- **Adverse events (AEs):** 74% of participants reported at least one AE, including:

  ◦ Fatigue (21.9%)

  ◦ Blurred vision or diplopia (21.3%)

  ◦ Cognitive effects such as confusion or dissociation (20.7%)

  ◦ Nausea (16.6%) and dizziness (13.6%)

- **Serious AEs:** Minimal; liver enzyme elevations occurred in a few cases but were unrelated to IN ketamine use.

Clinical implications

- **Acute rescue therapy:** IN ketamine effectively alleviates acute headaches for patients with limited options.

- **Bridge to other treatments:** It may serve as a transitional therapy during medication changes or before procedural interventions.

Recommendations for practice

- **Patient selection:**

  ◦ Ideal candidates include those with rCM unresponsive to standard treatments and significant functional impairment.

  ◦ Screening for contraindications, such as active substance use disorders, is essential.

- **Dosage and administration:**

  ◦ Initiate with 1-2 sprays per nostril, titrating to effect while adhering to safety limits.

  ◦ Educate patients on proper technique and risks, including the potential for AEs and dependence.

- **Safety monitoring:**

  ◦ Regular follow-ups to assess efficacy, adherence, and side effects.

  ◦ Conduct baseline and periodic liver function tests for long-term users.

- **Integration into care:**

  ◦ Combine with other preventive or abortive treatments for holistic management.

  ◦ Avoid use as a standalone therapy to minimize misuse or overuse risks.

Key takeaways

☑ IN ketamine offers rapid and effective relief for rCM, particularly in patients unresponsive to other therapies.

☑ While generally safe and well-tolerated, close monitoring is critical to manage AEs and prevent misuse.

☑ Its role as a rescue therapy rather than a primary treatment should be emphasized in clinical practice.

☑ Further research is needed to validate these findings and expand accessibility.

Additional recommended reading:

1. Yuan H, Natekar A, Park J, et al. Real-world study of intranasal ketamine for use in patients with refractory chronic migraine: A retrospective analysis. *Reg Anesth Pain Med.* 2023;48:581-587.

2. Afridi SK, Giffin NJ, Kaube H, et al. A randomized controlled trial of intranasal ketamine in migraine with prolonged aura. *Neurology.* 2013;80:642-647.

3. Petersen AS, Barloese MC, Jensen RH. Intranasal ketamine for acute cluster headache attacks: Results from a proof-of-concept trial. *Headache.* 2022;62:26-35.

Greater occipital nerve block with methylprednisolone and lidocaine for episodic cluster headaches

07

Why this topic is important

Cluster headaches (CH) are a rare but severely disabling type of primary headache disorder characterized by excruciating, unilateral pain typically concentrated around the orbital or temporal regions. Episodic cluster headache (ECH), the most common form, occurs in bouts (cluster periods) lasting weeks to months and significantly impacts quality of life. Managing ECH is particularly challenging due to the lack of universally effective preventive or transitional treatments.

Greater occipital nerve blocks (GONBs) have been increasingly utilized as a transitional preventive treatment for CH. These minimally invasive injections combine corticosteroids and local anesthetics to target inflammation and nociceptive pathways. The ANODYNE study by Chowdhury et al. (2024) is the first double-blind, randomized trial to rigorously assess the efficacy and tolerability of GONB with methylprednisolone and lidocaine in ECH patients. This update explores their findings and clinical implications for adopting GONB as a standard transitional therapy for ECH.

Objectives of this update

- Evaluate the efficacy of GONB with methylprednisolone and lidocaine for reducing attack frequency and severity in ECH.

- Assess the safety and tolerability of GONB as a transitional treatment.

- Provide clinical recommendations for integrating GONB into ECH management protocols.

What is new

The ANODYNE study presents key advancements:

- Demonstrates significant reduction in attack frequency and duration in ECH patients receiving GONB compared to placebo.

- Highlights GONB's safety, with transient and mild adverse effects observed in both active and placebo groups.

- Provides evidence that GONB induces remission earlier and in a higher proportion of patients than oral corticosteroids.

Methodology

- The study randomized 40 patients with ECH (diagnosed using ICHD-3 criteria) to receive either:

  - **Active GONB:** 2 mL methylprednisolone (80 mg) and 2 mL 2% lidocaine.

  - **Placebo:** 4 mL saline.

- Outcomes were assessed over a 4-week double-blind treatment phase, focusing on weekly attack frequency reduction, remission rates, and patient-reported outcomes.

- The primary endpoint was the change in weekly attack frequency from baseline to Week 4.

Results

Efficacy

Primary outcomes:

- Weekly attack frequency reduction was significantly greater in the active GONB group:

  - Active group: Mean reduction of 11.1 attacks.

  - Placebo group: Mean reduction of 7.7 attacks.

  - Mean difference: -3.4 attacks.

Secondary outcomes:

- **Complete remission rates:**

  - Day 4-Week 1: 52.6% (active) vs. 20% (placebo).

  - Day 4-Week 2: 73.7% (active) vs. 30% (placebo).

- **Attack duration and severity:**

  - Significant reductions were observed in the active group at Weeks 1-4 compared to placebo.

  - Active GONB also reduced cranial autonomic symptoms (CAS) and restlessness across attacks.

Safety

- Both groups reported mild and transient adverse events equally (90%).

- The most common adverse effects were injection-site pain and bleeding.

- No serious adverse events were observed, and no patients discontinued the study due to treatment-related side effects.

Limitations

This study's scope is a significant limitation, as it did not incorporate a direct comparison with oral corticosteroids. This omission restricts the ability to fully evaluate how the intervention measures against a widely used alternative in managing similar conditions. Further research is needed to compare the two treatment modalities.

Implications for clinical practice

Role of GONB in ECH management

- **Rapid onset:** Active GONB provided relief as early as Week 1, a crucial advantage for transitional treatment.

- **High remission rates:** Over 70% of patients experienced complete remission by Week 2, highlighting its effectiveness as a bridging therapy.

- **Alternative to oral steroids:** GONB demonstrated comparable efficacy to oral corticosteroids without the risk of systemic side effects or rebound headaches.

Practical recommendations

- **Patient selection:**

  - Ideal for patients with frequent, severe ECH attacks refractory to standard preventive medications.

  - Should be initiated within the first 10 days of cluster periods to maximize benefits.

- **Technique considerations:**
  - Administer injections at a standardized location, with equal distribution of the solution medially, centrally, and laterally.
- **Monitoring and follow-up:**
  - Regular assessment of attack frequency and duration is essential to evaluate treatment response.
  - Follow-up GONB or preventive medications (e.g., verapamil) may be necessary for patients with incomplete remission.

Key takeaways

☑ GONB with methylprednisolone and lidocaine significantly reduces attack frequency and duration in ECH patients compared to placebo.

☑ The treatment is well-tolerated, with only mild and transient side effects reported.

☑ GONB offers a rapid and effective transitional preventive option, potentially replacing oral corticosteroids in some cases.

☑ Early initiation during cluster periods maximizes efficacy, and careful patient monitoring is essential for optimizing outcomes.

Additional recommended reading:

1. Chowdhury D, Rao SK, Nagane R, et al. A double-blind randomized trial of greater occipital nerve block for episodic cluster headache. *Cephalalgia*. 2024;44(10):1-11.

2. Ambrosini A, Vandenheede M, Rossi P, et al. Suboccipital injection with rapid- and long-acting steroids in cluster headache: A placebo-controlled study. *Pain*. 2005;118:92-96.

3. Leroux E, Valade D, Taifas I, et al. Steroid injections for transitional treatment in cluster headache: A randomized controlled trial. *Lancet Neurol*. 2011;10(10):891-897.

OnabotulinumtoxinA injections targeting the sphenopalatine ganglion for refractory headache disorders

08

Why this topic is important

Chronic migraine (CM) and chronic cluster headache (CCH) are debilitating conditions that impose substantial physical, emotional, and socioeconomic burdens. Despite advances in migraine and headache treatments, patients with refractory forms of these disorders often experience limited relief, necessitating innovative approaches.

The sphenopalatine ganglion (SPG), a key relay center in headache pathophysiology, has emerged as a promising intervention target. Novel techniques for delivering OnabotulinumtoxinA (BTA) to the SPG have shown significant potential for managing refractory CM and CCH. The open-label study by Simmonds et al. (2024) provides critical insights into the safety and efficacy of this approach, highlighting its transformative role in headache management.

Objectives of this update

- Examine the efficacy of SPG-targeted OnabotulinumtoxinA injections in reducing headache frequency and severity.

- Review safety and tolerability data from repeated injections.

- Discuss clinical implications and recommendations for incorporating this technique into practice.

What is new

This study introduces and validates key advancements:

- **High responder rates:** First-time injections resulted in ≥ 50% improvement in 81% of CM patients and 69% of CCH patients.

- **Sustained efficacy:** Repeated injections demonstrated consistent benefits, particularly for CCH patients.

- **Favorable safety profile:** Adverse events were mild, transient, and largely related to localized injection effects.

Study highlights

Patient population

The study included 43 patients with refractory CM (n=12) and CCH (n=31) who had failed multiple prior preventive treatments. At baseline, the CM group had a mean of 15.3 moderate-to-severe headache days per month, while CCH patients experienced a mean of 17.9 weekly attacks.

Injection protocol

- **Procedure:** Percutaneous injections targeting the SPG were performed using a lateral approach under surgical navigation.

- **Dosage:** 25 units of OnabotulinumtoxinA suspended in 0.5 mL saline were delivered ipsilaterally (CCH) or bilaterally (CM).

- **Frequency:** Patients received injections every three months or based on symptom recurrence.

Results

Efficacy

- **Chronic migraine**

  - **Initial response:** 81% of CM patients achieved ≥ 50% reduction in headache days by weeks 5-8 post-injection.

  - **Repeated treatments:** Responder rates remained high (67-80%) across up to four consecutive injections.

  - **Onset and duration:** Maximal benefit occurred 2-3 months post-injection, with diminishing effects by month 4, supporting a 3-month reinjection interval.

- **Chronic cluster headache**

  - **Initial response:** 69% of CCH patients achieved ≥ 50% reduction in attack frequency after the first injection.

  - **Sustained efficacy:** Responder rates peaked at 89% after the third injection, with consistent benefits through subsequent treatments.

  - **Extended duration:** Unlike CM, benefits in CCH often lasted beyond three months for many patients.

Safety

123 adverse events (AEs) were reported across 261 treatments, with no discontinuations due to side effects.

- **Mild and transient AEs:**

  - Jaw pain or chewing difficulties (24 cases in CM; 11 in CCH).

  - Visual disturbances like blurring or diplopia (23 cases in CCH; 5 in CM).

  - Local swelling or discomfort at the injection site.

- **Serious AEs:** Only one serious AE (facial asymmetry) occurred, resolving entirely within 12 weeks.

Implications for clinical practice

Role in refractory headache management

SPG-targeted BTA injections offer a viable option for patients with limited responses to conventional treatments. The procedure is particularly beneficial for:

- CM patients unresponsive to oral preventives, CGRP monoclonal antibodies, or intra-muscular BTA.

- CCH patients with severe attack frequencies unmitigated by first-line therapies like verapamil.

Advantages of the SPG-targeted approach

- **Localized action:** Direct delivery of BTA to the SPG minimizes systemic exposure and associated risks.

- **Rapid onset:** Quick response times make this technique suitable as a transitional or crisis intervention.

- **Longer intervals for CCH:** Patients may experience sustained relief, reducing the need for frequent reinjections.

Practical recommendations

- **Patient selection:**

  - Ensure refractory status by documenting the failure of at least three preventive treatments for CM or two for CCH.

  - Prioritize patients with significant functional impairment or frequent, severe attacks.

- **Procedure optimization:**

  - Utilize surgical navigation tools to enhance precision and minimize procedural risks.

  - Consider bilateral injections for CM patients and ipsilateral injections for CCH, with adjustments based on side-shifting attacks.

- **Monitoring and follow-up:**

  - Maintain headache diaries to assess response and guide reinjection timing.

  - Monitor for transient AEs, particularly in the first few weeks post-injection.

Key takeaways

☑ SPG-targeted BTA injections are a promising treatment for refractory CM and CCH, with high efficacy and tolerable safety profiles.

☑ The procedure offers rapid and sustained relief, particularly for CCH patients, supporting its transitional or adjunctive therapy role.

☑ Careful patient selection, precise injection techniques, and ongoing monitoring are essential for optimizing outcomes.

Additional recommended reading:

1. Simmonds L, Jamtøy KA, Aschehoug I, et al. Open-label experience of repeated OnabotulinumtoxinA injections targeting the sphenopalatine ganglion in chronic migraine and chronic cluster headache. *Cephalalgia*. 2024;44(8):1-10.

2. Bratbak DF, Stovner LJ, Tronvik E, et al. Pilot study of sphenopalatine injection of OnabotulinumtoxinA for intractable headache. *Cephalalgia*. 2016;36(5):503-509.

3. Robbins MS, Robertson CE, Kaplan E, et al. The sphenopalatine ganglion: Anatomy, pathophysiology, and therapeutic targeting in headache. *Headache*. 2016;56(2):240-258.

Epidural blood or fibrin patches for post-dural puncture headache

09

Why this topic is important

Post-dural puncture headache (PDPH) is a frequent and debilitating complication of accidental dural puncture (ADP) during epidural anesthesia, especially in obstetric patients. The condition, caused by cerebrospinal fluid (CSF) leakage, can lead to orthostatic headaches and neurological symptoms, severely impacting patients' quality of life. Epidural blood patches (EBP) have long been the gold standard for treating PDPH. Yet, their efficacy remains inconsistent, and they can be associated with complications such as lumbar pain, radiculopathy, and infection.

Epidural fibrin patches (EFP) represent a novel alternative, offering enhanced adhesiveness and viscosity. They potentially provide better and faster relief with fewer side effects. However, EFP efficacy has not been extensively studied in a controlled setting. This randomized study by López-Millán et al. (2024) offers critical insights by directly comparing EBP and EFP for treating PDPH in obstetric patients.

Objectives of this update

- Assess the relative efficacy of EBP and EFP in achieving PDPH relief.

- Compare secondary outcomes such as recurrence, hospital stay duration, need for rescue analgesia, and patient satisfaction.

- Provide evidence-based recommendations for choosing between EBP and EFP in clinical practice.

What is new

This study delivers pivotal findings:

- **Superior efficacy of EFP:** EFP resolved PDPH faster and more completely than EBP, with fewer recurrences.

- **Enhanced patient satisfaction:** EFP patients reported higher satisfaction scores and shorter hospital stays.

- **Reduced complications:** EFP had fewer adverse events and required smaller injection volumes than EBP.

Methods

- **Design:** Prospective, randomized, open-label, parallel-group study.

- **Participants:** 70 postpartum women with PDPH refractory to conventional analgesic treatments, randomized to receive EBP (n=35) or EFP (n=35).

- **Interventions:**

  - EBP: 15 mL autologous blood.

  - EFP: 6 mL fibrin sealant (Tissucol Duo®).

  - Both were administered under surgical conditions, with follow-up at 2 hours, 12 hours, and 30 days.

Results

Primary efficacy outcomes

- **Immediate relief:**

  - EFP achieved complete PDPH relief in 97.1% of patients within 2 hours, compared to 54.3% in the EBP group.

  - By 24 hours, all EFP patients experienced complete resolution, versus 65.7% of EBP patients.

- **Need for rescue analgesia:**

  - EFP patients required significantly less rescue analgesia at 2 hours (2.9% vs. 48.6%) and 24 hours (0% vs. 37.1%).

Secondary outcomes

- **Recurrence rates:**

  - One EBP patient (2.9%) experienced a recurrence of PDPH, requiring a second patch. No recurrences occurred in the EFP group.

- **Hospital stay:**

  - The mean length of stay was shorter with EFP (3.9 days) compared to EBP (5.9 days).

- **Patient satisfaction:**

  - EFP patients reported significantly higher satisfaction on a Likert scale (mean: 4.7 vs. 3.0).

  - Extreme satisfaction was achieved in 68.6% of EFP patients, compared to none in the EBP group.

Safety outcomes

- **Adverse events:**

  - EFP demonstrated fewer adverse events, such as lumbar discomfort (88.2% with EBP vs. 80.0% with EFP).

  - No severe complications, such as meningitis or allergic reactions, occurred in either group.

Implications for clinical practice

Choosing between EBP and EFP

- **EFP as first-line treatment:**

  - EFP is highly effective in providing rapid and complete relief, making it the superior choice for patients with severe PDPH or those requiring expedited recovery.

- **EBP for resource-limited settings:**

  - While EFP is preferred, EBP remains an effective and accessible alternative when fibrin sealants are unavailable.

- **Considerations for patient selection:**

  - When choosing between EFP and EBP, evaluate patients' history, risk of complications, and need for rapid recovery.

Optimizing treatment outcomes

- **Early intervention:**

  - Prompt administration of EFP or EBP after PDPH onset improves outcomes and reduces the likelihood of chronic symptoms.

- **Post-procedure care:**
  - ○ Ensure patients remain supine for adequate clot stabilization and monitor for symptom recurrence.

- **Patient education:**
  - ○ To improve satisfaction and adherence, clearly explain the benefits, risks, and expected outcomes for each treatment option.

Key takeaways

☑ EFP outperforms EBP in achieving rapid, complete, and sustained relief of PDPH in obstetric patients.

☑ EFP leads to shorter hospital stays, less need for rescue analgesia, and higher patient satisfaction.

☑ Fewer adverse events and smaller injection volumes make EFP a safer and more tolerable option.

☑ While EBP remains a viable alternative, EFP should be prioritized when resources and expertise permit.

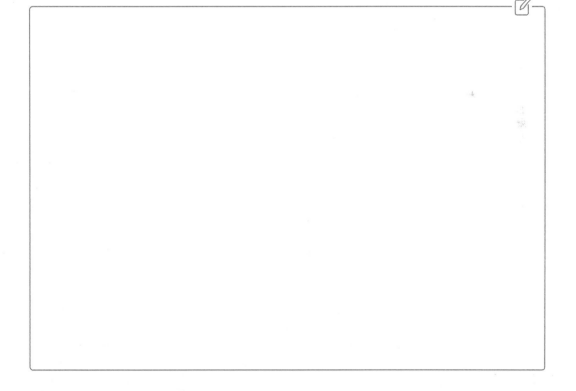

Additional recommended reading:

1. López-Millán JM, Ordóñez Fernández A, Muriel Fernández J, et al. Differential efficacy with epidural blood and fibrin patches for the treatment of post-dural puncture headache. *Pain Pract.* 2024;24:440-448.

2. Gupta A, Magnuson A, Van de Velde M, et al. Management practices for postdural puncture headache in obstetrics: A prospective, international cohort study. *Br J Anaesth.* 2020;125(6):1045-1055.

3. Paech MJ, Doherty DA, Christmas T, et al. The volume of blood for epidural blood patch in obstetrics: A randomized, blinded clinical trial. *Anesth Analg.* 2011;113(1):126-133.

Radiofrequency ablation of the occipital nerves for occipital neuralgia and chronic headaches

10

Why this topic is important

Occipital neuralgia and associated chronic headaches are common yet debilitating conditions that affect quality of life and functional capacity. Conventional pharmacological and non-pharmacological treatments often fail to provide long-term relief, leaving many patients with refractory symptoms. Radiofrequency ablation (RFA), a minimally invasive procedure that disrupts nociceptive pathways, has emerged as a promising alternative. Based on Abd-Elsayed et al. (2024), this update evaluates the efficacy and safety of RFA for occipital neuralgia and chronic headache management, offering new insights into its clinical potential.

Objectives of this update

- Assess the effectiveness of RFA for pain reduction in occipital neuralgia and chronic headaches.

- Highlight the duration of symptom relief and patient-reported outcomes.

- Provide clinical considerations for incorporating RFA into headache management strategies.

What is new

- **Significant pain reduction:** RFA reduced pain scores from 5.57 to 2.39 on the Visual Analog Scale (VAS), representing a 63.5% improvement.

- **Sustained relief:** On average, patients experienced 254 days of symptom relief, with some reporting benefits lasting nearly a year.

- **Robust sample size:** This study analyzed outcomes from 277 patients, making it one of the largest evaluations of RFA for occipital neuralgia to date.

- **Improved patient selection:** Insights into demographics and symptom patterns associated with better outcomes can refine patient selection for RFA.

Study design

This retrospective study analyzed the medical records of 277 patients treated with RFA for occipital neuralgia or chronic headaches at U.S. pain clinics from 2015 to 2022. Patients had a confirmed diagnosis of chronic headache originating from occipital neuralgia and completed at least one follow-up post-RFA.

- Patients were positioned prone with the cervical spine flexed.
- Target nerves were localized via sensory stimulation.
- Thermal RFA was performed at 80°C for 180 seconds after injecting 2% lidocaine.

Outcome measures

- Pain intensity was assessed using VAS before and after the procedure.
- Patient-reported improvement and duration of symptom relief were recorded during follow-ups.

Key findings

Pain reduction

- Pre-procedure mean pain score: 5.57.
- Post-procedure mean pain score: 2.39.
- Among patients reporting improvement, post-procedure scores further dropped to 1.71.

Patient-reported improvement

- Average symptom improvement: 63.5%.
- Among responders, improvement reached 75.6%.

Duration of relief

- Mean duration: 254 days.
- Patients with sustained improvement experienced relief for nearly 300 days on average.

Safety

- No severe complications were reported.
- Minor adverse effects, such as transient local pain and swelling, resolved without intervention.

Mechanisms of RFA

- RFA reduces nociceptive signaling by targeting small pain-specific fibers while sparing motor function.
- Emerging evidence suggests RFA may modulate neuroinflammatory pathways, enhancing its analgesic effects.

Comparative efficacy

- Compared to nerve blocks, RFA provides longer-lasting relief with fewer re-treatment requirements.
- While occipital nerve stimulation offers controlled pain relief, RFA avoids complications such as lead migration.

Ideal candidates

- Patients with refractory occipital neuralgia and consistent headache patterns are most likely to benefit.
- Prior positive response to nerve blocks may predict favorable RFA outcomes.

Clinical implications

- **Enhanced patient selection**
  - Use diagnostic nerve blocks to identify suitable candidates for RFA.
- **Integration into practice**
  - RFA should be considered for patients with refractory occipital neuralgia after conservative treatments fail.
- **Long-term management**
  - Educate patients about the expected duration of relief and the possibility of re-treatment.
- **Safety considerations**
  - Ensure procedural precision to minimize risks, particularly given the proximity of occipital nerves to critical structures.

Key takeaways

☑ RFA significantly reduces pain and improves quality of life for patients with occipital neuralgia and refractory headaches.

☑ The procedure offers a mean pain relief duration of approximately eight months, outperforming conventional therapies.

☑ With its minimally invasive nature and favorable safety profile, RFA represents a viable alternative to pharmacological and surgical treatments.

☑ Proper patient selection and procedural expertise are critical for maximizing outcomes and minimizing risks.

Additional recommended reading:

1. Abd-Elsayed A, Yapo SA, Cao NN, et al. Radiofrequency ablation of the occipital nerves for treatment of neuralgias and headache. *Pain Pract.* 2024;24(1):18-24. doi:10.1111/papr.13276.

2. Orhurhu V, Huang L, Quispe RC, et al. Use of radiofrequency ablation for the management of headache: A systematic review. *Pain Physician.* 2021;24(7):E973-87.

3. Hoffman LM, Abd-Elsayed A, Burroughs TJ, et al. Treatment of occipital neuralgia by thermal radiofrequency ablation. *Ochsner* J. 2018;18(3):209-14.

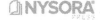

Cervical stabilization training for headache management

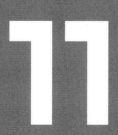

Why this topic is important

Headaches, particularly migraines, tension-type headaches (TTH), and cervicogenic headaches (CGH), are common and debilitating conditions with a significant global health burden. Up to 73% of migraine patients and 90% of those with TTH report concurrent neck pain, highlighting a strong association between cervical musculoskeletal dysfunction and headache pathophysiology. Emerging evidence suggests that targeted interventions could improve headache outcomes by addressing these dysfunctions.

Cervical stabilization training (CST) focuses on enhancing the strength, endurance, and coordination of cervical muscles, improving posture, and reducing neck pain. The study by Kacar et al. (2024) demonstrates the potential of CST to reduce headache frequency, intensity, and duration while improving quality of life, sleep, and mood. This update synthesizes these findings and their clinical implications for integrating CST into comprehensive headache management.

Objectives of this update

- Summarize the role of CST in addressing cervical musculoskeletal dysfunction in headache patients.

- Highlight the effects of CST on headache characteristics, neck pain, and associated quality of life metrics.

- Provide practical recommendations for implementing CST in clinical practice.

What is new

This study provides robust evidence supporting CST as an effective intervention for headache management:

- **Reduced headache burden:** CST significantly reduces headache frequency, intensity, and duration compared to standard medical treatment alone.

- **Improvement in cervical function:** Enhancements in deep cervical muscle activation and endurance translate to better pain outcomes.

- **Holistic benefits:** CST improves disability levels, quality of life, sleep quality, and mood, addressing physical and psychosocial aspects of headache disorders.

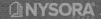

Study design

This single-blinded, randomized controlled trial included 90 female patients diagnosed with migraines, TTH, or CGH. Participants were randomized into a CST group (n=45) or a control group (n=45), with the intervention lasting eight weeks.

- **CST protocol:** Supervised CST sessions, per-formed thrice weekly, targeted cervical muscle activation, posture, and dynamic stabilization.

- **Control group:** Patients continued standard medical treatment without additional physical therapy.

Primary and secondary outcomes

- ○ **Pain metrics:** Headache frequency, duration, intensity, and neck pain intensity.

- ○ **Cervical function:** Forward head posture (FHP), activation of deep cervical flexors, and cervical muscle endurance.

- ○ **Quality of life:** Disability, sleep quality, mood, and general health metrics.

Results

Headache outcomes

CST significantly reduced headache burden compared to the control group:

- **Frequency**: Reduced from 7.4 to 3.9 attacks per week (CST group), with no significant change in controls.

- **Intensity (VAS):** Decreased by 2.65 points in the CST group versus negligible improvement in controls.

- **Duration:** Shortened by an average of 9.7 minutes in the CST group, with minimal changes in controls.

- **Medication use:** The number of drugs consumed per week decreased significantly in the CST group, further highlighting the intervention's impact on overall headache management.

Neck pain and cervical function

- **Neck pain:** Reduced by 4.81 points (VAS) in the CST group compared to no meaningful improvement in controls.

- **Forward head posture:** Significant improvement in craniovertebral angle (mean increase of 6.3° in CST group).

- **Muscle activation and endurance:**

  - ○ Activation of deep cervical flexors improved by 3.87 mmHg, meeting clinical significance thresholds.

  - ○ Cervical flexor and extensor endurance increased by 25.97 and 33.23 seconds, respectively, with moderate-to-strong correlations to reduced pain.

Holistic improvements

- **Disability levels:** Migraine Disability Assess-ment (MIDAS) scores improved significantly in the CST group.

- **Quality of life:** SF-36 scores revealed marked gains in both physical and mental health domains.

- **Sleep and mood:** Pittsburgh Sleep Quality Index and Beck Depression Inventory scores demonstrated significant enhancements, reflecting broader psychosocial benefits.

Implications for clinical practice

Role of CST in headache management

CST provides an effective, non-invasive strategy for addressing headache disorders, particularly in patients with coexisting neck pain. The strong correlation between improved cervical function and reduced headache burden supports using CST as a foundational therapy.

Recommendations for implementation

- **Patient selection:**
  - Ideal candidates include individuals with chronic headaches, cervical musculoskeletal dysfunction, and poor posture.
  - CST is particularly beneficial for patients with migraines, TTH, or CGH reporting neck pain.

- **Training protocol:**
  - Supervise sessions three times weekly for eight weeks.
  - Focus on progressive exercises targeting deep cervical flexors, extensor muscles, and dynamic stabilization.
  - Incorporate educational sessions on head and neck anatomy, posture, and lifestyle modifications.

- **Multidisciplinary integration:**
  - Combine CST with pharmacological treatments for optimized outcomes.
  - Regularly reassess cervical function and headache metrics to monitor progress and adjust therapy.

Key takeaways

- ☑ CST significantly reduces headache frequency, intensity, and duration, particularly in patients with coexisting neck pain.

- ☑ Improvements in cervical muscle activation and endurance are key mediators of pain relief.

- ☑ Holistic benefits include enhanced quality of life, sleep quality, and mood, emphasizing CST's broad therapeutic impact.

- ☑ Multidisciplinary approaches incorporating CST into routine care can optimize outcomes in headache management.

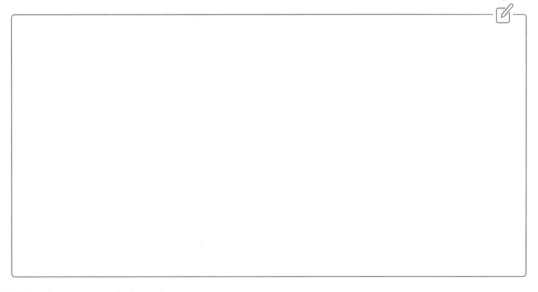

Additional recommended reading:

1. Kacar H, Ozkul C, Baran A, Guclu-Gunduz A. Effects of cervical stabilization training in patients with headache: A single-blinded randomized controlled trial. *Eur J Pain.* 2024;28:633-648.

2. Jull G, Hall T. The role of exercise in the management of cervicogenic headache. *Curr Pain Headache* Rep. 2018;22(4):27.

3. Fernandez-de-Las-Penas C, Cuadrado ML, Pareja JA. Physical therapy for headaches. *Cephalalgia.* 2016;36(12):1130-1140.

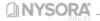

Surgical treatments for trigeminal neuralgia

12

Why this topic is important

Trigeminal neuralgia (TN) is a chronic pain disorder characterized by intense, episodic facial pain along the trigeminal nerve's distribution. Described as electric shocks or stabbing pain, it significantly impairs quality of life and daily functioning. While antiepileptic drugs such as carbamazepine and oxcarbazepine are first-line treatments, many patients develop refractory symptoms or intolerable side effects, requiring surgical intervention.

The three most common surgical modalities are microvascular decompression (MVD), percutaneous radiofrequency rhizotomy (RFR), and stereotactic radiosurgery (SRS). Each technique has distinct mechanisms, efficacy profiles, and risk-benefit ratios, yet limited head-to-head evidence comparing their long-term outcomes exists. Altamirano et al. (2024) conducted a quasi-experimental study to compare these interventions, offering valuable insights into their effectiveness, recurrence rates, quality of life impact, and patient satisfaction.

Objectives of this update

- Compare the efficacy of MVD, RFR, and SRS in reducing pain for idiopathic TN.

- Examine recurrence rates and the durability of pain relief across these surgical modalities.

- Highlight the implications of these findings for personalized treatment selection.

What is new

This study provides important advancements in understanding TN treatment:

- **MVD leads to long-term pain relief:** Most effective at achieving sustained pain control, with superior outcomes in pain-free survival.

- **Higher recurrence with RFR and SRS:** Ablative procedures demonstrated faster and higher recurrence rates than MVD.

- **Quality of life and satisfaction:** Despite differences in pain relief, patient-reported quality of life and satisfaction were comparable across groups.

Methods

- **Design:** Quasi-experimental, long-term study.

- **Participants:** 52 patients with idiopathic TN unresponsive to pharmacologic treatment:

  ○ MVD (n=33), RFR (n=10), SRS (n=9).

  ○ Inclusion criteria: Patients > 18 years with TN refractory to at least one first-line medication.

- **Outcomes measured:**

  ○ Pain relief (numerical rating scale [NRS], Barrow Neurological Institute [BNI] scale).

  ○ Recurrence rates and time to recurrence.

  ○ Quality of life (SF-36 scores) and satisfaction (Patient Global Impression of Change [PGIC]).

Results

Pain relief

- **MVD group:**

  ○ Most effective modality for immediate and sustained pain relief.

  ○ Pain-free rates were 93.9% immediately post-surgery, 72.7% at 1 year, and 50% at 2 years.

  ○ Median pain-free duration exceeded that of RFR and SRS.

- **RFR and SRS groups:**

  ○ Lower immediate pain relief and higher recurrence rates.

  ○ Pain-free rates at 1 year: RFR (22.2%) and SRS (11.1%).

  ○ Both methods provided temporary relief, with diminishing efficacy by the second year.

Recurrence and long-term outcomes

- **Recurrence rates:**

  ○ RFR (hazard ratio [HR]: 3.15) and SRS (HR: 4.26) had significantly higher recurrence risks compared to MVD.

  ○ The SRS group had the shortest median time to recurrence, followed by RFR, with MVD demonstrating the longest durability.

Quality of life and patient satisfaction

- **Quality of life (SF-36 scores):**

  ○ Comparable across all groups, despite differences in pain relief.

  ○ Significant improvements in physical and emotional functioning were reported post-treatment in all modalities.

- **Patient satisfaction (PGIC):**

  ○ High satisfaction levels were reported across all groups, likely influenced by reduced procedural morbidity in RFR and SRS.

Adverse events

- **MVD complications:**

  ○ Notable risks included cerebrospinal fluid leaks (6%), cranial nerve palsies (15%), and mild motor weakness (3%).

- **RFR and SRS complications:**

  ○ Both demonstrated favorable safety profiles, with transient facial hypoesthesia being the most common adverse event (22% in SRS cases).

Implications for clinical practice

Treatment selection

Microvascular decompression (MVD):

- **When to choose:** Ideal for patients seeking long-term pain relief and those with neurovascular compression detected on MRI.

- **Advantages:** Most effective at achieving sustained pain control and minimizing recurrence.

- **Considerations:** Involves craniotomy, necessitating careful patient selection due to higher procedural risks.

Radiofrequency rhizotomy (RFR):

- **When to choose:** Suitable for patients contraindicated for craniotomy or those requiring rapid symptom relief.

- **Advantages:** Minimally invasive, well-tolerated, with low complication rates.

- **Considerations:** Temporary pain relief with higher recurrence rates; may require repeat procedures.

Stereotactic radiosurgery (SRS):

- ◦ **When to choose:** Non-invasive option for elderly or high-risk patients unwilling or unable to undergo invasive procedures.

- ◦ **Advantages:** Outpatient procedure with minimal morbidity.

- ◦ **Considerations:** Offers slower pain relief compared to MVD and RFR, with the highest recurrence rates.

Multidisciplinary management

- **Surgical and pharmacological synergy:** Combining surgical interventions with optimized pharmacological management may enhance outcomes, particularly for patients experiencing recurrence.

- **Psychological support:** Incorporate counseling and coping strategies, as quality of life improvements may depend on emotional and mental well-being beyond pain relief.

Recommendations

- **Comprehensive evaluation:**

  - ◦ Assess patient-specific factors such as age, comorbidities, and neurovascular imaging findings to determine the most suitable intervention.

- **Follow-up care:**

  - ◦ Regular monitoring post-procedure to detect early recurrence and guide secondary interventions, especially in RFR and SRS patients.

- **Patient education:**

  - ◦ Provide clear guidance on each modality's benefits, risks, and expected outcomes, emphasizing realistic expectations.

Key takeaways

- ☑ **MVD** is the gold standard for durable pain relief, with superior long-term outcomes but higher procedural risks.

- ☑ **RFR and SRS** are safer alternatives for patients contraindicated for MVD, offering less invasive options but with higher recurrence rates.

- ☑ Quality of life and satisfaction outcomes underscore the importance of patient-centered care, even when pain relief differs across modalities.

- ☑ Personalized, multidisciplinary approaches ensure optimal outcomes, balancing efficacy with safety for each patient.

Additional recommended reading:

1. Altamirano JM, Jimenez-Olvera M, Moreno-Jimenez S, et al. Comparison of microvascular decompression, percutaneous radiofrequency rhizotomy, and stereotactic radiosurgery in the treatment of trigeminal neuralgia: A long-term quasi-experimental study. *Pain Pract.* 2024;24:514-524.

2. Holste K, Chan AY, Rolston JD, et al. Pain outcomes following microvascular decompression for drug-resistant trigeminal neuralgia: A systematic review and meta-analysis. *Clin Neurosurg.* 2020;86:182-190.

3. Zakrzewska JM, Linskey ME. Trigeminal neuralgia. *BMJ Clin Evid.* 2014;10:1207.

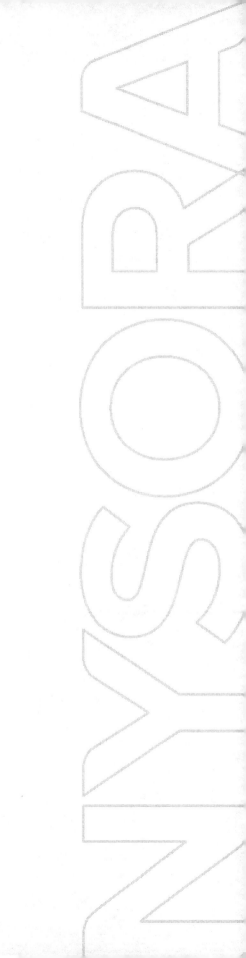

DSA-guided ethanol rhizotomy for trigeminal neuralgia

13

Why this topic is important

Trigeminal neuralgia (TN) is a chronic condition characterized by intense, episodic facial pain that significantly impairs quality of life. Traditional first-line treatments, such as anticonvulsant medications, often lose effectiveness over time or are poorly tolerated due to side effects, necessitating alternative interventions. Percutaneous procedures, including radiofrequency thermocoagulation (RF) and ethanol rhizotomy (ER), are second-line options for patients with refractory TN.

Ethanol rhizotomy, a less commonly used method, has been refined through digital subtraction angiography (DSA) guidance to enhance its precision and efficacy. This advanced technique enables visualization of Meckel's cave and associated structures, ensuring optimal placement of the ethanol injection and minimizing complications. This study by Van et al. (2023) compares outcomes between DSA-guided ER and RF in patients with TN, providing valuable insights into their relative benefits and risks.

Objectives of this update

- Compare the efficacy of DSA-guided ER and RF in achieving pain relief for TN.

- Evaluate recurrence rates, complications, and quality-of-life impacts for both methods.

- Highlight clinical considerations for selecting between ER and RF in treating TN.

What is new

This study provides several notable findings:

- **Superior efficacy of ER:** ER resulted in significantly higher rates of complete pain relief after a single intervention than RF.

- **Longer pain-free duration:** ER demonstrated lower recurrence rates over six years of follow-up.

- **Complication profiles:** ER was associated with more numbness and reduced corneal reflex, while RF had a higher incidence of burning dysesthesia.

Methods

- **Design:** Retrospective, single-center study with a minimum six-year follow-up.

- **Participants:** 33 patients with typical TN refractory to first-line medical management, treated with RF (n=10) or DSA-guided ER (n=23).

- **Outcomes measured:** Pain relief (complete or partial), recurrence rates, complications, and sensory/motor function changes.

Techniques

- **Radiofrequency thermocoagulation (RF):**

  ○ Conducted under fluoroscopic guidance with the patient in a supine position.

  ○ A 21-gauge RF needle was inserted through the foramen ovale following Hartel's trajectory, confirmed via submental and lateral fluoroscopic views.

  ○ Sensory testing was performed at 50 Hz, gradually increasing voltage to ensure appropriate placement targeting the painful nerve distribution.

  ○ After verification, the needle was heated to 80°C for 90 seconds to ablate the targeted nerve fibers.

- **Ethanol Rhizotomy (ER):**

  ○ Similar initial setup to RF, using a 25-gauge needle to access the foramen ovale.

  ○ Digital subtraction angiography (DSA) was employed to visualize Meckel's cave and confirm needle positioning.

  ○ After injecting 0.2 mL of lidocaine to test for numbness, 0.3 mL of absolute ethanol was slowly administered.

  ○ The patient remained supine for at least 10 minutes to allow ethanol distribution, targeting the Gasserian ganglion and trigeminal root canal.

Results

Efficacy

- **Initial pain relief:**

  ○ ER achieved complete pain relief in 95.7% of patients after the first intervention, compared to 60% for RF.

  ○ Fewer ER patients required repeat interv-entions (4.3% vs. 40%).

- **Recurrence rates:**

  ○ ER had a significantly lower recurrence rate (17.4% vs. 40%).

  ○ Time to recurrence was longer in the ER group, indicating better long-term durability.

Complications

- **Numbness:**

  ○ ER induced complete numbness in 30.4% of patients and partial numbness in 69.6%.

  ○ RF resulted in no complete numbness but caused partial numbness in 80% of patients.

- **Corneal reflex loss:**

  ○ ER patients experienced more frequent loss of corneal reflex (47.8%) compared to none in the RF group.

- **Burning dysesthesia:**

  ○ Occurred in 50% of RF patients, compared to 17.4% in the ER group.

- **Masseter weakness:**

  ○ Detected in both groups, with no significant difference (95.7% in ER vs. 90% in RF).

Implications for clinical practice

Treatment considerations

- **Ethanol rhizotomy (ER):**

  - Ideal for patients seeking longer-lasting pain relief with fewer repeat interventions.

  - Best suited for cases where complete trigeminal ganglion coverage is desired despite a higher risk of numbness.

- **Radiofrequency thermocoagulation (RF):**

  - Appropriate for patients who prioritize minimal sensory changes, particularly those concerned about corneal reflex preservation.

  - Suitable for targeting specific divisions of the trigeminal nerve, although it may require repeat procedures.

Recommendations

- **Patient selection:**

  - ER may be preferred for patients with severe, diffuse TN who are willing to accept a higher risk of numbness.

  - RF is advantageous for patients with localized TN or those at higher risk of corneal complications.

- **Procedure optimization:**

  - Utilize DSA guidance for ER to improve targeting accuracy and minimize complications.

  - Ensure precise needle placement and thorough patient counseling about potential side effects of RF.

- **Post-procedure care:**

  - Monitor sensory changes and corneal reflex recovery, especially in ER-treated patients.

  - Provide long-term follow-up to detect and manage recurrences promptly.

Key takeaways

- ☑ DSA-guided ER achieves superior pain relief and lower recurrence rates than RF but carries a higher risk of sensory complications.

- ☑ RF remains a valuable alternative for patients who prioritize minimal sensory alterations, though its pain relief may be less durable.

- ☑ Tailored patient selection and procedure-specific techniques are essential to optimize outcomes and minimize risks.

Additional recommended reading:

1. Van GB, Nguyen KD, Nguyen TC, et al. Refined percutaneous rhizotomy with DSA-guided ethanol for the second-line treatment of trigeminal neuralgia. *Interventional Pain Medicine.* 2023;2:100372.

2. Noorani I, Lodge A, Vajramani G, et al. Comparing percutaneous treatments of trigeminal neuralgia: 19 years of experience in a single center. *Stereotact Funct Neurosurg.* 2016;94(2):75-85.

3. Texakalidis P, Xenos D, Tora MS, et al. Comparative safety and efficacy of percutaneous approaches for the treatment of trigeminal neuralgia: A systematic review and meta-analysis. *Clin Neurol Neurosurg.* 2019;182:112-22.

Botulinum toxin for temporomandibular dysfunction-related myofascial pain

14

Why this topic is important

Temporomandibular disorder (TMD)-related myofascial pain (MFP) is a prevalent condition that significantly affects quality of life. It is characterized by chronic pain and muscle dysfunction, making it a challenging condition to manage, especially in patients with refractory symptoms. Although conservative therapies such as manual therapy, counseling, and occlusal splints remain first-line treatments, a subset of patients fail to achieve adequate relief.

Botulinum toxin type A (BoNT-A) has emerged as a potential therapeutic option due to its ability to reduce muscle hyperactivity and its analgesic properties. However, evidence for its efficacy in TMD-related MFP remains inconclusive, with some studies showing benefits and others demonstrating no superiority over placebo. This study by Sitnikova et al. (2024) investigates the clinical benefits and limitations of BoNT-A injections compared to placebo, contributing to the evidence base for its use in this context.

Objectives of this update

- Assess the efficacy of BoNT-A in reducing pain intensity and disability in patients with TMD-related MFP.

- Compare outcomes of BoNT-A to saline solution (SS) placebo injections.

- Highlight the implications for clinical practice, including recommendations for its use.

What is new

This randomized, placebo-controlled crossover trial provides several important insights:

- **Moderate dose evaluated:** A 50-unit dose of BoNT-A was used, revealing significant within-group improvements but no superiority over placebo.

- **Objective outcomes:** BoNT-A reduced muscle activity and bite force, indicating a strong muscle-relaxing effect.

- **Clinical relevance questioned:** The lack of significant differences between BoNT-A and placebo raises questions about the analgesic mechanism and its utility for MFP.

Methodology

- **Design:** A double-blinded, randomized, placebo-controlled crossover trial conducted in a tertiary care setting.

- **Participants:**

  ○ 66 patients with persistent TMD-related MFP.

  ○ Diagnostic criteria: Myalgia and myofascial pain per the Diagnostic Criteria for TMD (DC/TMD).

  ○ Exclusions: Prior BoNT-A use, medications affecting neuromuscular function, and systemic conditions such as arthritis or major psychiatric disorders.

- **Intervention:**

  ○ Sequence 1: BoNT-A first, SS placebo later.

  ○ Sequence 2: SS first, BoNT-A later.

  ○ Each injection was followed by assessments at 2, 11, and 16 weeks.

Results

Pain-related outcomes

- **Within-group improvements:**

  ○ BoNT-A significantly reduced pain intensity and pain-related disability at all follow-ups.

  ○ SS placebo also showed significant within-group improvements, suggesting a strong placebo effect.

- **Between-group comparisons:**

  ○ No significant differences in pain scores or disability reduction between BoNT-A and SS at any time point.

Objective outcomes

- **Muscle relaxation:** BoNT-A significantly reduced electromyographic (EMG) activity and bite force at all follow-ups compared to SS.

- **Number needed to treat (NNT):**

  ○ For a ≥ 30% reduction in pain, NNT for BoNT-A was 6.3 at 2 weeks but increased to 19.0 at 16 weeks, indicating diminishing clinical benefits over time.

Adverse effects

- Two minor adverse events were reported: one transient migraine attack and mild smile asymmetry, both resolving without intervention.

Implications for clinical practice

While BoNT-A demonstrated muscle-relaxing effects, its pain-relieving benefits were indistinguishable from placebo. This finding aligns with the hypothesis that MFP pain originates more from central pain modulation dysfunction than peripheral muscle hyperactivity.

Recommendations

- **Patient selection:**

  ○ Reserve BoNT-A for patients who fail conservative therapies and seek symptom relief from muscle-related factors.

  ○ Avoid using BoNT-A as a first-line treatment.

- **Dosage considerations:**

  ○ Moderate doses (50-100 U) may balance efficacy and side effects.

  ○ Higher doses may provide longer-lasting analgesia but risk muscle atrophy.

- **Treatment expectations:**

  ○ Set realistic expectations for patients, emphasizing limited evidence for significant pain relief.

  ○ Combine BoNT-A with multimodal therapies targeting central pain pathways for optimal outcomes.

Key takeaways

☑ BoNT-A provides significant muscle relaxation but does not outperform placebo in reducing pain intensity or disability in TMD-related MFP.

☑ Its use should be reserved for refractory cases, with caution regarding potential adverse effects such as muscle atrophy.

☑ Multimodal approaches addressing central pain modulation remain critical for managing TMD-related MFP.

Additional recommended reading:

1. Sitnikova V, Kämppi A, Kämppi L, et al. Clinical benefit of botulinum toxin for treatment of persistent TMD-related myofascial pain: A randomized, placebo-controlled, cross-over trial. *Pain Pract.* 2024;24:1014-1023.

2. Al-Moraissi EA, Conti PCR, Alyahya A, et al. The hierarchy of different treatments for myogenous temporomandibular disorders: A systematic review and network meta-analysis. *Oral Maxillofac Surg.* 2022;26(4):519-33.

3. Ramos-Herrada RM, Bellini-Pereira SA, Castillo AA, et al. Effects of botulinum toxin in patients with myofascial pain related to temporomandibular joint disorders: A systematic review. *Dent Med Probl.* 2022;59(2):271-80.

The relationship between insomnia and chronic orofacial pain

15

Why this topic is important

Chronic orofacial pain (OFP) encompasses a range of debilitating conditions such as temporomandibular disorders (TMD), neuropathic facial pain, and myofascial pain. Insomnia, a prevalent comorbidity in chronic pain populations, affects nearly 50% of these patients. The bidirectional relationship between sleep disturbances and pain exacerbates both conditions, creating a vicious cycle that worsens clinical outcomes.

Although significant advances have been made in understanding the role of sleep disturbances in chronic pain, insomnia remains underdiagnosed and undertreated in patients with OFP. The study by Alessandri-Bonetti et al. (2024) highlights the critical link between insomnia and pain intensity, psychological distress, and reduced quality of life in patients with OFP. Addressing insomnia alongside pain management is imperative to break the cycle of pain and poor sleep, offering a pathway to more effective, multidisciplinary care.

Objectives of this update

- Examine the associations between insomnia and pain intensity, psychological outcomes, and quality of life in chronic OFP patients.

- Explore differences in outcomes among insomnia subtypes, including sleep onset latency (SOL) and early morning awakening (EMA).

- Provide clinical recommendations for integrating insomnia management into OFP treatment protocols.

What is new

This study sheds light on critical insights for OFP management:

- **High prevalence:** Nearly half (45.1%) of OFP patients reported clinically significant insomnia.

- **Insomnia-pain interplay:** Insomnia is associated with increased pain intensity and interference, independent of pain duration.

- **Subtype-specific impacts:** SOL-insomnia correlates with more severe outcomes compared to EMA-insomnia.

- **Comprehensive impact:** Patients with insomnia exhibit worse mental health, lower satisfaction with life, and more medical comorbidities.

Methodology

Study design and setting

This study employed a cross-sectional design to investigate the relationship between insomnia symptomatology and pain, mental health, and physical health variables in patients seeking treatment for chronic orofacial pain (OFP). Data were retrospectively extracted from the medical records of patients evaluated at a university-affiliated tertiary OFP clinic.

Participants

Inclusion criteria:

- Adults aged between 18 and 80 years.

- Seeking treatment for an OFP complaint with a duration of more than 3 months.

- English-speaking and able to provide complete data at the baseline.

Exclusion criteria:

- Pain duration of less than 3 months.

- Age under 18 or over 80 years.

- Incomplete baseline data.

Demographics:

- The study included 450 patients.

- The mean age was 44.63 ± 15.98 years.

- Sex distribution:

  ◦ 82.2% were female (370 participants).

  ◦ 17.8% were male (80 participants).

Data collection

Patients completed standardized measures, including:

- **Insomnia Severity Index (ISI):** A 7-item questionnaire assessing insomnia severity over two weeks, with scores ranging from 0 to 28. Scores ≥ 11 indicated clinical insomnia.

- **Graded Chronic Pain Scale (GCPS):** Measured pain intensity (0-100) and pain interference (0-100) with daily activities.

- **Patient Health Questionnaire (PHQ-4):** Assessed anxiety and depression symptoms on a scale of 0-12.

- **Satisfaction with Life Scale (SWLS):** Evaluated life satisfaction on a scale of 5-35.

- **Medical Comorbidity Checklist:** Participants identified comorbidities from a list of 96 conditions confirmed during their clinical examination.

Results

Insomnia prevalence and associated outcomes

- **Pain intensity:** Patients with insomnia reported significantly higher mean pain intensity (60.7 vs. 44.2).

- **Pain interference:** Insomnia was associated with a threefold increase in pain interference scores (43.8 vs. 18.4).

- **Mental health:** Anxiety and depression scores were nearly double in patients with insomnia (5.5 vs. 2.7).

- **Quality of life:** Lower life satisfaction was observed in patients with insomnia (21.6 vs. 26.5).

- **Comorbidities:** Patients with insomnia had more medical conditions on average (6.7 vs. 4.4).

Insomnia subtypes

- **SOL-insomnia:** Patients with delayed sleep onset experienced significantly higher pain intensity (67.2 vs. 56.8) and interference (55.4 vs. 36.8) compared to those without SOL-insomnia.

- **EMA-insomnia:** Early morning awakenings did not significantly correlate with pain or psychological variables.

Implications for clinical practice

- **Routine screening:**
  Consider using validated tools, such as the Insomnia Severity Index (ISI), to assess insomnia symptoms in patients with chronic orofacial pain (OFP). Identifying insomnia subtypes, such as Sleep-Onset Latency (SOL) or Early Morning Awakening (EMA), may help guide individualized care approaches.

- **Multidisciplinary care:**
  Combining cognitive-behavioral therapy for insomnia (CBT-I) with standard OFP treatments could provide added benefits. Addressing factors such as bruxism, anxiety, or depression might also contribute to improved outcomes.

- **Personalized interventions:**
  - For patients with SOL-insomnia, incorporating relaxation techniques and sleep hygiene strategies may help manage hyperarousal.
  - For those with EMA-insomnia, approaches like maintaining consistent wake times and increasing exposure to bright light could be considered.

- **Monitoring progress:**
  Regularly reassessing sleep, pain, and psychological outcomes can help refine treatment plans and ensure they align with patient needs over time.

Key takeaways

☑ Insomnia is highly prevalent among OFP patients, significantly exacerbating pain, psychological distress, and overall health.

☑ Delayed sleep onset (SOL-insomnia) is associated with worse outcomes than early morning awakening (EMA-insomnia).

☑ Routine screening and management of insomnia can improve pain intensity, functional outcomes, and quality of life.

☑ Multidisciplinary approaches addressing both sleep and pain are essential for effective OFP management.

Additional recommended reading:

1. Alessandri-Bonetti A, Sangalli L, Boggero IA. Relationship between insomnia and pain in patients with chronic orofacial pain. Pain Med. 2024;25(5):319-326.

2. Smith MT, Finan PH, Buenaver LF, et al. Cognitive-behavioral therapy for insomnia comorbid with chronic pain: A systematic review. Sleep Med Clin. 2014;9(2):261-274.

3. Almoznino G, Haviv Y, Sharav Y, Benoliel R. Management of insomnia in patients with chronic orofacial pain. Oral Dis. 2017;23(8):1043-1051.

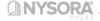

Spinal Pain

Delaying epidural steroid injections: Infection risks and platelet counts

16

Why this topic is important

Epidural steroid injections (ESIs) are widely used for treating radicular pain syndromes, offering substantial pain relief and functional improvement. However, two critical safety concerns arise in specific patient populations: infection risks during active or recent infections and bleeding risks in thrombocytopenic patients undergoing interlaminar epidural procedures. The absence of standardized guidelines leaves clinicians navigating these scenarios with limited evidence, raising questions about the timing and safety of ESIs under such conditions. This review by Zheng et al. (2024) consolidates current evidence and expert recommendations to guide clinicians in safely managing these complex cases while optimizing patient outcomes.

Objectives of this update

- Analyze the infection risk associated with ESIs in patients with active or recent infections.

- Evaluate the safety considerations for performing interlaminar ESIs in thrombocytopenic patients.

- Provide practical, evidence-informed guidance for managing these challenging scenarios in clinical practice.

What is new

This review presents a critical update on:

- Theoretical and observed infection risks of ESIs during systemic and localized infections, with insights on timing ESIs after antibiotic initiation.

- Evidence supporting the absence of a universally safe platelet cutoff for interlaminar ESIs, emphasizing patient-specific bleeding risk assessments.

- Recommendations for infection management and platelet threshold considerations, derived from multidisciplinary expertise and extrapolated data.

Infection risks with ESIs during active infections

- **Risk of infection due to systemic immuno-suppression:**

  - Corticosteroids suppress innate and adaptive immunity, impairing neutrophil migration, macrophage activation, and immunoglobulin production.

  - Large cohort studies report infection rates near 0%, but these often exclude patients with active infections, limiting applicability.

  - Transforaminal epidural steroid injections (TFESIs), by avoiding the central epidural space, may theoretically reduce the risk of central infections such as epidural abscess or meningitis.

- **Evidence summary:**

  - Three large studies involving over 50,000 ESIs found no major post-procedure infections; however, none explicitly studied patients with active infections.

  - Case reports document rare but severe infections, including epidural abscess and meningitis, in immunocompromised or medically complex patients.

- **Timing after antibiotics:**

  - Limited evidence suggests infections, such as uncomplicated cellulitis or UTIs, are largely sterilized after 3-5 days of antibiotic therapy. However, the optimal delay for ESIs post-antibiotic initiation remains undefined.

  - Delays of 24 hours or more after initiating antibiotics may reduce risk, though recommendations emphasize caution until complete resolution of infection-related symptoms.

  - In the case of TFESIs, the minimally invasive nature and targeted approach may allow for earlier consideration post-antibiotic initiation, provided robust infection control measures are implemented.

ESIs in thrombocytopenic patients

- **Bleeding risks and platelet function:**

  - While platelet count is a common marker of bleeding risk, it poorly predicts actual hemorrhage, as platelet function and coagulopathies also play significant roles.

  - Thrombocytopenia, defined as platelet counts < 150,000/mcL, may increase the risk of epidural hematoma in interlaminar procedures.

- **Findings from related populations:**

  - In obstetric populations, over 1,500 neuraxial procedures with platelet counts ≥ 70,000/mcL did not result in epidural hematomas.

  - Meta-analyses suggest a low hematoma risk with counts ≥ 70,000/mcL in patients without coagulopathy or anti-platelet therapy.

- **Extrapolated thresholds:**

  - Based on aggregated data, procedures are considered safer when platelet counts are ≥ 75,000/mcL, though definitive cutoff values remain elusive.

  - Routine pre-procedural platelet transfusions are not supported by evidence and should be avoided unless clinically indicated.

  - TFESIs, by accessing the epidural space through the neural foramen, may pose a lower bleeding risk than interlaminar approaches, particularly in thrombocytopenic patients.

Clinical guidance

- **Infection-related recommendations:**

  ○ Avoid ESIs during systemic or localized infections at the injection site until the infection is resolved and the patient is asymptomatic.

  ○ For infections remote to the injection site, assess the antibiotic response and delay the procedure until treatment completion whenever possible.

  ○ Engage infectious disease specialists for complex cases requiring nuanced decision-making.

  ○ For TFESIs, consider their reduced central epidural involvement as a potential advantage in cases of localized infections, provided adequate precautions are taken.

- **Thrombocytopenia-related recommendations:**

  ○ Assess bleeding risks based on platelet count, patient history, and concurrent medications.

  ○ Avoid interlaminar ESIs in patients with platelet counts < 70,000/mcL unless mitigating factors (e.g., platelet transfusions) are applied.

  ○ Involve hematologists when managing patients with severe thrombocytopenia or complex coagulopathies.

  ○ TFESIs may be a safer alternative for patients with platelet counts nearing lower thresholds, but a thorough risk-benefit analysis is essential.

Key takeaways

☑ **Infection risks during ESIs are low but significant in patients with active infections.** Therefore, it is advised to delay procedures until antibiotics are resolved or completed.

☑ **No absolute safe platelet cutoff exists for interlaminar ESIs,** though a threshold of ≥ 70,000/mcL is often recommended.

☑ **TFESIs, with their targeted approach, may pose lower risks of infection and bleeding,** making them a viable option in certain high-risk patients.

☑ **Patient-specific factors must guide procedural decisions,** with interdisciplinary collaboration for complex cases.

☑ **Evidence gaps highlight the need for further research** to optimize safety guidelines and clinical outcomes.

Additional recommended reading:

1. Zheng P, Hao D, Christolias G, et al. Delaying epidural steroid injections: Infection and safe platelet cutoff. *Interventional Pain Medicine.* 2024;3:100383.

2. Bauer ME, Arendt K, Beilin Y, et al. Neuraxial procedures in thrombocytopenic obstetric patients: A consensus statement. *Anesth Analg.* 2021;132(6):1531-44.

3. Hooten WM, Kinney MO, Huntoon MA. Epidural abscess and meningitis after epidural corticosteroid injection. *Mayo Clin Proc.* 2004;79(5):682-6.

Postpartum epidural steroid injections:

Lipomatosis and steroid safety

17

Why this topic is important

Epidural steroid injections (ESIs) are a cornerstone intervention for managing radicular pain caused by spinal stenosis, disc herniation, or degenerative changes. However, their potential to exacerbate spinal epidural lipomatosis (SEL) and concerns about systemic steroid effects in postpartum patients have raised important clinical questions. SEL, characterized by abnormal fat deposition in the epidural space, can lead to complications such as neurogenic claudication or cauda equina syndrome. In postpartum women, physiological changes in the hypothalamic-pituitary-adrenal (HPA) axis and lactation add layers of complexity to steroid use, particularly regarding infant exposure and maternal health. Understanding the intersection of these issues is essential to optimize patient safety and therapeutic outcomes. This update, based on the article by D'Souza et al. (2024), summarizes the evidence regarding these potential complications.

Objectives of this update

- Summarize the evidence linking ESIs to SEL development and progression.

- Discuss the safety profile of ESIs in postpartum patients, focusing on maternal and infant health.

- Provide recommendations for patient counseling, procedural planning, and follow-up care.

- Highlight research gaps and propose future directions to refine clinical guidelines.

What is new

This update synthesizes the latest data on:

- The association between repeated ESIs and the progression of SEL, with an emphasis on radiographic findings and clinical outcomes.

- Emerging considerations for administering ESIs postpartum, including their impact on lactation and infant health.

- Practical recommendations for managing risks associated with steroid administration in high-risk populations.

Epidural steroid injections and spinal epidural lipomatosis

- **Pathophysiology of SEL:**

  - SEL involves abnormal fat deposition within the epidural space, leading to thecal sac compression and potential neurological symptoms.

  - Key risk factors include systemic corticosteroid use, obesity, and idiopathic predisposition.

- **Evidence of ESI association with SEL:**

  - Observational studies and case reports suggest an association between repeated ESIs and SEL progression.

  - The largest study reviewed MRIs of 28,902 patients and identified SEL in 2.5% of cases, with prior ESIs being a significant risk factor.

- **Radiographic evidence:**

  - SEL severity correlates with the number of ESIs received, with studies showing a near 100% likelihood of SEL development after four or more injections.

  - Serial imaging demonstrates circumferential increases in SEL fat deposition after repeated ESIs.

- **Clinical outcomes in patients with pre-existing SEL:**

  - Limited evidence suggests mixed outcomes, with some patients experiencing short-term pain relief and others showing progression to neurological deficits.

  - Severe cases requiring surgical decompression underscore the need for cautious use of ESIs in SEL patients.

ESIs in postpartum patients

- **Physiological considerations:**

  - Postpartum changes in the HPA axis, including cortisol suppression and lactation-related prolactin elevation, may alter systemic responses to steroids.

  - These hormonal shifts can amplify side effects or prolong adrenal suppression.

- **Steroid transfer to breast milk:**

  - Corticosteroids are secreted into breast milk, though levels are generally low.

  - For example, methylprednisolone levels peak at 1.24 mg/L one hour after administration and decline rapidly within 8-12 hours.

  - While short-term "pump-and-dump" strategies have been suggested, robust evidence supporting this practice is lacking.

- **Impact on lactation and infant health:**

  - Case reports link high-dose corticosteroids to temporary milk production cessation, though effects appear dose-dependent.

  - No significant long-term effects on infant growth, development, or health have been observed in studies of lactating mothers receiving systemic steroids.

Clinical implications

- **Patient counseling:**

  - Discuss the risks and benefits of ESIs, particularly in patients with known SEL or during the postpartum period.

  - For lactating mothers, provide clear guidance on timing breastfeeding post-ESI to minimize infant exposure.

- **Risk mitigation strategies:**

  - Use the lowest effective corticosteroid dose to reduce systemic absorption and associated risks.

- Consider alternative interventional approaches, such as non-steroidal injections, in high-risk patients.

- **Monitoring and follow-up:**

  - Monitor neurological symptoms and consider serial imaging to assess progression for patients with SEL.

  - In postpartum patients, assess milk production and HPA axis recovery post-ESI.

- **Multidisciplinary collaboration:**

  - Engage endocrinologists, lactation consultants, and pediatricians to ensure comprehensive care when managing postpartum patients receiving ESIs.

Limitations and future directions

- **SEL evidence gaps:** Prospective studies are needed to establish causality between ESIs and SEL progression.

- **Postpartum steroid use:** Larger, well-designed studies are necessary to evaluate long-term maternal and infant outcomes following ESI during lactation.

- **Standardized guidelines:** The development of evidence-based protocols for steroid dosing and administration timing in high-risk populations remains a priority.

Key takeaways

☑ **SEL and ESIs:** Repeated ESIs are associated with increased SEL risk, emphasizing the need for judicious use in patients with predisposing factors.

☑ **Postpartum considerations:** While ESIs are generally safe for lactating women, careful maternal and infant health monitoring is recommended.

☑ **Risk reduction:** Minimize steroid dosage and use alternative therapies where appropriate to mitigate complications.

☑ **Patient education:** Clear communication about risks, benefits, and procedural options is essential for informed decision-making.

Additional recommended reading:

1. D'Souza RS, Zheng P, Christolias G, et al. Epidural steroid injections and spinal epidural lipomatosis: patient safety considerations. *Interventional Pain Medicine.* 2024;3:100408.

2. Holder EK, Raju R, Dundas MA, et al. Association of lumbosacral epidural lipomatosis with steroid injections: narrative review. *North Am Spine Soc J.* 2022;9:123-130.

3. Gunduz S, Gencler OS, Celik HT. Lactation interruption after high-dose steroid therapy: implications for breastfeeding mothers. *J Matern Fetal Neonatal Med.* 2016;29:3495-3501.

Cervical radicular pain: Diagnosis and management

18

Why this topic is important

Cervical radicular pain is a disabling condition that significantly impacts patients' quality of life and ability to perform daily activities. It manifests as radiating arm pain caused by nerve root compression or irritation, most commonly affecting the C7 and C6 nerve roots. The condition can arise from various causes, including disc herniation, foraminal stenosis, or degenerative changes in the cervical spine. While many cases resolve with conservative treatments such as physical therapy and medication, a subset of patients experiences persistent or severe symptoms requiring advanced diagnostic and interventional strategies. Given the substantial burden of cervical radicular pain on healthcare systems and individuals, accurate diagnosis and effective management are critical. This update , based on the article by Peene et al. (2024), synthesizes recent advancements to improve diagnostic accuracy and guide treatment decisions, aiming to optimize outcomes for patients with this challenging condition.

Objectives of this update

- Clarify diagnostic criteria and tools for cervical radicular pain, focusing on history, physical examination, and imaging.

- Review the effectiveness of conservative, pharmacologic, and interventional treatments.

- Discuss emerging evidence on advanced interventions, including pulsed radiofrequency and spinal cord stimulation.

What is new

Recent advances in understanding and managing cervical radicular pain have shifted clinical practice. Key updates include:

- Insights into the dynamic presentation of radicular pain, highlighting the importance of combining physical examination, history-taking, and imaging for accurate diagnosis.

- Evidence supporting pulsed radiofrequency (PRF) as an effective treatment for chronic cervical radicular pain that is refractory to epidural steroid injections (ESIs).

- Updated imaging recommendations, emphasizing MRI for soft tissue pathology and CT for evaluating osseous abnormalities.

Diagnostic approaches

- **Clinical presentation:**
  Cervical radicular pain typically presents as sharp, shooting, or electric-like pain that radiates from the neck into the arm, often along a dermatomal distribution. Commonly affected areas include the C7 and C6 dermatomes, which may also exhibit sensory deficits, paresthesia, and motor weakness. Depending on the nerve root affected, motor deficits may involve grip strength or triceps reflex. Early recognition of these patterns is critical to avoid misdiagnosis and ensure timely management.

- **Provocative maneuvers:**
  Physical examination techniques, such as Spurling's test and the shoulder abduction test, are valuable for identifying cervical radicular pain. Spurling's test involves compressing the cervical spine while the neck is extended and rotated toward the affected side, eliciting radiating pain in positive cases. Although these tests demonstrate high specificity, their moderate sensitivity necessitates using a combination of maneuvers to improve diagnostic accuracy.

- **Imaging:**
  MRI is the gold standard for diagnosing cervical radicular pain, particularly for identifying soft tissue causes like herniated discs or nerve root compression. CT scans are valuable when osseous abnormalities, such as osteophytes, are suspected. Imaging is recommended for patients with symptoms persisting beyond 4-6 weeks or when red-flag signs, such as myelopathy or malignancy, are present. Diagnostic nerve root blocks may also help confirm the pain source, especially in multilevel degenerative changes.

Treatment options

- **Conservative therapies:**
  Noninvasive treatments remain the cornerstone of managing cervical radicular pain, particularly in the acute phase. Physical therapy focusing on posture correction, cervical stabilization exercises, and gentle stretching has effectively alleviated symptoms and improved function. Manual therapy and mechanical traction may offer additional benefits, although evidence supporting traction is limited. Pharmacologic treatments, including NSAIDs and acetaminophen, provide symptomatic relief. For neuropathic pain, agents like pregabalin or gabapentin are commonly used, though results are inconsistent. Short courses of oral corticosteroids can reduce inflammation and pain, particularly in acute flare-ups, but their long-term benefits are limited.

- **Epidural corticosteroid injections (ESIs):** ESIs are effective for acute and subacute radicular pain, with interlaminar injections preferred over transforaminal due to safety concerns. These injections deliver corticosteroids and anesthetics to the epidural space, reducing inflammation and alleviating nerve root compression. However, evidence regarding their long-term efficacy is mixed, and repeated injections should be carefully considered to minimize risks.

- **Pulsed radiofrequency (PRF):**
  PRF is emerging as a promising treatment for chronic cervical radicular pain. Unlike continuous radiofrequency ablation, PRF delivers low-intensity energy to modulate nerve conduction without causing permanent damage. Studies show significant pain reduction and functional improvement with PRF adjacent to the dorsal root ganglion (DRG). Its safety profile and effectiveness make it an appealing option for patients unresponsive to conservative therapies or ESIs.

- **Spinal cord stimulation (SCS):**
  SCS is a last-resort option for patients with refractory cervical radicular pain. By delivering electrical impulses to the spinal cord, SCS modulates pain perception. Although evidence for its use in cervical radiculopathy is limited, it may benefit select patients in specialized pain management centers.

Key takeaways

☑ **Comprehensive assessment** combining history, physical examination, and imaging is crucial for accurate diagnosis.

☑ **ESIs are first-line interventional treatments** for acute to subacute cervical radicular pain, while PRF is emerging as a key modality for chronic cases.

☑ **Physical therapy and exercise** remain foundational for most patients, with manual therapy providing added benefit.

☑ **Interdisciplinary approaches optimize outcomes,** especially for refractory or chronic cases.

Additional recommended reading:

1. Peene L, Cohen SP, Brouwer B, et al. Cervical radicular pain: Diagnosis and treatment. *Pain Practice.* 2024;24:800-817.

2. Bogduk N. Advances in the diagnosis and management of neck pain. *BMJ.* 2017;358.

3. .Van Zundert J, Huntoon M, Lataster A, et al. Pulsed radiofrequency for chronic cervical radicular pain. *Pain.* 2007;127:123-132.

Minimizing risks with cervical epidural injections

19

Why this topic is important

Cervical epidural injections are a cornerstone in managing cervical radicular pain and other neck-related conditions. These injections, which include both interlaminar and transforaminal techniques, can provide significant relief to patients suffering from nerve root irritation caused by disc herniation, spondylosis, or other degenerative conditions. However, the procedure carries inherent risks, including the potential for neurological injury, spinal cord damage, and vascular complications. The proximity of the cervical epidural space to critical structures such as the spinal cord and vertebral arteries necessitates meticulous technique and adherence to safety protocols.

This review synthesizes evidence from Holder et al. (2024) and related literature, providing updated strategies to minimize risks while optimizing outcomes. Emphasizing proper patient selection, imaging, procedural techniques, and awareness of anatomical variations is a practical guide for clinicians to perform cervical epidural injections safely.

Objectives of this update

- Highlight key safety concerns associated with cervical epidural injections, focusing on both interlaminar and transforaminal approaches.

- Provide evidence-based recommendations for minimizing risks through imaging, procedural planning, and sedation protocols.

- Discuss patient-centered decision-making, including considerations for anticoagulation management and procedural necessity.

What is new

This update incorporates recent advancements, including:

- **Preferred injection levels:** Evidence supports performing cervical interlaminar epidural steroid injections (CILESIs) at C6-C7 or below to minimize risks.

- **Sedation recommendations:** Strong emphasis on minimizing sedation to allow for patient feedback during the procedure.

- **Enhanced imaging protocols:** Contralateral oblique (CLO) fluoroscopic views are utilized to improve the safety and accuracy of needle placement.

Key safety considerations

Needle placement and anatomical insights

- **Preferred levels for interlaminar injections:**

  - The dorsal epidural space is more capacious at lower cervical levels (C6-C7 or C7-T1), making these sites safer for needle access.

  - Needle placement at higher levels increases the risk of spinal cord injury due to the reduced distance between the ligamentum flavum (LF) and the spinal cord.

- **Midline ligamentum flavum gaps:**

  - Gaps in the LF, particularly at the midline, are common in the cervical spine and can lead to diminished tactile feedback during loss-of-resistance (LOR) techniques.

  - A paramedian approach is recommended to avoid midline LF gaps, reducing the risk of inadvertent dural puncture or spinal cord injury.

- **Imaging guidance:**

  - Multiplanar imaging is crucial for safe needle placement. The CLO view offers superior visualization of the needle tip compared to the lateral view, reducing the risk of aberrant placement.

Sedation considerations

- Deep sedation is strongly discouraged due to its association with catastrophic complications such as spinal cord injury.

- To enhance safety, minimal sedation, ensuring the patient can provide verbal feedback, is recommended. This allows clinicians to monitor for signs of nerve irritation or intrathecal placement during the procedure.

Vascular risks and transforaminal injections

Importance of preprocedural imaging

- The vascular anatomy of the cervical spine is highly variable, with the vertebral artery occasionally occupying positions that increase the risk of inadvertent puncture.

- Preprocedural MRI or CT imaging is recommended to identify anatomical variations, such as vertebral artery loops or anomalous segmental arteries, which can guide safer needle trajectories.

Technical recommendations

- The use of non-particulate steroids reduces the risk of embolic complications during transforaminal injections.

- Digital subtraction imaging (DSI) is preferred over standard fluoroscopy to detect vascular uptake and prevent inadvertent arterial injections.

Managing anticoagulation

- Cervical epidural injections carry a risk of epidural hematoma, particularly in patients on anticoagulants or antiplatelet therapy.

- Current guidelines recommend withholding anticoagulants before the procedure whenever possible, but this decision must be balanced against the risks of thrombotic events.

- Collaboration with the prescribing physician is essential to determine the safest approach for each patient.

Patient-centered decision-making

Cervical epidural injections are elective procedures and should be reserved for patients with clear indications and a likelihood of benefit. Clinicians should weigh the procedural risks against the patient's condition, ensuring that the intervention aligns with the patient's goals and clinical scenario.

Key takeaways

☑ Perform cervical interlaminar injections at C6-C7 or below, with C7-T1 being the preferred site for safety.

☑ Avoid deep sedation; use the least necessary sedation to allow for patient feedback.

☑ Use advanced imaging techniques, including CLO views and DSI, to enhance procedural accuracy and safety.

☑ Consider preprocedural imaging to identify vascular anomalies and guide needle trajectory.

☑ Carefully manage anticoagulation therapy in collaboration with the prescribing physician.

☑ Emphasize patient-centered care, ensuring that the procedure's benefits outweigh the risks.

Additional recommended reading:

1. Holder EK, Lee H, Raghunandan A, et al. Minimizing risks with cervical epidural injections. *Interventional Pain Medicine*. 2024;3:100430.

2. Rathmell JP, Benzon HT, Dreyfuss P, et al. Safeguards to prevent neurologic complications after epidural steroid injections. *Anesthesiology*. 2015;122(5):974-84.

3. Gitkind AI, Olson TR, Downie SA. Vertebral artery anatomical variations as they relate to cervical transforaminal epidural steroid injections. *Pain Med*. 2014;15(7):1109-14.

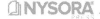

The safety of cervical transforaminal epidural steroid injections

20

Cervical TFESI and its clinical role

- **Prevalence of cervical radicular pain:** Affects approximately 83 per 100,000 individuals in the United States, often due to disc herniation or spondylosis.

- **Therapeutic goals:** Cervical TFESIs target inflammation and nerve root compression to reduce radicular symptoms and delay or prevent surgical intervention.

- **FDA warning (2014):** Highlighted neurological risks primarily linked to particulate steroids, emphasizing the importance of technique refinements and safer steroid choices.

Study design and methodology

1. **Retrospective analysis:**
   - 6,241 cervical TFESIs were identified through procedural coding (CPT 64479) performed between 2004 and 2021 at a single academic institution.
   - Non-particulate steroids were predominantly used after the mid-2000s.

2. **Detailed safety review:**
   - Catastrophic complications were assessed by querying performing physicians and department directors.
   - A subset of 200 consecutive procedures underwent chart review to capture minor side effects, including immediate recovery observations and follow-up clinic notes.

Key results

1. **Catastrophic complications:**
   - Across 6,241 cervical TFESIs, no cases of stroke, spinal cord injury, or death were reported.
   - Physicians and department directors corroborated the absence of major adverse events.

2. **Pain outcomes:**
   - Among 200 consecutive cases, 85.5% of patients reported pain reduction, with an average pain score decrease of 3.7 points.
   - 75.5% achieved at least a 2-point reduction in pain, and 62.5% had a 3-point or greater reduction.

3. **Minor complications:**
   - Transient pain increase: 7 patients (3.5%), with 5 experiencing a pain increase $\geq$ 3 points.
   - Other isolated complications: headache (2 cases), insomnia (1 case), transient numbness (1 case), elevated glucose > 500 (1 case), hypertension (1 case), and localized rash (1 case).

Clinical implications

1. **Safety profile:**
   - The findings strongly support the safety of cervical TFESIs when using non-particulate steroids, consistent with consensus guidelines.
   - Proper needle placement, fluoroscopic guidance, and live contrast visualization further mitigate risks.

2. **Technique optimization:**
   - Employing a modified oblique approach minimizes the likelihood of vascular or neural injury.
   - Incorporating digital subtraction angiography (DSA) enhances vascular flow detection, particularly for avoiding radiculomedullary artery injection.

3. **Patient counseling:**
   - Educate patients about the low risk of complications and high likelihood of pain relief.
   - Emphasize the transient nature of most side effects, such as minor pain increases or headaches.

4. **Future considerations:**
   - Adoption of standardized protocols for needle positioning, steroid type, and imaging guidance can further improve safety and outcomes.

Limitations

- **Retrospective design:** Relies on physician recall and chart documentation, which may underreport minor complications.

- **Lack of control group:** Comparative outcomes with other cervical epidural approaches (e.g., interlaminar) were not evaluated.

- **Incomplete steroid data:** J-codes were unavailable for all cases, limiting verification of steroid type in the early years of the study.

Future directions

- **Prospective trials:** Rigorous studies comparing cervical TFESIs with other techniques (e.g., interlaminar injections) are warranted.

- **Patient selection refinement:** Identifying anatomical or clinical predictors of poor response or complications could optimize outcomes.

- **Long-term follow-up:** Tracking pain relief durability and delayed complications will enhance understanding of cervical TFESI safety.

Key takeaways

☑ **Cervical TFESIs with non-particulate steroids are safe,** with no catastrophic complications reported across 6,241 procedures.

☑ **Pain relief is achieved in 85.5% of patients,** with an average pain score reduction of 3.7 points.

☑ **Minor complications are rare and self-limiting,** emphasizing the importance of technique and steroid choice.

☑ Continued refinement of safety protocols and procedural standards is essential for further risk reduction.

Additional recommended reading:

1. Backworth WJ, Ghanbari GM, Lamas-Basulto E, Taylor B. Safety of cervical transforaminal epidural steroid injections: a retrospective review. *Interventional Pain Medicine.* 2024;3:100420.

2. Rathmell JP, Benzon HT, Dreyfuss P, et al. Safeguards to prevent neurologic complications after epidural steroid injections: consensus opinions from a multidisciplinary working group and national organizations. *Anesthesiology.* 2015;122(5):974-984.

3. Gill B, Cheney C, Clements N, et al. Radiofrequency ablation for zygapophyseal joint pain. *Phys Med Rehabil Clin N Am.* 2022;33(2):233-249.

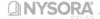

Cervical transforaminal epidural steroid injections for cervical radicular pain

21

Why this topic is important

Cervical radiculopathy, a condition characterized by radiating arm pain due to nerve root compression in the cervical spine, significantly affects patient quality of life. Cervical transforaminal epidural steroid injections (CTFESIs) are an established treatment option for refractory radicular pain, providing targeted delivery of corticosteroids to reduce inflammation. Despite its widespread use, long-term effectiveness data for CTFESIs are sparse, leaving questions about their sustained impact on pain relief, function, and health-related quality of life. This prospective cohort study by Conger et al. (2024) addresses these gaps by evaluating pain, disability, and healthcare utilization outcomes over 12 months, providing critical insights into the long-term value of CTFESIs.

Objectives of this update

- Assess the effectiveness of CTFESIs for clinically meaningful improvements in pain and disability in cervical radiculopathy patients.

- Evaluate the durability of these outcomes over a 12-month follow-up period.

- Explore secondary outcomes such as quality of life, sleep interference, healthcare utilization, and surgical avoidance rates.

What is new

This study provides important updates by:

- Demonstrating that **58-65% of patients achieved ≥ 50% reduction in arm pain scores** at 12 months, with similar improvements in neck disability indices (NDI-5).

- Showing **91% of participants required only one injection,** with a low surgical rate of 18% over the year.

- Highlighting improvements in secondary outcomes, including personal goal achievement, health-related quality of life, and reduced pain-related sleep disturbances.

Understanding cervical radiculopathy and CTFESIs

- **Pathophysiology:**

  - Cervical radiculopathy is commonly caused by disc herniation, osteophyte formation, or foraminal stenosis.

  - Transforaminal injections deliver corticosteroids directly to the affected nerve root, targeting inflammation and neural irritation.

- **Study population and design:**

  - This prospective cohort study enrolled 33 patients (63.6% female, mean age 51.2 years) with unilateral cervical radiculopathy lasting 6 weeks to 6 months.

  - Participants had significant arm pain (≥ 4/10), and the primary causes included disc herniation (33%) and foraminal stenosis (27%).

Results

1. **Primary outcomes:**
   - **Arm pain relief:**
     - At 12 months, **64.5% of participants** reported ≥ 50% reduction in arm pain, with an average pain decrease of 4.6 points.
   - **Disability improvement:**
     - The percentage achieving ≥ 30% improvement in NDI-5 scores ranged from 60.6% (1 month) to 71.0% (12 months).

2. **Secondary outcomes:**
   - **Quality of life:** Significant improvements in EQ-5D scores.
   - **Sleep quality:** 17-40% reported ≥ 30% improvement in Chronic Pain Sleep Inventory (CPSI) scores.
   - Personal goal achievement: 33-56% restored at least three of four key activities (e.g., work, self-care).

3. **Healthcare utilization:**
   - Only 9% of participants underwent surgery after the first month, with **91% requiring a single injection** during the study period.

4. **Adverse effects:**
   - No severe complications, such as infection or nerve injury, were reported.

Clinical implications

- **Efficacy of CTFESIs:**

  - Results confirm the long-term effectiveness of CTFESIs for reducing arm pain and disability in carefully selected patients.

  - Pain relief and functional improvements are maintained for up to one year, supporting CTFESIs as a viable alternative to surgical interventions.

- **Importance of patient selection:**

  - Strict inclusion criteria, such as unilateral symptoms and MRI-confirmed pathology, are crucial for optimizing outcomes.

  - Individuals with severe depression or other comorbidities may experience less favorable results.

- **Role in surgical avoidance:**

  - Low surgical conversion rates highlight the value of CTFESIs in delaying or preventing more invasive interventions.

Limitations

- **Small sample size:** The cohort size limited subgroup analyses and may restrict the generalizability of findings.

- **The absence of a control group** means that the study cannot separate treatment effects from the natural history of cervical radiculopathy.

- **Enrollment challenges:** Strict criteria resulted in low recruitment rates, potentially introducing selection bias.

Key takeaways

☑ **CTFESIs provide sustained pain relief and disability reduction** for up to one year in carefully selected cervical radiculopathy patients.

☑ **Secondary benefits include improved quality of life, personal goal achievement, and reduced healthcare utilization.**

☑ **No serious adverse effects** were reported, affirming the safety of CTFESIs.

☑ Strict **patient selection criteria are critical** for optimizing treatment success and minimizing surgical conversion rates.

Additional recommended reading:

1. Conger AM, Randall DJ, Sperry BP, et al. The effectiveness of cervical transforaminal epidural steroid injections for the treatment of cervical radicular pain: a prospective cohort study reporting 12-month outcomes. *Interventional Pain Medicine*. 2024;3:100379.

2. Dreyfuss P, Baker R, Bogduk N. Comparative effectiveness of cervical transforaminal injections with particulate and nonparticulate corticosteroid preparations for cervical radicular pain. *Pain Med*. 2006;7(3):237-42.

3. Kesikburun S, Aras B, Kelle B, et al. The effectiveness of cervical transforaminal epidural steroid injection for neck pain due to cervical disc herniation: long-term results. *Pain Manag*. 2018;8(5):321-6.

Ultrasound-guided medial branch blocks to select patients for cervical facet joint radiofrequency neurotomy

22

Why this topic is important

Cervical transforaminal epidural steroid injections (TFESIs) are a widely utilized intervention for managing cervical radicular pain caused by disc herniation or cervical spondylosis. While these injections offer substantial pain relief and improved quality of life, concerns about severe adverse events, such as spinal cord injury, stroke, and death, have persisted. These risks, highlighted by the FDA's 2014 safety warning, were predominantly associated with the use of particulate steroids. Advances in technique and the transition to non-particulate steroids have significantly enhanced safety, but ongoing skepticism among some practitioners warrants rigorous examination. This review by Backworth et al. (2024) analyzes safety outcomes for cervical TFESIs performed with non-particulate steroids, aiming to provide clarity on their risk profile and support evidence-based clinical decision-making.

Objectives of this update

- Evaluate the incidence of catastrophic complications associated with cervical TFESIs using non-particulate steroids.

- Analyze the frequency and severity of immediate and delayed minor side effects following the procedure.

- Offer practical recommendations to enhance safety during cervical TFESIs, informed by the study findings.

What is new

This study, one of the largest retrospective reviews of cervical TFESIs, highlights the following key insights:

- Over 6,241 cervical TFESIs were analyzed, with **no catastrophic complications** (e.g., spinal cord injury, stroke, or death) reported.

- Among 200 consecutive procedures examined for minor side effects, **85.5% of patients experienced a reduction in pain,** with an average pain score drop of 3.7 points.

- Minor complications were rare and included transient pain increases (3.5%), headaches (1%), and isolated cases of transient numbness, hypertension, and elevated glucose.

- Findings confirm the **safety of cervical TFESIs when performed with non-particulate steroids** and appropriate safety protocols.

Why this topic is important

Cervical facet joint pain is a common cause of chronic neck pain, often presenting with reduced range of motion, localized tenderness, and referred pain patterns. For patients with refractory symptoms, cervical facet joint radiofrequency neurotomy (CRFN) is a minimally invasive procedure that can provide significant and prolonged pain relief by denervating the medial branches of the dorsal rami. Selecting suitable candidates for CRFN relies on diagnostic medial branch blocks (MBBs), traditionally performed under fluoroscopic guidance (FLB).

Although fluoroscopy has been the gold standard for MBBs, ultrasound-guided blocks (USBs) are emerging as a viable alternative. USBs offer several potential advantages, including the absence of ionizing radiation, reduced cost, and greater accessibility. However, concerns about the accuracy and reliability of USBs compared to FLBs have limited their widespread adoption. This update reviews findings from Burnham et al. (2024), a matched retrospective cohort study that evaluates the validity of USBs in predicting CRFN outcomes. The study provides evidence supporting USBs as a safe and effective method for selecting patients for CRFN, offering essential implications for clinical practice.

Objectives of this update

- Compare the validity of USBs and FLBs in predicting outcomes after CRFN.

- Highlight the safety and efficiency benefits of USBs.

- Explore practical recommendations for implementing USBs in clinical practice.

What is new

This study presents key advancements:

- Demonstrates that USBs are as valid as FLBs in predicting CRFN outcomes, with comparable pain relief and quality-of-life improvements.

- Highlights the safety advantages of USBs, including reduced vascular injury rates and no radiation exposure.

- Establishes the potential for USBs to be integrated into routine practice, particularly in settings with limited access to fluoroscopy.

Study design

The study analyzed data from 27 patients (58 CRFNs) who underwent USBs and 38 patients (58 CRFNs) who underwent FLBs. Matching criteria included demographics, pain duration, diagnostic block outcomes, and CRFN number (first or repeat). Pain and disability were assessed using the numeric rating scale (NRS) and the Pain Disability Quality-of-Life Questionnaire-Spine (PDQQ-S). Outcomes were evaluated 3 months post-CRFN.

Key results

- Both USB and FLB groups experienced significant improvements in pain and function:
  - NRS pain reduction: 45% (USB) vs. 51% (FLB).
  - PDQQ-S reduction: 42% (USB) vs. 49% (FLB).
  - Proportions achieving ≥ 50% pain relief: 59% (USB) vs. 60% (FLB).
- Retrospective estimates of pain relief magnitude and duration were similar:
  - Pain relief: 79% (USB) vs. 84% (FLB).
  - Relief duration: 10.0 months (USB) vs. 10.4 months (FLB).

Clinical implications

- USBs are comparably valid to FLBs in predicting CRFN outcomes, supporting their use as a diagnostic tool.
- Comparable pain and functional outcomes between the groups affirm USBs' reliability in clinical practice.

Safety and efficiency

- **Safety:**
  USBs eliminate radiation exposure, reducing risks for patients and clinicians. Additionally, USBs demonstrated lower rates of vascular breaches, enhancing procedural safety.

- **Efficiency:**
  - USBs required less time than FLBs, streamlining procedural workflows.
  - Real-time visualization with Doppler ultra-sound aids in avoiding vascular structures and confirming injectate placement, minimizing complications.

Practical considerations

- **Operator expertise:**
  - Proficiency in ultrasound-guided interventions is essential. The study highlighted the steep learning curve for USBs, emphasizing the role of training and experience.

- **Anatomical limitations:**
  - Challenges in visualizing lower cervical facet joints (C6-T1) were noted, making USBs less suitable for some patients. Clear visualization of target structures should guide case selection.

- **Resource optimization:**
  - USBs offer a cost-effective alternative to fluoroscopy, particularly in outpatient or resource-limited settings.

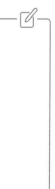

Key takeaways

☑ **USBs are a valid alternative** to FLBs for selecting CRFN candidates, with comparable pain relief and functional outcomes.

☑ **Safety and efficiency advantages** make USBs attractive in settings where fluoroscopy is unavailable or impractical.

☑ **Operator expertise and case selection** are critical for successful USB implementation.

☑ USBs can potentially expand access to diagnostic and interventional pain management, particularly in resource-limited environments.

Additional recommended reading:

1. Burnham R, Trow R, Smith A, et al. Can ultrasound-guided medial branch blocks be used to select patients for cervical facet joint radiofrequency neurotomy? *Pain Medicine.* 2024;25(11):671-674.

2. Finlayson RJ, Gupta G, Tran DQ. Ultrasound-guided cervical medial branch block: A novel technique. *Reg Anesth Pain Med.* 2012;37(2):219-223.

3. Hurley RW, Adams MCB, Barad M, et al. Consensus practice guidelines on interventions for cervical spine (facet) joint pain. *Reg Anesth Pain Med.* 2022;47(1):3-59.

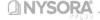

Epidural steroid injections in lumbar spinal stenosis

23

Why this topic is important

Lumbar spinal stenosis (LSS) is a common and challenging condition that predominantly affects older adults, arising from degenerative changes in the lumbar spine. It is characterized by a spinal canal narrowing, leading to nerve roots and spinal cord compression. This results in hallmark symptoms such as neurogenic claudication, which manifests as pain, numbness, or weakness in the lower extremities, often worsened by standing or walking and relieved by sitting or leaning forward. Radicular pain, or shooting pain radiating from the lower back to the legs, is another debilitating symptom of LSS. These symptoms impair physical functionality and diminish quality of life, limiting independence and increasing reliance on healthcare systems.

Conservative treatments, including physical therapy, activity modification, and medications like NSAIDs, remain the first-line approach for managing LSS. However, for patients whose symptoms persist or worsen, epidural steroid injections (ESIs) play a pivotal role in the interventional management pathway. ESIs aim to deliver corticosteroids directly into the epidural space to reduce inflammation and alleviate pain. They provide significant short-term relief, particularly for neurogenic claudication and radicular pain, enabling patients to engage in physical therapy and delay or avoid surgical interventions.

Despite their widespread use, ESIs have been scrutinized for their safety in patients with severe or multilevel stenosis. A significant concern is the potential for injectate volume to exacerbate neural compression within an already narrowed epidural space, theoretically worsening symptoms or causing neurological complications. This has fueled debates among practitioners, particularly regarding optimal injection techniques and safety protocols for high-risk patients.

This update synthesizes recent findings from clinical studies, including a 2024 review by Christolias et al. (2024), which addresses these concerns and provides evidence-based recommendations for the safe and effective use of ESIs in LSS. It emphasizes the importance of targeting the most stenotic levels, using appropriate injectate volumes, and adopting procedural techniques that enhance outcomes. These insights are critical for guiding clinical decision-making and optimizing patient care in this challenging population.

Objectives of this update

- Evaluate the safety of ESIs in patients with severe lumbar spinal stenosis, particularly concerning volume effects.

- Review the clinical efficacy of ESIs in managing pain and functional limitations in LSS.

- Provide recommendations for ESI use in the context of imaging findings, injectate volume, and procedural techniques.

What is new

This update highlights key advancements and practical insights:

- **Safety evidence:** No documented cases of neurological injury directly attributable to volume effects, even in patients with severe stenosis.

- **Targeted injections:** Better outcomes are achieved when ESIs are performed at the most stenotic level, emphasizing the importance of accurate imaging and procedural planning.

- **Updated techniques:** Careful selection of injectate volume enhances both safety and efficacy, reducing the risk of complications.

Lumbar spinal stenosis: Clinical and diagnostic overview

- **Pathophysiology and presentation**

  LSS commonly results from degenerative changes such as disc bulging, ligamentum flavum hypertrophy, and facet joint osteoarthritis. These changes narrow the spinal canal, compressing nerve roots and reducing the capacity of the neural structures to adapt to mechanical stress during movement. Patients frequently report neurogenic claudication, distinguishing LSS from other causes of low back and leg pain.

  The symptoms often worsen with activities like walking or prolonged standing and are alleviated by positions that increase spinal canal dimensions, such as forward flexion or sitting. Advanced cases may present with significant motor deficits, sensory loss, or bowel and bladder dysfunction, necessitating urgent intervention.

- **Imaging considerations**

  MRI remains the gold standard for diagnosing LSS, providing detailed visualization of soft tissue structures, including the degree of canal narrowing and nerve root impingement. Cross-sectional imaging, particularly in axial views, is critical for identifying the most stenotic levels, guiding precise ESI placement, and minimizing procedural risks. CT scans can supplement MRI when evaluating osseous contributions to stenosis, such as osteophytes.

Safety of epidural steroid injections

- **Concerns regarding volume effects:**

  - The theoretical risk of worsening neural compression due to added volume in the epidural space is a common concern.

  - However, injectate typically disperses along the path of least resistance, mitigating significant localized pressure increases.

- **Evidence summary:**

  - Large cohort studies involving over 69,000 ESIs report no documented cases of neurological injury directly linked to injectate volume effects.

  - Studies using injectate volumes of up to 20 mL (caudal approach) and 8 mL (interlaminar approach) have demonstrated no adverse effects, even in patients with severe stenosis.

- **Complication rates:**

  - Rare complications, such as cerebrospinal fluid leakage, hematoma, and localized infection, were reported at rates < 1%.

  - When ESIs were performed at the level of maximal stenosis, no increased risk of symptom exacerbation or neurological compromise was observed.

Efficacy of epidural steroid injections

- **Clinical outcomes**

  - ESIs provide significant short-term relief for neurogenic claudication and radicular symptoms, with 50-70% of patients reporting pain reduction and improved function. Targeting the most stenotic levels has been associated with better outcomes, likely due to the direct delivery of anti-inflammatory agents to the affected nerve roots.

- **Comparison of techniques**

  - Interlaminar ESIs: Preferred for delivering larger volumes, offering broad coverage of the epidural space.

  - Transforaminal ESIs: Provide targeted delivery to specific nerve roots, often with a faster onset of relief.

  - Caudal ESIs: Useful when direct access to the lumbar region is challenging, though higher volumes may be required for effectiveness.

- **Durability of relief**

  - The benefits of ESIs are transient, typically lasting weeks to months. Combining ESIs with physical therapy and structured exercise programs can enhance long-term outcomes by addressing the underlying biomechanical contributors to pain. However, repeated injections should be approached cautiously due to diminishing returns and potential risks.

Key takeaways

- ☑ **ESIs are safe and effective** for managing lumbar spinal stenosis, even in severe cases, when performed with appropriate technique and injectate volume.

- ☑ **Targeting the most stenotic level** improves clinical outcomes, reducing pain and enhancing function.

- ☑ **Interdisciplinary management,** combining ESIs with physical therapy, offers the best chance of long-term relief.

- ☑ **Close monitoring during procedures** is crucial, with immediate cessation of injection upon worsening symptoms to minimize risks.

Additional recommended reading:

1. Christolias G, Raghunandan A, Schneider BJ, et al. Epidural steroid injection in lumbar spinal stenosis: A patient safety review. *Interventional Pain Medicine.* 2024;3:100444.

2. Milburn J, Freeman J, Steven A, et al. Interlaminar epidural steroid injection for degenerative lumbar spinal canal stenosis: Does the intervertebral level of performance matter? *Ochsner J.* 2014;14(1):62-6.

3. Sencan S, Celenlioglu AE, Yolcu G, et al. Comparative outcomes of lumbar central stenosis patients treated with epidural steroid injections: Interlaminar versus bilateral transforaminal approach. *Korean J Pain.* 2020;33(3):226-33.

The timeline of pain relief after epidural steroid injections

24

Why this topic is important

Epidural steroid injections (ESI) are a cornerstone treatment for managing radicular pain associated with spinal conditions, offering potential relief for millions of patients worldwide. However, patients often ask: *"How soon will I feel better?"* or *"How will I know if this treatment worked?"* Until now, there has been limited research detailing the precise timeline of symptom improvement after ESI, leaving clinicians to rely on general guidelines or anecdotal experience. This update, based on the article by Schneider et al. (2024), addresses this gap by providing evidence-based insights into the temporal response of patients following ESI, enhancing clinical decision-making and patient communication.

Objectives of this update

- Summarize the key findings of a recent study tracking pain relief timelines after ESI.

- Provide clinicians with actionable insights to predict treatment outcomes within days rather than weeks.

- Clarify implications for follow-up care, including repeat injections or alternative therapies.

What is new

This study followed 134 patients over three weeks post-ESI to determine how quickly pain relief occurred and its predictive value for long-term success. It demonstrated that patient responses on day 4 and beyond are highly predictive of their outcomes at three weeks. The results challenge previous assumptions, suggesting that waiting two weeks to assess ESI efficacy may only sometimes be necessary.

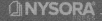

Study design and approach

- Conducted at a single academic spine center, this prospective study tracked pain relief in 134 patients using detailed follow-ups every three days post-ESI for 21 days.

- Pain relief was measured using a numeric pain score and subjective reports of percentage pain reduction.

- Both cervical and lumbar ESIs were included, utilizing a variety of corticosteroids and injection techniques.

Key outcomes

1. **Timeline of pain relief:**

   ◦ Of the patients who achieved ≥ 50% pain relief at three weeks, 94% had already reported significant relief by day 4.

   ◦ A small subset achieved delayed relief after day 4, highlighting a minority with slower responses.

2. **Predictive value of early response:**

   ◦ Pain relief on day 4 strongly predicted three-week outcomes. Sustained relief by day 7 or day 10 further solidified this likelihood.

   ◦ Negative responses on day 4 were equally predictive of poor outcomes, allowing early identification of non-responders.

Clinical implications

- **Patient counseling:**

  ◦ Clinicians can inform patients that most will know by day 4 if the ESI is effective.

  ◦ By day 7, outcomes are highly predictable, making prolonged waiting unnecessary.

- **Repeat injection timing:**

  ◦ While Medicare guidelines recommend waiting 14 days before repeating a failed ESI, the study suggests this could be reconsidered for patients with early negative responses.

- **Understanding variability:**

  ◦ 46% of patients experienced some variability in relief during the three weeks, emphasizing the need for comprehensive follow-up.

Limitations

- The study only extended up to three weeks, leaving long-term predictive patterns unexamined.

- Due to small subgroup sizes, it was underpowered to analyze differences based on steroid type or injection technique.

- Post-injection medication adjustments, though monitored, may have influenced results.

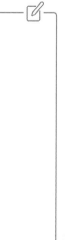

Key takeaways

☑ Most patients (94%) who will achieve significant pain relief post-ESI experience it by day 4.

☑ Early pain relief (by day 4) strongly predicts sustained success at three weeks.

☑ Negative responses by day 4 are equally reliable indicators of poor outcomes.

☑ Clinicians do not need to wait two full weeks to evaluate ESI efficacy.

☑ This data challenges current Medicare recommendations for waiting 14 days before considering repeat ESIs.

Additional recommended reading:

1. Schneider BJ, Chukwuma VU, Fechtel BM, Kennedy DJ. How soon after an epidural steroid injection can you predict the patient's response? *Interventional Pain Medicine.* 2024;3:100435.

2. Smith CC, McCormick ZL, Mattie R, MacVicar J, Duszynski B, Stojanovic MP. The effectiveness of lumbar transforaminal injection of steroid for the treatment of radicular pain: a comprehensive review of the published data. *Pain Med.* 2020;21(3):472-487.

3. El-Yahchouchi C, Wald J, Brault J, et al. Lumbar transforaminal epidural steroid injections: does immediate post-procedure pain response predict longer-term effectiveness? *Pain Med.* 2014;15(6):921-928.

Lumbosacral radicular pain: Diagnosis and management

25

Why this topic is important

Lumbosacral radicular pain is a prevalent and debilitating condition characterized by radiating pain along the lumbar or sacral dermatomes, often accompanied by sensory or motor deficits. Common causes include lumbar disc herniation and degenerative spinal changes, such as foraminal stenosis or ligamentum flavum hypertrophy. This condition affects 9.9% to 25% of the general population annually, making it one of the most frequent causes of neuropathic pain.

Despite its prevalence, diagnosing lumbosacral radicular pain remains challenging due to the overlap of symptoms with other conditions like facet joint or sacroiliac joint pain. Accurate identification is critical to guide appropriate management, which ranges from conservative therapies to advanced interventional techniques such as epidural steroid injections (ESIs), pulsed radiofrequency (PRF), and spinal cord stimulation (SCS). This update synthesizes findings from Peene et al. (2024) and highlights evidence-based diagnostic criteria, management strategies, and emerging innovations in the field.

Objectives of this update

- Summarize current diagnostic standards for lumbosacral radicular pain.

- Review the evidence supporting conservative, pharmacologic, and interventional treatments.

- Explore the utility of advanced interventions for refractory cases, including PRF and SCS.

What is new

Recent insights have enhanced the understanding and management of lumbosacral radicular pain:

- **Diagnostic clarity:** Standardized tools like dermatomal mapping and selective nerve root blocks improve diagnostic accuracy.

- **Tailored interventions:** Evidence supports pulsed radiofrequency adjacent to the dorsal root ganglion (DRG) as effective for chronic cases unresponsive to conservative therapy.

- **Evolving technologies:** High-frequency SCS and epidural adhesiolysis demonstrate potential for improved outcomes in refractory cases.

Diagnosis

Clinical presentation

Lumbosacral radicular pain often manifests as sharp, shooting, or burning pain radiating from the lower back into the legs. Patients may also report paresthesia or motor weakness in a dermatomal pattern, with symptoms exacerbated by activities like sitting or bending. Associated conditions, such as lumbar spinal stenosis, may cause neurogenic claudication, characterized by leg pain and weakness during walking, relieved by sitting or bending forward.

Physical examination

- **Straight leg raise (Lasègue test):** High sensitivity (92%) but low specificity (28%) for identifying nerve root irritation due to lumbar disc herniation.
- **Crossed straight leg raise:** High specificity (90%) but lower sensitivity (28%).
- **Reflex and motor tests:** L4 involvement may reduce patellar reflex, while S1 deficits affect Achilles reflex and plantar flexion.

Imaging

- **MRI:** Gold standard for visualizing nerve root compression or disc herniation.
- **CT myelography:** Useful when MRI is contraindicated.
- **Electrodiagnostic studies:** Aid in differentiating radiculopathy from peripheral neuropathy.

Treatment options

Conservative management

- **Physical therapy and exercise:**
  - Improves functionality and reduces pain, though evidence for long-term benefits is mixed.
  - Manual therapy combined with supervised exercise yields better outcomes than exercise alone.

- **Pharmacological treatments:**
  - **NSAIDs:** Modest short-term pain relief in acute radicular pain but less effective for chronic cases.
  - **Corticosteroids:** Systemic corticosteroids may provide temporary relief but are not recommended for long-term use.
  - **Neuropathic agents:** Mixed evidence for gabapentinoids and tricyclic antidepressants in chronic pain.
  - **Opioids:** Limited role due to significant risks and minimal long-term efficacy.

Interventional therapies

- **Epidural steroid injections (ESIs):**
  - **Transforaminal approach:** Offers targeted delivery to inflamed nerve roots, providing superior pain relief compared to interlaminar or caudal approaches.
  - **Interlaminar and caudal ESIs:** May be appropriate for patients with bilateral symptoms or challenging anatomy.
  - **Benefits:** Short-term pain relief and improved mobility, particularly in subacute cases.

- **Pulsed radiofrequency (PRF):**
  - Targets the DRG to modulate nerve activity and reduce chronic pain.
  - Provides significant relief in refractory cases, with reported effectiveness lasting several months.

- **Epidural adhesiolysis:**
  - Utilized for breaking up scar tissue and enhancing the spread of analgesics.
  - May benefit patients with epidural fibrosis or failed back surgery syndrome (FBSS).

- **Spinal cord stimulation (SCS):**
  - Effective for neuropathic pain and FBSS, with newer high-frequency and burst stimulation modalities offering paresthesia-free pain relief.

Surgical options

Surgery may be necessary for severe cases with significant neurological deficits or refractory pain. Indications include large disc herniations, cauda equina syndrome, or persistent pain despite exhaustive conservative and interventional management.

Key takeaways

☑ Comprehensive assessment combining history, physical examination, and imaging is essential for accurate diagnosis.

☑ Conservative treatments, including physical therapy and NSAIDs, are first-line options for subacute cases.

☑ Transforaminal ESIs and PRF are effective interventional strategies for managing pain and improving function.

☑ When applied judiciously in specialized settings, SCS and epidural adhesiolysis offer hope for refractory cases.

☑ A multimodal approach integrating pharmacologic, interventional, and psychological therapies optimizes patient outcomes.

Additional recommended reading:

1. Peene L, Cohen SP, Kallewaard JW, et al. Lumbosacral radicular pain: Update of evidence-based interventional pain medicine. *Pain Practice.* 2024;24:525-552.

2. Bogduk N. The clinical anatomy of lumbosacral radicular pain. *Pain.* 2009;139:9-12.

3. Manchikanti L, Hirsch JA, Falco FJ, et al. A systematic review of mechanical lumbar disc decompression techniques for chronic low back pain. *Pain Physician.* 2014;17-E557.

Lumbar transforaminal or interlaminar epidural steroid injections

26

Why this topic is important

Lumbar radicular pain, commonly associated with intervertebral disc herniation or spinal stenosis, is a debilitating condition frequently managed with epidural steroid injections (ESIs). Transforaminal (TFESI) and interlaminar (ILESI) approaches are the two main techniques for delivering corticosteroids to the epidural space, yet their comparative efficacy remains a topic of debate. The transforaminal approach, with its precision in targeting ventral epidural pathology, has been hypothesized to offer superior pain relief for radicular symptoms. Conversely, the interlaminar approach is valued for its simplicity and broader medication distribution. This study by Haring et al. (2024) leverages a robust clinical registry to directly compare the effectiveness of these approaches, providing clarity for clinicians and improving patient outcomes.

Objectives of this update

- Compare the effectiveness of TFESI and ILESI in reducing radicular, claudicatory, and axial low back pain significantly.

- Analyze patient-specific factors influencing outcomes to identify subgroups most likely to benefit from each approach.

- Offer evidence-based recommendations for tailoring ESI approaches based on presenting symptoms and pathology.

What is new

This study, drawn from a prospective clinical registry, provides new insights by:

- Demonstrating that **TFESI is significantly more effective** than ILESI for radicular and claudicatory leg pain, achieving ≥ 50% pain reduction in 57% versus 30% of patients, respectively.

- Finding **no significant differences between TFESI and ILESI** in managing axial back pain, reinforcing current guidelines that recommend against ESIs for isolated axial pain.

- Highlighting that the **type of steroid used (particulate or non-particulate)** does not significantly influence outcomes for either approach.

Understanding TFESI and ILESI

- **Pathophysiological considerations:**

  ○ TFESI offers targeted delivery of corticosteroids to the ventral epidural space, making it ideal for pathologies such as disc herniation.

  ○ ILESI provides broader corticosteroid distribution but may be less effective for specific nerve root compression.

- **Key procedural differences:**

  ○ TFESI requires precise fluoroscopic guidance and poses a higher technical demand.

  ○ ILESI is generally faster and requires less expertise, making it more accessible in varied practice settings.

Study design and methods

- **Population:** 73 patients from a single academic registry who underwent either TFESI (n=51) or ILESI (n=22) between 2011 and 2017.

- **Outcomes measured:** Pain reduction was assessed using the 11-point Numeric Rating Scale (NRS) at baseline and 3 months post-procedure.

- **Primary endpoint:** $\geq$ 50% reduction in pain scores for leg pain, with secondary outcomes including back pain reduction and the influence of steroid type.

Results

- **TFESI versus ILESI for leg pain:**

  ○ For radicular or claudicatory leg pain, TFESI was associated with significantly higher odds of achieving $\geq$ 50% pain reduction than ILESI.

  ○ Adjusted analyses confirmed TFESI's superiority.

- **Back pain outcomes:**

  ○ No significant differences were observed between TFESI and ILESI in reducing axial back pain, which is consistent with evidence against ESIs for isolated back pain.

- **Steroid type:**

  ○ The choice of particulate (e.g., triamcinolone) versus non-particulate (e.g., dexamethasone) corticosteroids did not significantly influence pain outcomes for either approach.

- **Repeat injections:**

  ○ 34% of patients received repeat injections within the 3-month follow-up, with no significant differences in repeat rates or outcomes between the groups.

Clinical implications

- **Approach selection based on symptoms:**

  ○ TFESI should be preferred for patients with radicular or claudicatory leg pain due to its targeted delivery and superior outcomes.

  ○ ILESI may still be viable for patients with mixed symptoms or when technical constraints limit TFESI feasibility.

- **Guidance for axial pain:**

  ○ Neither TFESI nor ILESI showed significant efficacy for isolated axial back pain, underscoring the need for alternative therapies for this population.

- **Standardization of steroid type:**

  ○ Since steroid type did not influence outcomes, clinicians can focus on other factors such as cost, availability, and safety when selecting particulate and non-particulate options.

Limitations

- **Small sample size:** Despite its strengths, the study included only 73 patients, limiting subgroup analyses.

- **Non-randomized design:** The injection approach was not randomized, potentially introducing selection bias.

- **Single-center data:** Findings may not be generalizable to diverse practice settings or patient populations.

Future directions

- **Prospective trials:** Randomized studies are needed to validate the findings and explore outcomes for specific subgroups, such as patients with degenerative stenosis.

- **Long-term outcomes:** Evaluating the durability of pain relief beyond 3 months would provide valuable insights.

- **Comparative safety:** Further research should investigate TFESI and ILESI complication rates, particularly in high-risk populations.

Key takeaways

☑ **TFESI provides superior pain relief** for radicular and claudicatory leg pain compared to ILESI.

☑ **Neither approach is effective for isolated axial back pain,** highlighting the need for alternative management strategies.

☑ **Steroid type does not significantly affect outcomes,** allowing flexibility in corticosteroid selection.

☑ **Approach selection should be tailored** to patient symptoms and procedural feasibility.

Additional recommended reading:

1. Haring RS, Kennedy DJ, Archer KR, et al. Comparing the clinical outcomes of lumbar transforaminal vs interlaminar epidural steroid injections in a registry cohort. *Interventional Pain Medicine.* 2024;3:100396.

2. Smith CC, McCormick ZL, Mattie R, et al. The effectiveness of lumbar transforaminal injection of steroid for the treatment of radicular pain: a comprehensive review. *Pain Med.* 2020;21(3):472-487.

3. Friedly JL, Comstock BA, Turner JA, et al. A randomized trial of epidural glucocorticoid injections for spinal stenosis. *N Engl J Med.* 2014;371(1):11-21.

4. Peene L, Cohen SP, Kallewaard JW, et al. 1. Lumbosacral radicular pain. Pain Pract. 2024;24(3):525-552.

Pain originating from the lumbar facet joints

27

Why this topic is important

Lumbar facet joint pain is a common and challenging cause of chronic lower back pain. The facet joints, synovial structures connecting the vertebrae, contribute to spinal stability and flexibility but are prone to degeneration due to mechanical stress, aging, and biomechanical factors like disc degeneration and obesity. Pain associated with these joints can significantly impair function and quality of life.

Diagnosis and management of lumbar facet joint pain remain controversial, with estimates of prevalence ranging from 4.8% to over 50%, depending on the diagnostic criteria. This variation reflects the lack of definitive clinical signs and limited specificity of imaging techniques. Interventional strategies, particularly medial branch blocks (MBBs) and radiofrequency ablation (RFA) are cornerstone treatments but are also subject to debate regarding efficacy, safety, and appropriate patient selection.

This update summarizes the findings of Van den Heuvel et al. (2024), providing evidence-based guidance on the diagnosis and management of lumbar facet joint pain.

Objectives of this update

- Clarify diagnostic criteria for lumbar facet joint pain, including clinical features and the role of imaging.

- Review the evidence for interventional treatments, focusing on medial branch blocks and radiofrequency ablation.

- Provide practical recommendations for managing lumbar facet joint pain using a multimodal approach.

What is new

This update integrates recent advancements:

- Recognition of the limited diagnostic value of imaging findings like facet degeneration, emphasizing the necessity of diagnostic/prognostic blocks.

- Evidence supporting single MBBs with ≥ 50% pain relief as a reliable threshold for proceeding to RFA.

- Innovations in RFA techniques, such as cooled and pulsed modalities, may improve outcomes for selected patients.

Diagnosis

Clinical presentation

Patients with lumbar facet joint pain typically describe aching, axial low back pain that may radiate to the flank, hip, or posterior thigh but rarely below the knee. Pain often worsens with extension, rotation, or prolonged static postures and improves with rest. Morning stiffness may also be present.

Physical examination

Although no single test reliably diagnoses facet joint pain, paraspinal tenderness, and pain exacerbation during extension or lateral bending can provide clues. Like Revel's criteria, standardized criteria combine multiple clinical signs but show variable accuracy.

Imaging

- **MRI and CT:** Commonly reveal degenerative changes like joint space narrowing, subchondral sclerosis, and hypertrophy. However, these findings are also prevalent in asymptomatic individuals, limiting their diagnostic utility.
- **SPECT imaging:** May identify active joint inflammation and has modest predictive value for interventional outcomes but requires further validation.

Diagnostic/prognostic blocks

The gold standard for diagnosing facet joint pain is MBBs, targeting the dorsal rami's medial branches. Single diagnostic blocks with low volumes of local anesthetic (< 0.5 mL) and ≥ 50% pain relief are recommended as thresholds for proceeding to RFA. False positives can occur due to placebo effects or non-specific spread of anesthetic.

Treatment options

Conservative management

- **Pharmacologic therapy:**
  - **NSAIDs:** Provide modest short-term relief.
  - **Duloxetine:** Effective for chronic musculoskeletal pain.
  - **Muscle relaxants and topical agents:** May offer supplementary benefits.
- **Physical therapy:**
  - Core stabilization and aerobic exercises reduce mechanical stress on the lumbar spine.
  - Manual therapy combined with therapeutic exercise shows better outcomes than therapy alone.
- **Lifestyle modifications:**
  - Weight loss and ergonomic adjustments can mitigate exacerbating factors.

Interventional therapies

- **Medial branch blocks (MBBs):**
  - Used diagnostically and prognostically to select candidates for RFA.
  - Routine therapeutic use is not recommended due to limited efficacy beyond placebo.
- **Radiofrequency ablation (RFA):**
  - Conventional RFA disrupts nociceptive pathways by heating targeted nerves.
  - **Cooled RFA:** Creates larger lesions, potentially improving outcomes for patients with anatomical variability.
  - **Pulsed RFA:** Offers an alternative with reduced tissue damage but shows less efficacy for chronic lumbar facet pain.
  - Studies report ≥ 50% long-term pain relief in well-selected patients following RFA.
- **Intra-articular (IA) injections:**
  - May provide short-term relief in cases of active joint inflammation but are generally less effective than RFA.

Innovations and future directions

- **Advanced imaging-guided techniques:** Using ultrasound and CT for precise needle placement is expanding, though fluoroscopy remains the gold standard.
- **Combination therapies:** Research is exploring the integration of biologics, such as platelet-rich plasma, with interventional techniques.
- **Individualized treatment:** Incorporating psychosocial assessments and biomarkers could improve patient selection and outcomes.

Key takeaways

☑ Clinical features and imaging findings are insufficient to definitively diagnose lumbar facet joint pain. MBBs are essential for confirming the pain source and guiding treatment.

☑ A single MBB with ≥ 50% pain relief is a reliable threshold for proceeding to RFA, which remains the most effective intervention for lumbar facet joint pain.

☑ Conservative therapies should be trialed for at least three months before considering invasive procedures.

☑ Innovations in RFA techniques and multimodal strategies offer promising avenues for improving patient outcomes.

Additional recommended reading:

1. Van den Heuvel SAS, Cohen SP, Kallewaard JW, et al. Pain originating from the lumbar facet joints: Update of evidence-based interventional pain medicine. *Pain Practice.* 2024;24:160-176.

2. Cohen SP, Bhaskar A, Bhatia A, et al. Consensus practice guidelines on interventions for lumbar facet joint pain. *Reg Anesth Pain Med.* 2020;45(6):424-467.

3. Knezevic NN, Candido KD, Vlaeyen JWS, et al. Low back pain: A clinical review. *Lancet.* 2021;398:78-92.

Osteoarthritis of zygapophysial joints as a cause of back and neck pain

28

Why this topic is important

Osteoarthritis (OA) of the zygapophysial joints (facet joints) has long been considered a potential cause of chronic back and neck pain. These small, synovial joints play a crucial role in spinal movement and stability, and their degeneration is often implicated in mechanical spinal pain syndromes. Radiological findings of OA, such as joint space narrowing and osteophyte formation, are frequently observed in individuals with spinal pain, leading to the assumption that these changes are causally linked to the pain.

This belief has significant implications for clinical practice and patient care. When facet joint OA is viewed as the primary cause of pain, treatment efforts may focus on addressing the arthritic changes through interventions like joint injections or radiofrequency neurotomy. However, if OA is not directly responsible for pain, these approaches could misdirect resources and delay more effective treatments. Furthermore, medicolegal and insurance decisions often rely on attributing pain to degenerative findings, potentially affecting coverage and access to care.

Bogduk et al. (2024) conducted a comprehensive scoping review to evaluate whether the current evidence supports a causal relationship between facet joint OA and pain. This update summarizes their findings and discusses the clinical implications for diagnosing and managing spinal pain associated with facet joint degeneration.

Objectives of this update

- Assess whether OA of the facet joints is a proven cause of chronic back and neck pain.

- Evaluate the diagnostic and therapeutic relevance of facet joint OA in clinical practice.

- Provide evidence-based recommendations for interpreting imaging findings and managing suspected facet joint pain.

What is new

This scoping review challenges conventional assumptions and highlights critical insights:

- **Lack of evidence:** No definitive association between facet joint OA and spinal pain was identified across 18 population, diagnostic, and case-control studies.

- **Imaging limitations:** Radiographic findings of facet joint OA were equally prevalent in symptomatic and asymptomatic individuals, undermining their diagnostic utility.

- **Pathophysiological implications:** Pain in facet joints may be unrelated to visible OA, requiring diagnostic methods like controlled blocks for accurate identification.

Evidence from population studies

Population studies are foundational for identifying associations between diseases and symptoms. Of the 11 studies reviewed, none demonstrated a statistically significant link between the presence or severity of facet joint OA and pain. For example, data from the Framingham Heart Study revealed that while 63% of participants showed signs of lumbar facet joint OA on imaging, the prevalence of pain was identical in those with and without radiographic evidence of degeneration.

These findings suggest that OA is not a reliable predictor of facet joint pain. Similar observations have been made for other small joints, such as the interphalangeal joints of the hands, where degenerative changes are often asymptomatic.

Insights from diagnostic studies

Four diagnostic studies evaluated whether anesthetizing facet joints affected by OA could relieve pain. Results were consistently negative:

- Patients with radiographic evidence of facet joint OA did not experience greater pain relief than those without such findings.

- The prevalence of OA in joints proven to be painful (via diagnostic blocks) did not differ significantly from non-painful joints.

These results emphasize that pain in facet joints cannot be assumed to arise from OA. Rather than imaging findings, diagnostic blocks remain the gold standard for identifying painful joints.

Case-control studies

Three case-control studies compared the prevalence of facet joint OA in individuals with and without spinal pain. Again, the results were inconclusive:

- For lumbar facet joints, odds ratios for the association between OA and pain were weak and often not statistically significant.

- The prevalence of OA in cervical facet joints was similar in patients with and without neck pain, suggesting that the condition is a normal age-related change rather than a pathological driver of symptoms.

These findings further undermine the assumption that OA is a primary cause of facet joint pain.

Clinical implications

Diagnostic considerations

- **Imaging pitfalls:** Radiographic evidence of facet joint OA should not be interpreted as a definitive cause of pain. The high prevalence of asymptomatic OA necessitates caution when correlating imaging findings with clinical symptoms.

- **Role of diagnostic blocks:** Controlled medial branch blocks are essential for identifying the true source of facet joint pain. Imaging findings should guide, but not replace, these diagnostic procedures.

Therapeutic recommendations

- **Targeted interventions:**
  Treatments like radiofrequency neurotomy should be reserved for patients with confirmed facet joint pain through diagnostic blocks, regardless of radiographic findings.

- **Multimodal approaches:**
  Physical therapy and exercise should remain foundational for managing spinal pain, with interventional procedures used selectively.

Key takeaways

☑ Radiographic findings of facet joint OA are poor predictors of spinal pain and should not be relied upon for definitive diagnosis.

☑ Controlled diagnostic blocks are essential for identifying painful facet joints and guiding targeted treatments.

☑ Pain management strategies should prioritize patient-specific approaches, combining conservative care with validated interventional procedures.

Additional recommended reading:

1. Bogduk N, MacVicar J. Osteoarthritis of zygapophysial joints as a cause of back pain and neck pain: A scoping review. *Pain Medicine.* 2024;25:541-552.

2. Engel A, King W, Schneider BJ, et al. Effectiveness of cervical medial branch thermal radiofrequency neurotomy stratified by selection criteria. *Pain Medicine.* 2020;21(11):2726-2737.

3. MacVicar J, Bogduk N. Prevalence of "pure" lumbar zygapophysial joint pain in patients with chronic low back pain. *Pain Medicine.* 2021;22(1):41-48.

Sacroiliac joint pain: Diagnosis and management

29

Why this topic is important

Sacroiliac (SI) joint pain is a significant contributor to mechanical low back pain, with a prevalence of 15-30% among patients. Despite its impact, SI joint pain often remains underdiagnosed due to the complexity of its presentation and overlap with other conditions. Advances in diagnostic techniques and interventional therapies have improved management strategies, offering patients better pain relief and functional outcomes. This review by Szadek et al. (2024) synthesizes updated evidence on diagnosing and treating SI joint pain to guide clinical practice.

Objectives of this update

- Review current diagnostic criteria and tools for SI joint pain.

- Discuss conservative and interventional treatment options, emphasizing evidence-based strategies.

- Explore recent advances in radiofrequency ablation (RFA) and other interventional techniques.

What is new

This review highlights critical updates, including:

- Enhanced understanding of diagnostic tests, including the value of provocative maneuvers and imaging techniques.

- Evidence supporting **radiofrequency ablation (RFA)** as a highly effective interventional therapy, with newer lesioning techniques demonstrating improved outcomes.

- Insights into the role of **multidisciplinary approaches,** combining physical therapy, psychological support, and interventional treatments for optimal patient outcomes.

Diagnosis of SI joint pain

- **Clinical presentation:**

  - Pain localized to the gluteal region, often radiating to the lower lumbar area, groin, or lower limb.

  - Pain worsens with activities stressing the SI joint (e.g., prolonged standing, stair climbing, or transitioning from sitting to standing).

  - Common risk factors include leg length discrepancies, trauma, obesity, pregnancy, and lumbar fusion surgery.

- **Provocative maneuvers:**

  - Key recommended tests:

    - Compression test and thigh thrust test due to higher diagnostic reliability.

  - Comprehensive testing approach:

    - Use at least three provocation tests (e.g., compression, thigh thrust, distraction, Patrick's [FABER], and Gaenslen's tests) to increase sensitivity (78-94%) and specificity (79-85%).

    - Avoid relying solely on individual test results due to potential for false positives or negatives.

    - Ensure a detailed history evaluation, focusing on pain patterns (e.g., worsened pain upon rising from a seated position) and focal tenderness near the posterior superior iliac spine.

- **Imaging and diagnostic blocks:**

  - Imaging:

    - Primarily used to rule out alternative pathologies.

    - MRI can identify inflammatory changes (e.g., bone marrow edema) that support SI joint dysfunction when correlated with clinical findings.

  - Diagnostic blocks:

    - Controversial due to the risk of false positives or negatives.

    - Use fluoroscopic or CT guidance to improve the accuracy of intra-articular blocks.

    - Blind injections show a success rate of only 8-22% and are not recommended.

    - Lateral branch blocks can clarify posterior SI joint involvement and predict response to advanced treatments like radiofrequency ablation.

Treatment options

- **Conservative management:**

  - Initial therapies include physical therapy, NSAIDs, cognitive-behavioral therapy, and exercise programs.

  - Evidence supports manual therapy and targeted exercise for postural or gait-related SI joint dysfunction.

- **Corticosteroid injections:**

  - Provide significant pain relief in 50-70% of patients for up to 6 months.

  - Periarticular injections may offer comparable or superior benefits to intra-articular injections.

- **Radiofrequency ablation (RFA):**

  - RFA of the lateral branches and L5 dorsal ramus is effective for chronic SI joint pain.

  - Cooled RFA demonstrates enhanced outcomes, with 50-79% of patients reporting ≥ 50% pain relief at 3-6 months.

- **Surgical options:**

  - Minimally invasive SI joint fusion may benefit select patients, particularly those with degenerative or unstable joints.

  - Evidence supports its effectiveness but highlights the need for standardized diagnostic protocols.

Limitations

- **Diagnostic ambiguity:** False positives/negatives in tests and blocks complicate accurate diagnosis.

- **Variable study methodologies:** Inconsistent definitions of success and RFA techniques across studies hinder generalizability.

Key takeaways

☑ **A comprehensive diagnosis** is essential, combining history, provocative tests, and imaging.

☑ **RFA, particularly cooled RFA, offers robust pain relief** and should be considered for refractory cases.

☑ **Conservative treatments remain first-line,** emphasizing physical therapy and targeted exercise.

☑ A **multidisciplinary approach optimizes outcomes,** addressing both physical and psychological aspects of SI joint pain.

Additional recommended reading:

1. Szadek K, Cohen SP, de Andrés Ares J, et al. Sacroiliac joint pain: Diagnosis and treatment. *Pain Practice.* 2024;24:627-646.

2. Patel N, Gross A, Moreland A, et al. Comparative outcomes of cooled radiofrequency ablation versus traditional approaches for sacroiliac joint pain. *Anesth Analg.* 2020;130(4):1047-1056.

3. Cosman ER Jr, Gonzalez CD. Bipolar radiofrequency lesion geometry: implications for palisade treatment of sacroiliac joint pain. *Pain Pract.* 2011;11(1):3-22.

Persistent spinal pain syndrome type 2: Diagnosis and management

30

Why this topic is important

Persistent Spinal Pain Syndrome (PSPS) type 2, formerly known as Failed Back Surgery Syndrome (FBSS), represents a significant challenge in the management of chronic pain. It refers to persistent or recurrent pain that arises after spinal surgery, with symptoms that often include back pain, radicular pain, paresthesia, and functional impairment. PSPS type 2 can result from several causes, including technical failures during surgery, recurrent pathology, biomechanical changes, or complications like epidural fibrosis and arachnoiditis. The condition affects 10%-40% of spinal surgery patients, with higher rates observed in complex or repeat surgeries.

Effective management of PSPS type 2 is essential for improving affected individuals' quality of life and functionality. However, treatment outcomes are frequently suboptimal due to the condition's complex and multifactorial nature. This update, based on the article by Van de Minkelis et al. (2024), synthesizes the latest evidence, focusing on diagnostic challenges and therapeutic options, including advanced interventional techniques such as epidural adhesiolysis and spinal cord stimulation (SCS).

Objectives of this update

- Clarify the diagnostic criteria and tools for PSPS type 2.

- Review the efficacy of conservative and interventional treatments for managing pain and functional limitations.

- Highlight emerging evidence and techniques for optimizing outcomes in PSPS type 2.

What is new

Recent advancements in the management of PSPS type 2 include:

- Enhanced understanding of the etiological factors contributing to persistent pain after spinal surgery.

- Evidence supporting interventional approaches like pulsed radiofrequency (PRF), epidural adhesiolysis, and spinal endoscopy for selected patients.

- Refinements in spinal cord stimulation techniques, such as high-frequency stimulation and closed-loop systems, offering improved outcomes for neuropathic pain.

Diagnostic approach

Etiology and pathophysiology

The causes of PSPS type 2 are diverse and can be broadly categorized into:

- **Surgical complications:** Examples include wrong-level surgery, retained disc fragments, or instrumentation failure.
- **Biomechanical sequelae:** Adjacent segment disease, loss of spinal stability, or paraspinal muscle atrophy.
- **Recurrent pathology:** Disc herniation, epidural fibrosis, or scar tissue.
- **Other factors:** Psychological comorbidities, central sensitization, or unaddressed sacroiliac joint pain.

Diagnostic methods

- **Patient history:** Detailed documentation of symptom onset, evolution, and patterns can help identify underlying causes.
- **Physical examination:** Neurological tests, such as the straight leg raise or femoral stretch test, aid in assessing radicular pain. Signs of central sensitization (e.g., hypersensitivity or impaired conditioned pain modulation) should also be evaluated.
- **Imaging:** MRI with gadolinium contrast is preferred for distinguishing recurrent herniation from scar tissue, while CT scans are useful for evaluating hardware placement and bone fusion. CT myelography may be considered for patients with MRI-incompatible implants.

Treatment options

Conservative therapies

- **Physical rehabilitation:**
  - Exercise programs can improve functionality, although evidence for their long-term benefits in PSPS type 2 is limited.
  - Intensive rehabilitation appears more effective than mild regimens in the short term.
- **Pharmacological treatments:**
  - Evidence for medications such as NSAIDs, antidepressants, and gabapentinoids is mixed. Duloxetine has shown some benefit for mechanical back pain, while opioids offer modest short-term relief but carry significant risks.
  - Muscle relaxants and botulinum toxin may provide targeted relief in select cases.
- **Multidisciplinary approaches:**
  - Incorporating cognitive-behavioral therapy (CBT) or biofeedback into pain management programs addresses the psychological dimensions of chronic pain.

Interventional therapies

- **Epidural steroid injections (ESIs):**
  - ESIs are effective for short-term relief of radicular symptoms but show limited efficacy beyond six months.
  - Routine use in PSPS type 2 is not recommended for prolonged symptoms.
- **Pulsed radiofrequency (PRF):**
  - PRF targets the dorsal root ganglia (DRG) and may reduce pain in selected patients. Studies report over 50% pain reduction at six months in some cases.
- **Epidural adhesiolysis and spinal endoscopy:**
  - Adhesiolysis aims to free entrapped nerve roots and restore epidural blood flow.
  - Spinal endoscopy enhances visualization of epidural space, allowing targeted removal of scar tissue. Evidence suggests moderate efficacy for leg pain relief in PSPS type 2.
- **Spinal cord stimulation (SCS):**
  - Conventional tonic SCS provides pain relief in approximately 50% of patients.
  - High-frequency and burst stimulation systems offer superior outcomes for neuropathic back and leg pain, with long-term response rates exceeding 70% in some trials.
  - Closed-loop SCS automatically adjusts stimulation parameters based on real-time feedback, enhancing pain control.

Key takeaways

☑ **Thorough evaluation:** A comprehensive history, physical examination, and imaging are essential for an accurate diagnosis of PSPS type 2.

☑ **Multimodal management:** Combining conservative, pharmacological, and interventional therapies offers the best outcomes.

☑ **Targeted interventions:** Procedures like PRF, adhesiolysis, and SCS are effective for well-selected patients.

☑ **Continued research:** High-quality trials are needed to refine treatment approaches and improve long-term success rates.

Additional recommended reading:

1. Van de Minkelis J, Peene L, Cohen SP, et al. Persistent spinal pain syndrome type 2: Update of evidence-based interventional pain medicine. Pain Practice. 2024;24:919-936.

2. Amirdelfan K, Manchikanti L, Zundert JV, et al. A systematic approach to treating failed back surgery syndrome: What is the evidence? Pain Physician. 2017;20-S117.

3. North RB, Shipley J. Spinal cord stimulation for chronic, intractable pain: Superb outcomes in carefully selected patients. Pain Med. 2021;22-S24.

Musculoskeletal Pain & Regional Pain Syndromes

Local anesthetic chondrotoxicity and safety in stellate ganglion blocks

31

Why this topic is important

Local anesthetics are integral to many interventional pain management techniques, including intra-articular injections and stellate ganglion blocks. However, their potential chondrotoxic effects-particularly in joint applications-raise significant safety concerns. Chondrotoxicity varies between anesthetic agents, concentrations, and exposure durations. Additionally, stellate ganglion blocks, used for sympathetically mediated pain conditions, carry procedural risks that can be mitigated by imaging guidance. Understanding these risks and evidence-based safety strategies can improve patient outcomes. This update summarizes the evidence collected by Saffarian et al. (2023) regarding local anesthetic chondrotoxicity and stellate ganglion blocks.

Objectives of this update

- Summarize the chondrotoxic properties of commonly used local anesthetics and their clinical implications.

- Highlight safe practices in stellate ganglion blocks, including the advantages of imaging guidance.

- Provide recommendations to minimize complications related to local anesthetic use and nerve blocks.

What is new

A recent review by Saffarian et al. (2023) evaluated the chondrotoxic effects of local anesthetics and outlined safety strategies for stellate ganglion blocks. Key findings include:

- **Chondrotoxicity**: Bupivacaine at 0.5% or higher concentrations is the most chondrotoxic, while ropivacaine at ≤ 0.5% is the least toxic.

- **Risk mitigation in stellate ganglion blocks:** Ultrasound guidance offers improved visualization of vascular and soft tissue structures, reducing complications compared to fluoroscopy or blind techniques.

- **Impact of additives:** Combining local anesthetics with corticosteroids or epinephrine may increase cytotoxic effects, emphasizing the need for cautious formulation choices.

Local anesthetic chondrotoxicity

Mechanisms of toxicity

Local anesthetics can harm cartilage cells (chondrocytes) in a concentration- and time-dependent manner. Proposed mechanisms include increased apoptosis, mitochondrial dysfunction, and extracellular matrix damage. These effects may predispose cartilage to further degeneration, particularly in osteoarthritic joints.

Key findings from in vitro studies

- **Bupivacaine:** The most chondrotoxic ane-sthetic at concentrations of 0.5% or higher. Time-dependent toxicity is notable, with complete chondrocyte death occurring within 60 minutes of exposure to 0.5% bupivacaine in one study.

- **Lidocaine:** Shows significant chondro-toxicity at concentrations $\geq$ 1%. Toxic effects intensify with prolonged exposure.

- **Ropivacaine:** Demonstrates the lowest chondrotoxicity, especially at $\leq$ 0.5%. Higher concentrations ($\geq$ 0.75%) result in reduced cell viability but remain less harmful than bupivacaine or lidocaine.

- **Combination with corticosteroids:** Adding corticosteroids exacerbates chondrotoxicity. This practice may hasten joint deterioration and is under increasing scrutiny.

Safety in stellate ganglion blocks

Procedural risks

Stellate ganglion blocks are used for conditions like complex regional pain syndrome and refractory sympathetically mediated pain. However, blind techniques risk serious complications, including vascular injury, nerve damage, and unintentional intravascular or intrathecal injections.

Imaging guidance benefits

- **Ultrasound:** Provides real-time visualization of vascular and soft tissue structures, reducing risks of esophageal puncture, vascular injury, and hematoma.

- **Fluoroscopy:** Offers precise needle placement at the cervical vertebral levels but lacks visualization of soft tissues, increasing certain risks.

- **Improved outcomes:** Studies show lower complication rates and better pain relief with ultrasound-guided blocks compared to blind techniques.

Clinical implications

- **Selection of local anesthetic:**
  - Ropivacaine at concentrations $\leq$ 0.5% is preferred for intra-articular injections to minimize chondrotoxic effects.
  - Avoid bupivacaine at concentrations $\geq$ 0.5% in joint spaces due to its high chondrotoxicity.

- **Safety practices in nerve blocks:**
  - Use imaging guidance (ultrasound or fluoroscopy) for stellate ganglion blocks to enhance precision and minimize complications.
  - Administer small test doses of anesthetics to detect unintentional intravascular placement.

- **Formulation considerations:**
  - Avoid combining local anesthetics with corticosteroids when possible to reduce chondrotoxicity.
  - Be cautious with additives like epinephrine, which may have variable effects on chondrocyte viability.

Key takeaways

☑ Chondrotoxicity of local anesthetics is concentration- and time-dependent, with bupivacaine being the most harmful and ropivacaine the least.

☑ Ropivacaine at ≤ 0.5% is preferred for intra-articular use to minimize cartilage damage.

☑ Imaging-guided stellate ganglion blocks improve safety and effectiveness compared to blind techniques.

☑ Adding corticosteroids to local anesthetics increases cytotoxic risks and should be limited.

Additional recommended reading:

1. Saffarian M, Holder EK, Mattie R, et al. Local anesthetic chondrotoxicity and stellate ganglion blocks. *Interventional Pain Medicine.* 2023;2:100282. doi:10.1016/j.inpm.2023.100282.

2. Jayaram P, Kennedy DJ, Yeh P, Dragoo J. Chondrotoxic effects of local anesthetics on human knee articular cartilage: A systematic review. *PM&R.* 2019;11:379-400.

3. Narouze S. Ultrasound-guided stellate ganglion block: Safety and efficacy. *Curr Pain Headache Rep.* 2014;18:424.

Oral corticosteroids for complex regional pain syndrome

32

Why this topic is important

Complex regional pain syndrome (CRPS) is a chronic pain condition characterized by sensory, motor, and autonomic dysfunction, often triggered by injury or surgery. CRPS is associated with an exaggerated inflammatory response, including elevated pro-inflammatory cytokines and neuropeptides. While corticosteroids are widely used for their anti-inflammatory and immunosuppressive effects, their efficacy in CRPS remains debated. This update reviews a retrospective cohort study by van den Berg et al. (2024) that evaluated the impact of oral corticosteroids in CRPS management, focusing on clinical outcomes and safety.

Objectives of this update

- Summarize the findings on the effectiveness of oral corticosteroids for pain relief and symptom management in CRPS.

- Highlight corticosteroid therapy's safety profile and potential side effects in this context.

- Discuss factors influencing treatment response, including inflammation and disease duration.

What is new

This study assessed the outcomes of oral corticosteroid therapy in 27 CRPS patients treated at a specialized center. Key findings include:

- **Moderate efficacy:** 51.9% of patients responded positively to corticosteroids, reducing pain and improving inflammation-related symptoms.

- **Temporary benefits:** In some responders, the effects subsided shortly after discontinuing therapy.

- **Influence of disease stage:** Patients with shorter CRPS duration and signs of active inflammation (e.g., warmth) were more likely to respond.

- **Safety:** Side effects were mild and occurred in 17.9% of patients.

Study design and participants

The study analyzed 27 CRPS patients treated with oral corticosteroids at a tertiary care center from 2015 to 2020. CRPS diagnosis was based on the Budapest Criteria, and patients were included only if they presented clinical signs of inflammation and elevated soluble interleukin-2 receptor (sIL-2R) levels.

- **Demographics:** Most patients were female (92.6%), with a mean age of 41.5 years.

- **Treatment details:** Patients received an average daily dose of 28.9 mg prednisolone for a mean duration of 10.5 days.

Outcome measures

- **Responder definition:** Patients with significant pain reduction, symptom improvement, or functional gains were categorized as responders.

- **Global Perceived Effect (GPE):** Patients self-rated their condition post-treatment using a 7-point Likert scale, with scores of 1-3 indicating improvement.

Key findings

- **Pain and symptom relief**

  - 51.9% of patients (14/27) responded positively to corticosteroids. Improvements included pain reduction, reduced swelling, and better range of motion.

  - In many cases, symptom relief persisted only during treatment and relapsed afterward.

- **Disease stage and inflammation**

  - Responders were more likely to present with signs of active inflammation, such as warmth in the affected limb.

  - Nonresponders exhibited chronic disease features like colder extremities and nail changes, suggesting progression beyond an inflammatory phase.

- **Global Perceived Effect (GPE)**

  - Responders reported significantly lower GPE scores (median 3.0) than nonresponders (median 4.0), correlating with clinician-reported outcomes.

- **Safety profile**

  - Side effects were mild, including vomiting, dizziness, and minor wound issues. These occurred in 17.9% of patients, primarily among responders.

  - No severe complications were reported, such as adrenal insufficiency or immune suppression.

Clinical implications

- **Efficacy considerations**

  - Corticosteroids can provide meaningful relief in patients with early-stage CRPS and active inflammation.

  - Their role is limited in chronic stages, where inflammation has resolved, and structural or central nervous system changes predominate.

- **Patient selection**

  - Signs of active inflammation (e.g., warmth, swelling) and shorter disease duration may predict better outcomes.

  - Tailored, mechanism-based approaches are crucial, particularly in a disease as heterogenous as CRPS.

- **Safety and monitoring**

  - While side effects are generally mild, corticosteroids should be used judiciously and for short durations to minimize risks.

  - Regular monitoring of metabolic and immune markers can enhance safety.

- **Limitations of treatment**

  - The transient nature of benefits underscores the need for adjunctive or follow-up therapies to maintain improvements.

Key takeaways

☑ Oral corticosteroids effectively reduce pain and inflammation in approximately half of CRPS patients, particularly in early-stage disease with active inflammation.

☑ Short courses (7-21 days) at moderate doses (28.9 mg/day) are generally well-tolerated, with minimal side effects reported.

☑ Indicators of treatment success include signs of active inflammation, such as limb warmth and shorter disease duration.

☑ Symptom recurrence post-treatment highlights the need for comprehensive, multimodal management strategies.

Additional recommended reading:

1. van den Berg C, Huygen FJPM, Tiemensma J. The efficacy of oral corticoids in treating complex regional pain syndrome: A retrospective cohort study. *Pain Pract.* 2024;24:394-403. doi:10.1111/papr.13310.

2. Harden RN, Bruehl S, Perez R, et al. Validation of proposed diagnostic criteria (the "Budapest Criteria") for complex regional pain syndrome. *Pain.* 2010;150:268-274.

3. Dirckx M, Stronks DL, Groeneweg JG, et al. Inflammation in cold complex regional pain syndrome. *Acta Anaesthesiol Scand.* 2015;59:733-739.

Lumbar sympathetic blocks with thermographic monitoring for complex regional pain syndrome

33

Why this topic is important

Complex regional pain syndrome (CRPS) is a debilitating condition characterized by severe, chronic pain, often accompanied by autonomic dysfunction, motor impairment, and trophic changes. Treatments such as lumbar sympathetic blocks (LSBs) aim to alleviate symptoms by targeting autonomic dysregulation. However, the efficacy of LSBs remains inconsistent, with only about one-third of patients typically responding. Infrared thermography, when used as a procedural adjunct, may enhance the precision and effectiveness of LSBs. This update reviews a prospective study by Bovaira et al. (2023) assessing clinical outcomes of thermography-guided LSBs for CRPS.

Objectives of this update

- Evaluate the role of thermography as a real-time adjunct to fluoroscopic guidance in LSBs.

- Highlight the clinical outcomes and safety profile of LSBs in lower limb CRPS patients.

- Discuss factors predictive of treatment response to LSBs.

What is new

This study evaluated the impact of thermography-guided LSBs in 27 patients with lower limb CRPS. Key findings include:

- **Moderate response rate:** 37% of patients were categorized as responders, achieving at least a 30% reduction in pain along with the disappearance of resting pain.

- **Improvement in clinical variables:** Many patients' symptoms, such as tingling, edema, and vasomotor abnormalities, significantly improved.

- **Predictive factor:** Shorter immobilization time following injury was associated with a higher likelihood of response.

- **Safety:** The procedure demonstrated a favorable safety profile, with no major complications reported.

Design and participants

The study included 27 patients with CRPS diagnosed according to the Budapest criteria. Inclusion criteria required moderate-to-severe pain (≥ 5 on a 10-point visual analog scale [VAS]) persisting for less than two years and unresponsive to standard therapies, including pharmacological treatments and rehabilitation.

Procedure

All patients underwent a series of three LSBs spaced three weeks apart, performed at the L4 level. Local anesthetic (levobupivacaine 0.25%) combined with corticosteroid (triamcinolone) was used. Infrared thermography was employed to monitor temperature changes in the affected limb's plantar surface, confirming successful block placement.

Outcomes

Primary outcomes included pain relief ($\geq 30\%$ VAS reduction) and improved symptoms like tingling, edema, and vasomotor abnormalities. Assessments were conducted at baseline, one, three, and six months after the third block.

Key findings

- **Pain relief**
  - Average VAS scores significantly decreased at all follow-up points. For responders, the mean VAS score dropped from 7.9 at baseline to 2.8 at one month post-treatment.
  - Overall, 37% of patients achieved the response threshold of $\geq 30\%$ pain reduction with no resting pain.

- **Symptom improvement**
  - Significant improvements were observed in tingling, thermal asymmetry, edema, and sweating.
  - The Harden severity scale and the Lower Limb Functional Index also demonstrated notable gains, particularly at six months.

- **Predictors of response**
  - Logistic regression analysis identified immobilization time as the key predictor of treatment success. Patients with shorter immobilization periods were more likely to respond.

- **Safety and procedural success**
  - No major complications were reported, although 44% of patients had mild lumbar discomfort.
  - Infrared thermography confirmed proper block placement in 76.25% of cases on the first attempt, improving procedural accuracy.

Clinical implications

- **Optimizing procedural accuracy:**
  - Infrared thermography provides real-time confirmation of block efficacy, enhancing precision and reducing the need for repeated attempts.

- **Patient selection:**
  - Shorter immobilization time post-injury may predict better outcomes, guiding clinicians in selecting suitable candidates for LSBs.

- **Role of LSBs in CRPS management:**
  - While not a first-line treatment, LSBs can be effective for patients with clear autonomic dysfunction, particularly when monitored with advanced imaging tools like thermography.

- **Safety profile:**
  - The low complication rate supports using LSBs in experienced hands, particularly when standard therapies fail.

Key takeaways

☑ Infrared thermography enhances the precision and efficacy of lumbar sympathetic blocks for CRPS.

☑ A moderate response rate (37%) was observed, with significant improvements in pain and autonomic symptoms.

☑ Immobilization time is a critical predictor of treatment success, highlighting the need for early intervention.

☑ The procedure is safe, and no major complications have been reported, making it a viable option for refractory lower limb CRPS.

Additional recommended reading:

1. Bovaira M, Cañada-Soriano M, García-Vitoria C, et al. Clinical results of lumbar sympathetic blocks in lower limb complex regional pain syndrome using infrared thermography as a support tool. *Pain Pract.* 2023;23:713-723. doi:10.1111/papr.13236.

2. Cepeda MS, Lau J, Carr DB. Local anesthetic sympathetic blockade for complex regional pain syndrome. *Cochrane Database Syst Rev.* 2005;(4):CD004598. doi:10.1002/14651858.CD004598.pub2.

3. Van Eijs F, Stanton-Hicks M, Van Zundert J, et al. Evidence-based interventional pain medicine according to clinical diagnoses: Complex regional pain syndrome. *Pain Pract.* 2011;11(5):470-487.

Sympathetic blocks to predict ketamine infusion response in complex regional pain syndrome

34

Why this topic is important

Complex regional pain syndrome (CRPS) is a debilitating condition that presents significant challenges in diagnosis and management. Treatment options, such as ketamine infusions and sympathetic nerve blocks, are often used in clinical practice despite limited evidence for their long-term efficacy. These procedures are labor-intensive, costly, and not without risks, making it essential to identify predictors of treatment response. This study by Cohen et al. (2023) highlights the use of sympathetic blocks as a potential predictive tool for determining which patients with CRPS are likely to benefit from ketamine infusions. Such insights can help optimize resource allocation and improve patient outcomes.

Objectives of this update

- Explain the role of sympathetic blocks in predicting ketamine infusion response in CRPS patients.

- Outline the key findings from a recent multicenter study evaluating this association.

- Discuss the clinical implications of these findings for patient selection and personalized treatment strategies.

What is new

The study has provided evidence that the response to sympathetic blocks, defined by immediate pain relief and increased extremity temperature, correlates with ketamine infusion outcomes in CRPS patients. Key findings include:

- **Sympathetically maintained pain (SMP) as a predictor:** Patients with SMP, characterized by ≥ 50% immediate pain relief following sympathetic block, showed a higher likelihood of significant pain reduction after ketamine infusion. This contrasts with patients exhibiting sympathetically independent pain (SIP), who had lower success rates with ketamine.

- **Temperature increase significance:** A post-block temperature rise in the affected extremity was associated with better ketamine outcomes. On average, responders to ketamine had a greater temperature increase than non-responders.

- **Role of obesity:** Obese patients were significantly more likely to benefit from ketamine infusion. This finding aligns with emerging research suggesting that obesity may amplify the affective component of pain, which ketamine may target.

- **Lack of psychiatric influence:** Contrary to previous hypotheses, coexisting psychiatric conditions like depression or anxiety did not predict ketamine response.

Study design

The study evaluated 71 patients diagnosed with CRPS per the Budapest Criteria between 2011 and 2021. Patients underwent a sequence of interventions: sympathetic blocks (stellate ganglion or lumbar sympathetic blocks) followed by ketamine infusions. The effectiveness of sympathetic blocks was assessed by post-block pain relief and temperature changes. Ketamine infusion success was defined as a $\geq$ 30% pain reduction lasting over three weeks.

- **Sympathetic blocks:** Technically successful blocks were indicated by a $\geq$ 2°C temperature rise in the affected extremity. The presence of SMP was determined by $\geq$ 50% immediate pain relief.

- **Ketamine infusions:** Most infusions were outpatient procedures using mean doses of 174.54 mg, monitored for adverse effects like nausea or psychomimetic symptoms.

Key findings and clinical implications

- **Sympathetic blocks as screening tools:** Immediate pain relief and post-block temperature increases provide reliable indicators of ketamine infusion success. For patients considering the financial and physical burdens of ketamine therapy, sympathetic blocks can serve as an initial, less intensive test.

- **Impact of SMP:** Patients with SMP demonstrated a success rate of 61% with ketamine infusions compared to just 26.7% in SIP cases. These results suggest a strong physiological link between SMP mechanisms and ketamine's therapeutic effects, likely mediated by the affective-motivational aspects of pain.

- **Practical application of temperature metrics:** The degree of post-block temperature rise can guide clinicians in predicting outcomes. Higher temperature increases reflect more effective sympathetic blockade, potentially correlating with better ketamine responsiveness.

- **Obesity as a modifiable factor:** Obesity's role in amplifying the emotional and psychological dimensions of pain could make obese patients more amenable to ketamine's effects. Understanding this relationship could influence patient counseling and therapeutic choices.

- **Refuting psychiatric assumptions:** The absence of significant psychiatric influence suggests ketamine's efficacy may be less dependent on psychological factors than previously assumed. This reinforces its potential as a broad-spectrum analgesic for CRPS.

Limitations

- **Small sample size**
  With only seven RCTs and 433 participants, the findings have limited generalizability.

- **Heterogeneity**
  Variations in study design, prone protocols, and patient populations affect comparability.

- **Limited long-term data**
  Most studies focus on short-term outcomes, leaving gaps in long-term impact assessment.

- **Complications underreported**
  Adverse events like pressure ulcers and accidental extubation were sparsely reported.

- **Risk of publication bias**
  The small number of studies increases the potential for overestimating benefits.

- **Pediatric-specific challenges**
  Adult-derived ARDS criteria and ventilatory strategies may not fully apply to children.

Key takeaways

☑ Sympathetic blocks can effectively predict ketamine infusion success in CRPS patients, particularly when SMP is present or when post-block temperature rises are substantial.

☑ SMP is a robust predictor of positive ketamine outcomes, underscoring the need for thorough assessment during initial blocks.

☑ Obesity may enhance ketamine's efficacy, possibly through its impact on the affective dimensions of pain.

☑ Psychiatric conditions like depression and anxiety were not associated with ketamine response, suggesting a broader therapeutic applicability.

☑ Utilizing sympathetic blocks as a screening tool can help clinicians identify suitable candidates for ketamine therapy, reducing unnecessary procedures and expenses.

Additional recommended reading:

1. Cohen SP, Khunsriraksakul C, Yoo Y, et al. Sympathetic blocks as a predictor for response to ketamine infusion in patients with complex regional pain syndrome: A multicenter study. *Pain Med.* 2023;24(3):316-324. doi:10.1093/pm/pnac153.

2. Harden RN, Oaklander AL, Burton AW, et al. Complex regional pain syndrome: Practical diagnostic and treatment guidelines, 4th edition. *Pain Med.* 2013;14(2):180-229.

3. Connolly SB, Prager JP, Harden RN. A systematic review of ketamine for complex regional pain syndrome. *Pain Med.* 2015;16(5):943-969.

Perfusion index for monitoring response to intravenous ketamine in complex regional pain syndrome

35

Why this topic is important

Complex regional pain syndrome (CRPS) is a challenging chronic primary pain condition marked by severe pain, vasomotor disturbances, and diminished blood flow in affected limbs. Despite various treatments, many patients fail to achieve adequate relief. Ketamine, an N-methyl-D-aspartate (NMDA) receptor antagonist, is frequently used for CRPS, but its efficacy varies, and no objective tool exists to predict or monitor therapeutic responses. The perfusion index (PI), derived from pulse oximetry, reflects blood flow and may offer a reliable, non-invasive method to assess response to ketamine therapy. Its potential to quantify physiological changes related to vasomotor disturbances makes it a valuable tool for personalized treatment strategies in CRPS. Its use could also address limitations seen with other objective measures, such as skin temperature asymmetry, influenced by ambient conditions and may provide less consistent monitoring of therapeutic effects. A 2023 study by Hong et al. explored the PI's utility in CRPS patients undergoing intravenous ketamine therapy.

Objectives of this update

- Introduce the role of the PI in assessing CRPS-associated blood flow abnormalities.

- Summarize findings on PI changes in response to ketamine therapy.

- Discuss how PI can guide monitoring and predict treatment outcomes in CRPS patients.

- Explore practical challenges in integrating PI into CRPS management, including equipment standardization and patient-specific factors.

What is new

- **Lower PI in affected limbs:** Patients had significantly reduced PI in CRPS-affected limbs compared to contralateral limbs, indicating vasomotor dysfunction.

- **PI correlated with pain improvement:** Changes in PI during therapy were strongly linked to reductions in pain scores, suggesting its potential as an objective monitoring tool.

- **Threshold value for response prediction:** A 22.60% increase in PI was identified as an optimal threshold to distinguish responders (≥ 50-point reduction in pain scores) from non-responders, with high sensitivity (81%) and specificity (89%).

Study design and population

This prospective study evaluated 46 CRPS patients diagnosed via the Budapest criteria. Participants had unilateral CRPS affecting an arm or leg and had experienced intractable pain for ≥ 6 months. Patients with psychological disorders or conditions preventing PI sensor application were excluded.

Interventions and measurements

- **PI monitoring:** Two pulse oximetry sensors measured the PI of both affected and unaffected limbs before, immediately after, and 30 minutes post-ketamine infusion.

- **Ketamine therapy:** Patients received 1 mg/kg of ketamine in 500 mL Hartmann solution infused at 4 mL/kg/h. Pain was assessed using a visual analog scale (VAS) and the McGill Pain Questionnaire.

Key outcomes

- **Differences in PI between limbs:** The PI measured in the affected limb was significantly lower than that in the unaffected limb at all measured time points. Before the ketamine infusion, the perfusion index was 1.35 in the affected limb compared to 2.35 in the unaffected limb.

- **Improvement after therapy:** Both the PI and pain scores showed significant improvement following ketamine infusion therapy. Pain scores decreased markedly, from an average of 70 before the infusion to 20 thirty minutes afterward.

- **Correlation with pain relief:** A greater increase in the PI in the affected limb was strongly associated with larger reductions in pain scores, indicating a positive correlation.

Clinical implications

- **Objective response monitoring:** The PI offers a quantitative, real-time method to track physiological changes during ketamine therapy, addressing the limitations of subjective pain scales. Its ability to provide an unbiased measure of vasomotor changes makes it a potentially superior alternative to skin temperature asymmetry, which may be less reliable in variable environmental conditions.

- **Predicting treatment success:** An increase of 22.60% in the PI of the affected limb reliably predicts significant pain relief, enabling clinicians to identify patients who are likely to respond to therapy early in the treatment process.

- **Guiding treatment decisions:** Incorporating PI monitoring into CRPS management protocols can enhance personalized care by tailoring interventions based on physiological markers.

Key takeaways

- ☑ The PI is consistently lower in CRPS-affected limbs, reflecting vasomotor dysfunction.

- ☑ Ketamine therapy improves PI and reduces pain, with changes in PI strongly correlating with pain relief.

- ☑ A ≥ 22.60% increase in PI post-therapy is a reliable threshold for distinguishing responders from non-responders.

- ☑ PI monitoring provides an objective, non-invasive tool to evaluate and predict treatment outcomes in CRPS patients. Its integration into clinical practice requires addressing barriers such as equipment standardization, individual variability in responses, and comparisons with existing methods like skin temperature asymmetry.

- ☑ While these findings are promising, the study did not address potential limitations, such as individual variability in PI responses due to patient-specific vasomotor factors or the influence of external confounders like ambient temperature. Further research is needed to refine protocols and confirm these results.

Additional recommended reading:

1. Hong S-W, Hwang M-S, Kim JH, et al. Usefulness of the perfusion index for monitoring the response to intravenous ketamine infusion therapy in patients with complex regional pain syndrome. *Pain Pract.* 2023;23:535-542. doi:10.1111/papr.13215.

2. Harden RN, Bruehl S, Perez R, et al. Validation of proposed diagnostic criteria (the "Budapest criteria") for complex regional pain syndrome. *Pain.* 2010;150:268-74.

3. Zhao J, Wang Y, Wang D. The effect of ketamine infusion in the treatment of complex regional pain syndrome: A systemic review and meta-analysis. *Curr Pain Headache Rep.* 2018;22:12.

Patient outcomes following rehabilitation in early or persistent complex regional pain syndrome

36

Why this topic is important

Complex Regional Pain Syndrome (CRPS) is a chronic pain condition marked by severe pain, functional impairment, and psychological distress, often following injury or surgery. It is classified into early (symptoms < 1 year) and persistent (symptoms ≥ 1 year) stages. While international guidelines emphasize early intervention, little empirical evidence supports the assumption that early CRPS responds better to multidisciplinary rehabilitation programs than persistent CRPS.

This study by Lewis et al. (2024) addresses this gap, providing critical insights into how symptom duration impacts rehabilitation effectiveness. Understanding these dynamics can help clinicians optimize care strategies for patients at different stages of CRPS.

Objectives of this update

- Compare the outcomes of multidisciplinary rehabilitation in early versus persistent CRPS.

- Assess the sustainability of rehabilitation benefits over time.

- Challenge assumptions about the superiority of early CRPS outcomes and inform clinical practices.

What is new

- Both early and persistent CRPS show significant improvements in function, pain, and psychological health post-rehabilitation.

- Persistent CRPS demonstrates greater sustainability of rehabilitation benefits at three months, contrary to prior assumptions favoring early intervention.

- Highlights the importance of addressing psychological and social factors to sustain gains, especially in early CRPS.

Study design

This retrospective analysis examined patient-reported outcome measures (PROMs) from 218 individuals undergoing a standardized multidisciplinary rehabilitation program in the United Kingdom.

- **Early CRPS group:** 40 patients with symptom duration < 1 year.
- **Persistent CRPS group:** 178 patients with symptoms ≥ 1 year.
- PROMs were collected at three time points: pre-rehabilitation (T1), post-rehabilitation (T2), and three months post-rehabilitation (T3).

Post-rehabilitation outcomes

- **Pain reduction:**
  - Both groups showed moderate reductions in pain intensity (e.g., Numeric Rating Scale, Brief Pain Inventory).
  - Persistent CRPS achieved statistically significant sustained pain reduction at three months, while early CRPS saw worsening pain at follow-up.

- **Functional improvements:**
  - Early CRPS demonstrated small functional improvements, including mobility and daily activity engagement, which were not sustained at follow-up.
  - Persistent CRPS maintained functional gains (e.g., EuroQol-5D utility index, Quick Disabilities of the Arm, Shoulder, and Hand questionnaire).

- **Psychological health:**
  - Depression and anxiety scores improved in both groups immediately post-rehabilitation (e.g., Patient Health Questionnaire, Generalized Anxiety Disorder-7).
  - Persistent CRPS maintained reductions in psychological distress, while early CRPS did not.

- **Self-efficacy:**
  - Persistent CRPS patients reported sustained improvements in self-efficacy at three months, reflecting enhanced confidence in managing symptoms.

- **Kinesiophobia (fear of movement):**
  - Significant decreases in kinesiophobia were observed in both groups immediately post-rehabilitation. Persistent CRPS maintained this improvement.

Comparative analysis

- **Between-group differences:**
  - At three months, persistent CRPS patients outperformed early CRPS in key areas such as pain reduction and functional mobility.
  - Early CRPS patients experienced regression in pain and functional outcomes, underscoring the need for targeted follow-up strategies.

- **Influence of symptom duration:**
  - Persistent CRPS patients may benefit more from rehabilitation due to adaptations in coping mechanisms and physiological adjustments over time.
  - Early CRPS patients often exhibit unmet expectations of "cure," potentially hindering long-term adherence to self-management strategies.

Clinical implications

- **Tailored interventions:**
  - Early CRPS patients may require additional psychological support to address ambivalence about the condition and facilitate acceptance.
  - Persistent CRPS patients can benefit from sustained rehabilitation programs emphasizing long-term functional maintenance.

- **Family and social involvement:**

  - ◦ Engaging family members in education about CRPS may enhance support systems for early CRPS patients, reducing setbacks at home.

- **Setback planning:**

  - ◦ Incorporating relapse prevention and setback management into early CRPS rehabilitation can help sustain gains post-discharge.

- **Focus on psychological resilience:**

  - ◦ Persistent CRPS patients' sustained outcomes highlight the importance of bolstering resilience through psychological interventions during rehabilitation.

Key takeaways

- ☑ Multidisciplinary rehabilitation improves pain, function, and psychological health in CRPS regardless of symptom duration.

- ☑ Persistent CRPS patients maintain greater long-term benefits, challenging the assumption of superior outcomes in early CRPS.

- ☑ Early CRPS rehabilitation strategies should address psychological barriers and improve family engagement to enhance sustainability.

- ☑ Clinical practice should emphasize tailored approaches to maximize benefits for both early and persistent CRPS patients.

Additional recommended reading:

1. Lewis JS, Wallace CS, White P, et al. Early versus persistent Complex Regional Pain Syndrome: Is there a difference in patient-reported outcomes following rehabilitation? *Eur J Pain.* 2024;28:464-475.

2. Harden RN, Swan M, King A, et al. Treatment of complex regional pain syndrome: Functional restoration. *Clin J Pain.* 2006;22(5):420-424.

3. Bruehl S. Complex regional pain syndrome. *BMJ.* 2015;351:h2730.

Continuous peripheral nerve blocks for postamputation phantom and residual limb pain

37

Why this topic is important

Phantom limb pain (PLP) and residual limb pain (RLP) are challenging conditions affecting a significant number of amputees, often leading to debilitating physical and psychological consequences. These conditions remain difficult to treat, with conventional pharmacological and rehabilitative approaches frequently yielding suboptimal results. Continuous peripheral nerve blocks (CPNBs) offer a promising intervention, providing targeted analgesia and potentially improving pain outcomes for patients with established PLP and RLP.

This reanalysis by Ilfeld et al. (2023) focuses on patient-centered secondary outcomes from a multicenter randomized controlled trial, emphasizing the clinically meaningful benefits of CPNBs. The findings highlight their potential in alleviating PLP and RLP, offering amputees evidence-based options for improved quality of life.

Objectives of this update

- Evaluate the efficacy of CPNBs in reducing phantom and residual limb pain.

- Highlight patient-centered outcomes, including clinically relevant pain reductions and functional improvements.

- Provide insights for clinical decision-making and future research.

What is new

- CPNBs more than double the likelihood of clinically relevant improvements in phantom and residual limb pain compared to placebo.

- For the first time, patient-specific metrics for small, medium, and large improvements in pain and function are defined.

- Comprehensive insights into how baseline pain severity influences response rates.

Study design and population

- **Trial overview:**

  - Multicenter, double-blind, randomized trial comparing six-day continuous ropivacaine infusions versus saline placebo.

  - Participants: 144 patients with established PLP or RLP post-amputation, randomized into active treatment (n=71) and placebo (n=73).

- **Baseline characteristics:**

  - Patients were stratified based on mild (< 5), moderate (5-7), and severe (> 7) baseline pain scores using the Numeric Rating Scale (NRS).

Efficacy of continuous peripheral nerve blocks

- **Phantom limb pain:**

  - 57% of patients receiving CPNBs experienced clinically significant reductions (≥ 2-point improvement on the NRS) in average phantom limb pain compared to 26% in the placebo group.

  - CPNBs provided meaningful improvements in worst phantom pain for 49% of active-treatment participants versus 21% for placebo.

- **Residual limb pain:**

  - Similar trends were observed for RLP, with significant pain reductions achieved in 49% of active-treatment patients versus 21% of placebo group patients.

  - Patients with mild or moderate baseline pain showed the greatest improvements, while those with severe pain demonstrated smaller, yet still meaningful, benefits.

Functional and patient-centered outcomes

- **Global impressions of change:**

  - Participants rated their pain improvements on a seven-point Patient Global Impression of Change (PGIC) scale.

  - 53% of active-treatment patients reported self-described improvement, compared to 30% in the placebo group.

- **Pain interference:**

  - Changes in the Brief Pain Inventory (BPI) interference subscale reflected the impact of CPNBs on physical and emotional functioning.

  - Median improvements for small, medium, and large analgesic effects were 8, 22, and 39 points on the BPI scale, respectively.

- **Patient-defined thresholds:**

  - Median NRS reductions associated with small, medium, and large improvements in phantom pain were 2, 3, and 5 points, respectively.

Safety profile

- **Adverse events:**

  - The trial reported no severe adverse events related to CPNBs.

  - Transient side effects, such as localized pain or catheter-related issues, were manageable and resolved without lasting complications.

- **Clinical implications:**

  - CPNBs demonstrate a favorable safety profile, making them a viable option for patients with refractory PLP or RLP.

Clinical implications

- **Optimizing patient selection:**
  - Patients with mild-to-moderate baseline pain may experience the most substantial benefits from CPNBs.
  - Comprehensive pain assessments are essential for identifying candidates likely to benefit from this intervention.

- **Integration into multimodal care:**
  - CPNBs should complement, rather than replace, existing therapies such as physical rehabilitation, psychological support, and pharmacological interventions.

- **Focus on patient-centered care:**
  - Incorporating patient-defined outcomes into clinical practice ensures that treatment aligns with individual priorities and expectations.

Key takeaways

☑ Continuous peripheral nerve blocks are effective in significantly reducing phantom and residual limb pain, with benefits more than doubling those of placebo.

☑ Patient-defined metrics for clinically relevant pain and functional improvements provide actionable insights for individualizing care.

☑ The favorable safety profile of CPNBs supports their integration into multimodal pain management strategies for amputees.

Additional recommended reading:

1. Ilfeld BM, Khatibi B, Maheshwari K, et al. Patient-centered results from a multicenter study of continuous peripheral nerve blocks and postamputation phantom and residual limb pain: Secondary outcomes from a randomized clinical trial. *Reg Anesth Pain Med.* 2023;48:1-7.

2. Dworkin RH, Turk DC, Peirce-Sandner S, et al. Recommendations for chronic pain clinical trials: IMMPACT guidelines. *Pain.* 2010;149:177-93.

3. Bruel BM, Burton AW. Interventional techniques for the management of neuropathic pain in amputees. *Pain Med.* 2016;17:2404-21.

Radiofrequency thermocoagulation for chronic hip pain

38

Why this topic is important

Chronic hip pain significantly reduces mobility and quality of life, especially in older adults. Conservative treatments like physical therapy and analgesics often provide only temporary relief, while total hip replacement, though effective, carries risks, costs, and potential complications. For patients unfit for surgery or seeking to delay it, radiofrequency thermocoagulation (RFT) offers a minimally invasive alternative to alleviate pain and improve function. This update, based on the study by Karaoğlu et al. (2024), focuses on the effectiveness of RFT targeting the articular branches of the femoral and obturator nerves for managing chronic hip pain.

Objectives of this update

- Explain the technique and therapeutic impact of RFT for chronic hip pain.

- Summarize findings on its effects on pain relief, hip function, and quality of life.

- Highlight its role as an alternative for patients who cannot undergo surgery.

What is new

This study has provided compelling evidence of the benefits of RFT for chronic hip pain. Key findings include:

- **Significant pain relief:** RFT achieved substantial pain reduction, with the greatest improvement occurring within the first week post-procedure. Pain levels remained lower than baseline for six months.

- **Enhanced hip function:** Patients reported improved mobility and reduced stiffness on standardized arthritis indices like the Western Ontario and McMaster Universities Arthritis Index (WOMAC).

- **Improved physical quality of life:** Scores on the physical component of the Short-Form Health Survey-12 (SF-12) improved significantly, although mental health scores remained unchanged.

- **Minimal complications:** The procedure demonstrated a favorable safety profile, with only one case of transient motor deficit that resolved spontaneously.

Study design and population

The study enrolled 53 patients (48 completed the trial) suffering from chronic hip pain unresponsive to conservative treatments. The participants were aged 18 and older, with pain persisting for at least three months. Most had hip osteoarthritis (77.1%), while others had postoperative hip pain, malignancy-related pain, or avascular necrosis.

Patients with major psychiatric conditions, radiating lumbar pain, infections, or recent surgery were excluded. All participants provided informed consent before undergoing the procedure.

Interventions

RFT was performed under combined ultrasound and fluoroscopic guidance to ensure precise targeting of the femoral and obturator nerve articular branches. Thermal lesions were created at two sites per nerve at 80°C for 90 seconds each using a specially designed electrode. Patients received pre-procedure sedation and local anesthetics with corticosteroids to minimize discomfort and inflammation.

Outcome measures

- **Pain:** Assessed using the Verbal Pain Scale (VPS) at baseline, one week, and one, three, and six months post-procedure.

- **Hip function:** Evaluated using the WOMAC index, which measures pain, stiffness, and physical function.

- **Quality of life:** Measured using the SF-12 survey, focusing on both physical and mental components.

Key findings

- **Pain relief**
  - Patients reported a significant drop in pain scores. The average VPS decreased from 8.9 before the procedure to 2.4 within one week.

- While pain gradually increased over time, scores at six months (5.8) remained significantly lower than baseline.

- **Functional improvement**
  - WOMAC scores showed substantial improvements in pain, stiffness, and physical function after the procedure, maintained throughout the six-month follow-up.
  - These findings highlight RFT's ability to enhance daily mobility and reduce the disability associated with chronic hip pain.

- **Quality of life**
  - The physical component of the SF-12 survey improved significantly, reflecting better overall physical health. However, mental health scores did not show meaningful changes, potentially due to the psychological burden of chronic pain.

- **Safety and tolerability**
  - RFT was well-tolerated, with no major complications reported. A single patient experienced transient motor weakness, which resolved spontaneously within 12 hours.

Clinical implications

- **Effective pain management:**
  - RFT offers reliable and sustained pain relief, making it a suitable option for patients who cannot or prefer not to undergo surgery.
  - The procedure is particularly effective for those with advanced osteoarthritis or refractory hip pain.

- **Improved functional outcomes:**
  - Enhanced mobility and reduced stiffness allow patients to engage in daily activities more easily.
  - These functional benefits complement RFT's analgesic effects, offering a holistic approach to chronic hip pain management.

- **Safety and practicality:**

  ◦ RFT's minimally invasive nature, coupled with its low complication rate, makes it a safe and practical alternative for a wide range of patients.

  ◦ Combining ultrasound and fluoroscopic guidance ensures precise nerve targeting, reducing the risk of vascular or neural injury.

Key takeaways

☑ Radiofrequency thermocoagulation provides significant pain relief for up to six months in patients with chronic hip pain.

☑ The procedure enhances hip function and physical quality of life, making it a viable alternative for patients who are not surgical candidates.

☑ RFT is safe and well-tolerated, with minimal complications reported.

☑ Its minimally invasive nature and sustained efficacy position RFT as a promising option in the multimodal management of chronic hip pain.

Additional recommended reading:

1. Karaoğlu ŞS, Sari S, Ekin Y, et al. The effect of conventional radiofrequency thermocoagulation of femoral and obturator nerves' articular branches on chronic hip pain: A prospective clinical study. *Pain Med.* 2024;25(7):444-450. doi:10.1093/pm/pnae016.

2. Mariconda C, Megna M, Fari G, et al. Therapeutic exercise and radiofrequency in the rehabilitation project for hip osteoarthritis pain. *Eur J Phys Rehabil Med.* 2020;56(4):451-458. doi:10.23736/S1973-9087.20.06152-3.

3. Tran A, Reiter D, Wong PK-W, et al. Alternative treatment of hip pain from advanced hip osteoarthritis utilizing cooled radiofrequency ablation: A single-institution pilot study. *Skeletal Radiol.* 2022;51(5):1047-1054. doi:10.1007/s00256-021-03927-0.

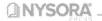

Polynucleotide, sodium hyaluronate, or crosslinked sodium hyaluronate for knee osteoarthritis

39

Why this topic is important

Knee osteoarthritis is one of the most common causes of chronic joint pain and functional disability, particularly in older populations. Traditional treatments include physical therapy, nonsteroidal anti-inflammatory drugs (NSAIDs), and intra-articular injections of corticosteroids or viscosupplements. Among these, hyaluronic acid and emerging alternatives like polynucleotide injections aim to improve joint lubrication and reduce pain. This update focuses on a multicenter, randomized study by Moon et al. (2023) comparing polynucleotide, classic hyaluronic acid, and crosslinked hyaluronic acid for their efficacy in relieving knee osteoarthritis pain.

Objectives of this update

- Present the comparative effectiveness of polynucleotide and two forms of hyaluronic acid for pain relief and functional improvement in knee osteoarthritis.

- Highlight the safety profile and practical applications of these therapies.

- Offer insights into how these treatments can be integrated into clinical practice.

What is new

- **Superior pain relief with polynucleotide:** Polynucleotide significantly reduced knee pain, with earlier and greater pain relief than both hyaluronic acid forms.

- **Early-onset effects:** Both polynucleotide and crosslinked hyaluronic acid showed rapid pain reduction, with improvements noted as early as one week.

- **Comparable functional improvement:** All three treatments improved knee function and quality of life, with no significant differences in functional measures.

- **Minimal adverse events:** All treatments were well-tolerated, with no severe adverse effects reported.

Design and participants

This multicenter, randomized, double-blind trial included 90 participants with moderate knee osteoarthritis, classified as Kellgren-Lawrence grades I to III. Eligible patients experienced chronic knee pain that was unresponsive to conservative management, including physiotherapy or pharmacotherapy, for at least three months.

Treatments

Participants were randomly assigned to one of three treatment groups:

- **Polynucleotide:** Three intra-articular injections at one-week intervals.
- **Classic hyaluronic acid:** Three intra-articular injections at one-week intervals.
- **Crosslinked hyaluronic acid:** A single injection followed by two saline injections.

Experienced physicians administered each treatment under ultrasound guidance using standardized aseptic techniques.

Outcome measures

The primary outcome was the change in pain intensity during weight-bearing activities at 16 weeks, measured using the visual analog scale (VAS). Secondary outcomes included pain intensity during walking and rest, functional disability, quality of life, and adverse events.

Key findings

- **Pain relief**
  - Polynucleotide achieved the largest reduction in weight-bearing knee pain (VAS decrease of 41 points) compared to classic (23.3 points) and crosslinked hyaluronic acid (20.2 points).
  - Polynucleotide and crosslinked hyaluronic acid reduced pain rapidly starting one week after treatment. Classic hyaluronic acid showed delayed effects, with improvements becoming significant only after 16 weeks.

- **Functional improvement**
  - All groups showed significant improvements in knee function and quality of life, as measured by the Western Ontario and McMaster Universities Arthritis Index and the EuroQol-5D questionnaire.
  - No significant differences were found between the groups regarding functional outcomes, except for better quality-of-life scores with polynucleotide compared to crosslinked hyaluronic acid at 16 weeks.

- **Safety and tolerability**
  - Mild, transient adverse events, such as knee swelling and procedural pain, were reported in nine patients across the three groups.
  - No severe adverse events or significant changes in vital signs occurred during the study.

Clinical implications

- **Efficacy and onset:**
  - Polynucleotide is highly effective for both early and sustained pain relief in knee osteoarthritis.
  - It may be particularly beneficial for patients seeking rapid symptom relief without compromising long-term outcomes.

- **Practical considerations:**
  - While polynucleotide requires multiple injections, it may provide greater pain relief and faster results than single injections of crosslinked hyaluronic acid.
  - All three options are viable, and patient preferences, cost considerations, and clinical presentation could guide treatment choices.

- **Safety profile:**
  - The minimal adverse events across all treatments highlight the safety of these intra-articular therapies and support their continued use in clinical practice.

Key takeaways

☑ Polynucleotide injections provide superior and faster pain relief compared to classic and crosslinked hyaluronic acid in patients with knee osteoarthritis.

☑ Functional improvement and quality of life are significantly enhanced with all three treatments.

☑ All therapies are well-tolerated, with no severe adverse events reported.

☑ Intra-articular viscosupplementation remains valuable for managing knee osteoarthritis when conservative treatments fail.

Additional recommended reading:

1. Moon JY, Kim J, Lee JY, et al. Comparison of polynucleotide, sodium hyaluronate, and crosslinked sodium hyaluronate for the management of painful knee osteoarthritis: A multicenter, randomized, double-blind, parallel-group study. *Pain Med*. 2023;24(5):496-506. doi:10.1093/pm/pnac155.

2. Vanelli R, Costa P, Rossi SM, et al. Efficacy of intra-articular polynucleotides in the treatment of knee osteoarthritis: A randomized, double-blind clinical trial. *Knee Surg Sports Traumatol Arthrosc*. 2010;18(7):901-7.

3. Bannuru RR, Osani MC, Vaysbrot EE, et al. OARSI guidelines for the non-surgical management of knee osteoarthritis. *Osteoarthritis Cartilage*. 2019;27(11):1578-89.

Genicular nerve radiofrequency ablation for chronic knee pain

40

Why this topic is important

Chronic knee pain, often due to osteoarthritis or post-surgical conditions, significantly impacts mobility and quality of life. While total knee arthroplasty is an effective solution for many, nonsurgical options are essential for patients who cannot undergo or prefer to avoid surgery. Genicular nerve radiofrequency ablation (GNRFA) has emerged as a promising minimally invasive treatment targeting sensory nerves to reduce pain. This update reviews findings from a large real-world cohort study by Caragea et al. (2023) that assessed the effectiveness and prognostic factors of GNRFA for chronic knee pain, providing valuable insights into patient selection and procedural optimization.

Objectives of this update

- Summarize the long-term outcomes of GNRFA for chronic knee pain.

- Identify key factors that predict treatment success.

- Highlight clinical implications for optimizing patient outcomes and procedural techniques.

What is new

- **Sustained pain relief:** Approximately half of the patients reported clinically meaningful pain relief, with 47.8% achieving ≥ 50% pain reduction at a mean follow-up of nearly two years.

- **Patient-reported improvements:** Nearly 60% of patients reported feeling "much improved" or better on the Patient Global Impression of Change (PGIC) scale.

- **Prognostic factors:** Success was associated with targeting more than three nerves and having advanced osteoarthritis (Kellgren-Lawrence grade 4). Conversely, baseline use of opioids or antidepressants predicted poorer outcomes.

Design and population

This observational study analyzed data from 134 patients treated at a tertiary care center for chronic knee pain between 2015 and 2021. Participants were required to meet the following criteria:

- Diagnosed knee osteoarthritis or persistent postsurgical pain.
- Minimum pain intensity of 3 on the numerical rating scale (NRS).
- ≥ 50% pain relief following a diagnostic nerve block.

Patients with uncontrolled systemic diseases or missing baseline data were excluded.

Intervention

GNRFA was performed using fluoroscopic guidance, targeting at least three genicular nerves, including the superior medial, superior lateral, and inferior medial nerves. Lesions were created using a cooled or conventional RFA system, with temperatures ranging between 60°C and 80°C depending on the probe type.

Outcomes

- **Pain reduction:** Evaluated using the NRS, with ≥ 50% reduction considered clinically significant.
- **Patient satisfaction:** Assessed via the PGIC scale, with scores ≥ 6 indicating a meaningful improvement.
- **Safety:** Adverse events were documented throughout follow-up.

Key findings

- **Pain relief**
  - The mean baseline NRS score was 6.2. At follow-up (mean 23 months), the average reduction was 2.9 points, with 61.2% of patients achieving at least a 2-point reduction.
  - Clinically significant pain relief (≥ 50% reduction in NRS) was reported by 47.8% of participants.

- **Patient-reported outcomes**
  - Nearly 60% of patients felt "much improved" or better on the PGIC scale, indicating high patient satisfaction.
  - However, outcomes were less favorable in patients with a history of total knee replacement.

- **Prognostic factors**
  - Targeting more than three nerves was associated with a 29% greater reduction in pain scores.
  - Advanced osteoarthritis (Kellgren-Lawrence grade 4) was linked to higher odds of achieving ≥ 50% pain relief.
  - Baseline use of opioids, antidepressants, or anxiolytics predicted poorer outcomes, likely due to underlying central sensitization or psychological comorbidities.

- **Safety**
  - No severe complications, such as infections or nerve damage, were reported. Minor adverse events included mild bruising and temporary discomfort at needle sites.

Clinical implications

- **Effectiveness of GNRFA:**
  - GNRFA provides significant, long-term pain relief for approximately half of patients with chronic knee pain, supporting its role as an alternative to surgery or pharmacological therapies.

- **Patient selection:**
  - Patients with advanced osteoarthritis and no opioid or antidepressant use are more likely to benefit. Careful pre-procedural evaluation can enhance success rates.

- **Technical considerations:**
  - Expanding the number of targeted nerves and optimizing lesioning protocols can improve outcomes. Emerging evidence suggests targeting up to five genicular nerves may enhance efficacy.

- **Safety assurance:**
  - The low incidence of adverse events highlights the safety of GNRFA in experienced hands, reinforcing its viability for a broad patient population.

Key takeaways

☑ GNRFA offers effective, sustained pain relief and improved quality of life for patients with chronic knee pain, particularly in cases of advanced osteoarthritis.

☑ Success is enhanced by targeting more than three genicular nerves and avoiding pre-procedural opioid or antidepressant use.

☑ The procedure is safe, with minimal risks and high patient satisfaction rates.

☑ Optimized patient selection and procedural protocols are crucial for maximizing therapeutic outcomes.

Additional recommended reading:

1. Caragea M, Woodworth T, Curtis T, et al. Genicular nerve radiofrequency ablation for the treatment of chronic knee joint pain: A real-world cohort study with evaluation of prognostic factors. *Pain Med.* 2023;24(12):1332-1340. doi:10.1093/pm/pnad095.

2. McCormick ZL, Walega DR, Cohen SP. Technical considerations for genicular nerve radiofrequency ablation: Optimizing outcomes. *Reg Anesth Pain Med.* 2021;46(6):518-523.

3. Chen AF, Mullen K, Casambre F, et al. Radiofrequency ablation for knee osteoarthritis: A systematic review. *J Am Acad Orthop Surg.* 2021;29(9):387-396.

Genicular nerve ablation for osteoarthritic and post-total knee arthroplasty pain

41

Why this topic is important

Chronic knee pain is a significant cause of disability, with osteoarthritis and post-surgical complications being major contributors. Genicular nerve radiofrequency ablation (GNRFA) is a minimally invasive procedure that targets sensory nerves to reduce pain. While its effectiveness in osteoarthritis-related knee pain is well-established, its role in managing pain after total knee arthroplasty (TKA) is unclear. This study by Shi et al. (2024) examines the efficacy of GNRFA for these two patient populations to guide clinical decision-making.

Objectives of this update

- Compare the outcomes of GNRFA for osteoarthritic and post-TKA knee pain.

- Highlight success rates and functional improvements across these conditions.

- Discuss the technical and clinical considerations unique to post-TKA patients.

What is new

- **Comparable efficacy:** Both groups experienced significant and similar pain relief and functional improvements at three and six months.

- **Success rates:** At three months, 81% of post-TKA patients and 80% of osteoarthritic patients reported at least 50% pain relief.

- **Safety:** The procedure demonstrated a favorable safety profile, with no severe complications reported.

Design and participants

This retrospective study included 73 patients (46 with osteoarthritic pain, 27 with post-TKA pain) treated with traditional thermal GNRFA. All patients had at least six months of chronic knee pain unresponsive to conservative treatments, including medications and physical therapy.

Interventions

GNRFA targeted up to nine genicular nerves based on the patient's pain distribution. Needle placement followed standard anatomical guidelines, confirmed by sensory testing. The ablation was performed at 85°C for 150 seconds. McCormick's standardized technique was used for needle positioning, leveraging specific anatomical landmarks to improve procedural accuracy.

Outcome measures

- **Pain relief:** Assessed using the numerical rating scale (NRS). A ≥ 50% reduction in pain was considered a successful outcome.

- **Functional improvement:** Evaluated using the patient-specific functional scale (PSFS) for activities like walking, standing, and stair negotiation.

- **Follow-up periods:** Outcomes were assessed at three and six months post-procedure.

Key findings

- **Pain relief**
  - At three months, both groups achieved significant pain reduction (median pain relief: 60%).
  - At six months, pain relief diminished slightly in both groups but remained clinically significant (median pain relief: 50%).

- **Functional improvement**
  - Both groups showed significant gains in PSFS scores at three and six months.

Improvements were comparable between osteoarthritic and post-TKA patients.

- **Success rates**
  - Success, defined as ≥ 50% pain reduction, was observed in 81% of post-TKA patients and 80% of osteoarthritic patients at three months.
  - At six months, success rates declined to 56% in both groups.

- **Safety**
  - No major complications were reported. Minor bruising at cannula entry sites was the only adverse event observed.

Clinical implications

- **Effectiveness across conditions:**
  - GNRFA provides similar levels of pain relief and functional improvement for osteoarthritic and post-TKA knee pain, supporting its use in both populations.

- **Challenges in post-TKA patients:**
  - Post-TKA anatomy presents technical challenges due to scar tissue and prosthetic hardware. Careful needle placement, using landmarks like the fibular head, is essential to avoid complications.

- **Patient selection and expectations:**
  - While GNRFA offers meaningful relief, pain reduction tends to diminish over time. Patients should be informed about the potential for recurrence and the need for repeat procedures.
  - Consider patient age and comorbidities, as these factors may influence outcomes and confound retrospective analyses.

- **Minimizing complications:**
  - Adherence to anatomical guidelines and sensory testing during needle placement enhances procedural safety.
  - Prospective studies are needed to refine safety protocols and validate the long-term benefits of GNRFA, particularly in post-TKA populations.

Key takeaways

☑ GNRFA provides comparable and effective pain relief for both osteoarthritic and post-TKA knee pain, with success rates exceeding 80% at three months.

☑ Functional improvements are significant and similar across patient groups.

☑ The procedure is safe, with no major complications reported in this study.

☑ Post-TKA cases may require advanced technical expertise due to altered anatomy and potential scar tissue.

☑ The study's retrospective design, broad patient demographics, and many confounders highlight the need for prospective, controlled studies to confirm findings.

Additional recommended reading:

1. Shi W, Vu T-N, Annaswamy T, et al. Effectiveness comparison of genicular nerve ablation for knee osteoarthritic versus post-total knee arthroplasty pain. *Interventional Pain Medicine.* 2024;3:100390. doi:10.1016/j.inpm.2024.100390.

2. McCormick ZL, Walker K, Wasan AD, et al. Technical considerations for genicular nerve radiofrequency ablation: Optimizing outcomes. *Regional Anesthesia and Pain Medicine.* 2021;46:518-23.

3. Tran J, Peng PW, Lam K, et al. Anatomical Study of the Innervation of Anterior Knee Joint Capsule: Implication for Image-Guided Intervention. *Regional Anesthesia & Pain Medicine* 2018;43:407-414.

4. Paula J Yu, Eldon Loh, Anne M R Agur, John Tran, Advanced three-dimensional anatomical mapping of saphenous and inferior medial genicular nerve branching: enhancing precision in knee joint denervation, *Pain Medicine, 2024;,* pnae102, https://doi.org/10.1093/pm/pnae102

5. Alomari A, Bhatia A. An update on radiofrequency denervation for arthritis-related knee joint pain: a synthesis of the current evidence. *BJA Educ.* 2024 May;24(5):164-172. doi: 10.1016/j.bjae.2024.01.007. Epub 2024 Mar 2. PMID: 38646452; PMCID: PMC11026924.

6. Ng TK, Lam KHS, Allam AE. Motor-Sparing Neural Ablation with Modified Techniques for Knee Pain: Case Series on Knee Osteoarthritis and Updated Review of the Underlying Anatomy and Available Techniques. Biomed Res Int. 2022 May 31;2022:2685898. doi: 10.1155/2022/2685898. PMID: 35686229; PMCID: PMC9173899.

Cooled and monopolar radiofrequency ablation for chronic knee pain

42

Why this topic is important

Knee osteoarthritis is a prevalent and debilitating condition, often leading to chronic pain and reduced mobility. While total knee arthroplasty offers definitive relief, many patients are not ideal surgical candidates due to comorbidities or preferences. Radiofrequency ablation (RFA) of sensory nerves in the knee is a minimally invasive alternative for managing pain. Based on a recent randomized controlled trial by Vallejo et al. (2023), this update evaluates the comparative efficacy of cooled radiofrequency ablation (CRFA) and monopolar radiofrequency ablation (MRFA) in providing long-term pain relief and improving functionality.

Objectives of this update

- Compare the long-term pain relief CRFA and MRFA provide for chronic knee pain.

- Assess the effects of these treatments on knee functionality and quality of life.

- Explore their safety profiles and clinical implications for patient care.

What is new

- **Sustained pain relief:** Both CRFA and MRFA significantly reduced pain for up to 52 weeks, with CRFA demonstrating slightly better durability.

- **Functional improvements:** Significant enhancements in knee function were observed across both groups, with better outcomes in unilateral cases treated with CRFA.

- **Patient satisfaction:** Over 50% of patients treated with CRFA reported a very good or good global perceived effect at 52 weeks, compared to 38% for MRFA.

- **Safety:** Both techniques were well-tolerated, with no severe treatment-related adverse events.

Design and participants

The trial included 75 patients aged 18 and older with chronic knee pain lasting more than six months and radiologic evidence of osteoarthritis graded 2 to 4 on the Kellgren-Lawrence scale. Participants were required to have stable medication regimens and at least 50% pain reduction with diagnostic nerve blocks. Exclusion criteria included prior total knee replacement, BMI over 40, and uncontrolled systemic diseases.

Interventions

Participants were randomly assigned to receive either CRFA or MRFA. Using standard fluoroscopic and ultrasound guidance, both procedures targeted the sensory branches of the superior medial, superior lateral, and inferior medial genicular nerves.

- **CRFA:** Applied for 150 seconds at 80°C with a cooled active tip.

- **MRFA:** Applied for 90 seconds at 80°C using a monopolar active tip.

Pain and functionality were evaluated at 1, 4, 12, 24, and 52 weeks post-treatment.

Outcome measures

- **Pain:** Measured using a 100 mm visual analog scale (VAS).

- **Knee functionality:** Assessed with the Western Ontario and McMaster Universities Arthritis Index (WOMAC) and the Oxford Knee Score (OKS).

- **Patient satisfaction:** Evaluated through the Global Perceived Effect questionnaire.

- **Adverse events:** Documented and classified based on severity and relation to treatment.

Key findings

- **Pain relief**
  - Both treatments significantly reduced knee pain.
  - At 24 weeks, CRFA reduced VAS scores by 42 mm, while MRFA achieved a 39 mm reduction.
  - At 52 weeks, CRFA sustained pain relief (41 mm reduction), whereas MRFA showed a slight decline (31 mm reduction).

- **Functional improvement**
  - Significant enhancements in WOMAC and OKS scores were observed in both groups.
  - CRFA demonstrated better long-term functionality in unilateral cases, with OKS scores higher at 52 weeks than MRFA (32.7 vs. 26.0).

- **Patient satisfaction**
  - 51% of CRFA-treated patients reported very good or good outcomes at 52 weeks, compared to 38% in the MRFA group.

- **Safety profile**
  - A total of 70 adverse events were recorded, most unrelated to treatment.
  - Only three mild, treatment-related events (increased post-procedural knee pain) were reported. No serious adverse events were linked to either technique.

Limitations

- Retrospective design with potential selection bias.

- Small sample size and single-center scope limit generalizability.

- Wide age range and comorbidities add variability.

- Diagnostic blocks may lead to selection bias.

- Shorter ablation duration for MRFA might underestimate efficacy.

- Limited nerve targets could underrepresent outcomes.

- Industry funding may introduce bias despite disclosures.

Cooled and monopolar radiofrequency ablation for chronic knee pain

Clinical implications

- **Effective long-term pain management:**

  - CRFA provides slightly more sustained pain relief than MRFA, particularly at 52 weeks.

  - Both techniques are effective non-surgical options for managing knee osteoarthritis pain.

- **Improved functionality:**

  - Both CRFA and MRFA significantly enhance physical function and mobility, making daily activities easier for patients.

  - CRFA shows superior benefits in patients with unilateral knee pain.

- **Practical considerations:**

  - CRFA's extended application time (150 seconds) and cooling system increase procedural costs, which its longer-lasting benefits may justify.

  - Patient preferences, cost constraints, and clinical presentation should guide the choice between CRFA and MRFA.

- **Safety assurance:**

  - Both CRFA and MRFA are safe with minimal risk of severe complications, supporting their use in a broad patient population.

Key takeaways

- ☑ Both CRFA and MRFA are effective for long-term pain relief and functional improvement in patients with chronic knee osteoarthritis.

- ☑ CRFA provides slightly more durable pain relief and functional benefits, particularly in unilateral cases.

- ☑ Over half of CRFA-treated patients report significant satisfaction, making it a strong choice for chronic knee pain management.

- ☑ Both techniques are safe and minimally invasive, offering valuable alternatives to surgical interventions.

Additional recommended reading:

1. Vallejo R, Benyamin R, Orduña-Valls J, et al. Long-term efficacy of cooled and monopolar radiofrequency ablation for chronic knee pain related to osteoarthritis: A randomized controlled trial. *Interventional Pain Medicine*. 2023;2:100249. doi:10.1016/j.inpm.2023.100249.

2. Davis T, Loudermilk E, DePalma M, et al. Twelve-month outcomes of cooled radiofrequency ablation for knee osteoarthritis: A multicenter trial. *Reg Anesth Pain Med*. 2019;44(5):533-540. doi:10.1136/rapm-2018-100051.

3. Chen AF, Khalouf F, Zora K, et al. Cooled radiofrequency ablation vs. hyaluronic acid injection for knee osteoarthritis: 12-month results. *J Bone Joint Surg Am*. 2020;102(17):1501-1510. doi:10.2106/JBJS.19.00935.

4. Belba A, Vanneste T, Kallewaard JW, et al. Cooled versus conventional radiofrequency treatment of the genicular nerves for chronic knee pain: 12-month and cost-effectiveness results from the multicenter COCOGEN trial. *Reg Anesth Pain Med*.

Cooled or conventional radiofrequency treatment of the genicular nerves for chronic knee pain

43

Why this topic is important

Chronic knee pain, frequently caused by osteoarthritis (OA) or persistent postsurgical pain (PPSP) after total knee arthroplasty (TKA), is a significant contributor to disability and reduced quality of life globally. With the aging population and rising obesity prevalence, the burden of these conditions is escalating. While conservative treatments like physiotherapy and pharmacological interventions are often insufficient, radiofrequency (RF) treatment of the genicular nerves offers a promising minimally invasive option for pain relief.

Two primary modalities of RF-conventional and cooled-are widely used, yet direct comparisons of their efficacy and safety remain limited. This pilot trial (COCOGEN) by Vanneste et al. (2023) aimed to address this gap by evaluating the effectiveness of both approaches in patients with OA or PPSP, providing critical insights into optimizing treatment for chronic knee pain.

Objectives of this update

- Compare pain reduction and functional outcomes of conventional and cooled RF in chronic knee pain.

- Assess safety profiles and adverse events associated with both modalities.

- Explore the implications of this study for clinical practice and future research.

What is new

- Cooled RF showed a trend toward higher pain reduction (≥ 50%) compared to conventional RF, though statistical significance was not achieved.

- Both modalities resulted in significant pain relief and functional improvement, with no serious adverse events reported.

- This pilot study highlights the need for a larger, adequately powered trial to confirm findings and refine recommendations.

Study design and patient population

The COCOGEN trial was a multicenter, double-blind, randomized pilot study with a non-inferiority design. Patients with chronic anterior knee pain (NRS > 4) lasting more than 12 months due to OA (Kellgren-Lawrence grades II-IV) or PPSP post-TKA were included. 49 patients were randomized into conventional RF and cooled RF groups.

- **Baseline demographics:** Similar across groups, with mean ages of 62 and 65 years in OA and PPSP subgroups, respectively.

- **Exclusions:** To ensure homogeneity, patients with systemic infection, widespread chronic pain, or recent intra-articular injections were excluded.

Primary outcomes

- **Pain reduction (≥ 50%):**

  - At three months, 33% of patients in the cooled RF group achieved ≥ 50% pain reduction compared to 17% in the conventional RF group.

  - Though not statistically significant, the trend suggests potential superiority of cooled RF.

- **Sustained pain relief:**

  - Pain reduction remained stable at six months, with 37.5% of cooled RF patients achieving ≥ 50% relief versus 18.2% in the conventional RF group.

Secondary outcomes

- **Numerical Rating Scale (NRS):**

  - Both modalities significantly reduced mean NRS scores from baseline at three and six months ($p < 0.05$).

  - Cooled RF showed slightly greater reductions than conventional RF at all time points.

- **Functional improvement:**

  - Oxford Knee Score (OKS): Both groups improved significantly, with no significant differences between modalities.

  - Timed Up and Go (TUG) test: Comparable improvements in mobility were observed in both groups.

- **Quality of life:**

  - EQ-5D-3L scores increased, reflecting better health-related quality of life post-treatment.

Safety profile

- **Adverse events (AEs):**

  - No severe AEs were reported.

  - Conventional RF: Five cases of transient pain exacerbation.

  - Cooled RF: Three subcutaneous hematomas, one case of infrapatellar hypoesthesia, and two transient pain increases.

- **Patient satisfaction:**

  - Over 80% of patients remained blinded to their treatment allocation, ensuring unbiased outcomes.

Clinical implications

- **Treatment selection:**

  - Cooled RF may offer better pain relief outcomes in OA and PPSP patients, though additional studies are needed to confirm its superiority.

  - Both modalities provide significant pain and functional improvements, supporting their use as viable options for chronic knee pain.

- **Safety considerations:**

  - Both conventional and cooled RF are safe and have low complication rates.

  - Monitoring for transient pain increases or minor complications like hematomas is essential.

- **Optimization of protocols:**

  - Future trials should explore the impact of targeting additional genicular nerves to improve efficacy.

Key takeaways

☑ Cooled RF showed a promising trend toward greater pain reduction compared to conventional RF, though further studies are needed to confirm this.

☑ Both modalities significantly improve pain, function, and quality of life in patients with OA or PPSP.

☑ Both treatments are safe, with no serious adverse events reported in this trial.

☑ This pilot study underscores the need for more extensive, well-designed trials to refine recommendations for RF treatment of chronic knee pain.

Additional recommended reading:

1. Vanneste T, Belba A, Kallewaard JW, et al. Comparison of cooled versus conventional radiofrequency treatment of the genicular nerves for chronic knee pain: A multicenter non-inferiority randomized pilot trial. *Reg Anesth Pain Med.* 2023;48:197-204.

2. Chen AF, Khalouf F, Zora K, et al. Cooled radiofrequency ablation for chronic knee pain: Clinical trial demonstrating greater efficacy. *J Bone Joint Surg Am.* 2020;102:1501.

3. McCormick ZL, Korn M, Reddy R, et al. Cooled radiofrequency ablation of genicular nerves for chronic pain: Six-month outcomes. *Pain Med.* 2017;18:1631-41.

Cryoneurolysis for chronic knee pain

44

Why this topic is important

Chronic knee pain, often associated with conditions like osteoarthritis or post-surgical complications, poses a significant challenge in pain management. Traditional treatments, such as pharmacological interventions and physical therapy, may not always yield satisfactory outcomes. Cryoneurolysis, a minimally invasive technique that uses extreme cold to temporarily disrupt nerve conduction, offers a promising alternative. It targets specific nerves to relieve pain while preserving their connective tissue for eventual regeneration. This update explores the review by Diep et al. (2023) supporting cryoneurolysis for non-cancer-related knee pain and its potential to enhance patient care.

Objectives of this update

- Provide an overview of cryoneurolysis and its application in managing chronic knee pain.

- Summarize findings on its effectiveness, safety, and technical variations.

- Highlight its role as an adjunct or alternative to existing pain management strategies.

What is new

- **Significant pain relief:** Improvements in pain scores were consistently observed across studies, often exceeding thresholds for clinical significance.

- **Functional gains:** Enhanced knee function and reduced stiffness were documented, particularly in patients with osteoarthritis or perioperative pain.

- **Opioid-sparing effects:** Cryoneurolysis significantly reduced opioid use in multimodal pain management regimens.

- **Favorable safety profile:** Adverse events were typically mild and self-limiting, such as bruising or temporary numbness.

- **Variation in techniques:** Considerable differences in nerve targets, freeze parameters, and diagnostic approaches highlight the need for standardization.

Overview of cryoneurolysis

Cryoneurolysis involves percutaneous insertion of a cryoprobe to expose peripheral nerves to temperatures between −20°C and −100°C. This induces reversible axonotmesis (temporary nerve injury) while sparing the nerve's connective tissue, allowing regeneration at a rate of 1-2 mm/day.

Study design

The review analyzed 868 patients from 14 studies, including those with chronic osteoarthritis, non-specific knee pain, and perioperative pain following total knee arthroplasty (TKA).

- **Intervention details:** Most studies used fluoroscopic or ultrasound guidance to target the infrapatellar branch of the saphenous nerve and/or the anterior femoral cutaneous nerve. Treatment parameters, such as freeze cycles and probe temperature, varied widely.

- **Control groups:** Comparators included sham cryoneurolysis, standard therapy, or no intervention.

Key findings

- **Pain relief**
  - Cryoneurolysis demonstrated statistically and clinically significant reductions in pain scores.
  - In one high-quality RCT, cryoneurolysis outperformed sham interventions in reducing Western Ontario and McMaster Universities Arthritis Index (WOMAC) pain scores by 7.12 points at 30 days, exceeding the minimum clinically important difference (MCID).

- **Functional improvement**
  - Patients experienced enhanced physical function and reduced stiffness, as reflected in WOMAC subscale improvements.
  - Benefits were sustained for up to three months in most studies and for up to one year in some perioperative cohorts.

- **Reduced opioid use**
  - Several studies highlighted opioid-sparing benefits, with reductions in morphine equivalents of up to 45% when cryoneurolysis was integrated into perioperative pain protocols.

- **Safety**
  - Most adverse events were mild, including bruising, local numbness, and swelling. Severe complications were rare but included two cases of dysesthesia (persistent nerve discomfort) and one case of myonecrosis.

- **Technical considerations**
  - Nerve targets varied, with most studies focusing on cutaneous innervation (e.g., infrapatellar branch) rather than deeper genicular branches responsible for intra-articular pain.
  - Diagnostic nerve blocks were inconsistently reported, with only a few studies using them to confirm nerve involvement before treatment.

Clinical implications

- **Efficacy and patient selection**
  - Cryoneurolysis offers a viable option for patients unresponsive to conservative therapies or those seeking alternatives to pharmacological interventions.
  - It is particularly effective for mild-to-moderate osteoarthritis and as part of multimodal perioperative pain management.

- **Safety assurance**
  - The favorable safety profile of cryoneurolysis supports its use across diverse patient populations, though careful patient selection and procedural precision are essential.

- **Technical standardization**
  - To optimize outcomes, practitioners should consistently target relevant nerves and appropriate cryoprobe parameters.

- **Limitations**
  - Variations in technique and study quality underscore the need for high-quality RCTs to establish standardized protocols and long-term efficacy.

Key takeaways

☑ Cryoneurolysis is an effective and minimally invasive option for managing chronic knee pain, with benefits in pain relief, functionality, and opioid reduction.

☑ Its safety profile makes it a viable alternative or adjunct to existing pain management strategies.

☑ Variations in techniques and nerve targets necessitate further research to develop standardized approaches and enhance reproducibility.

Additional recommended reading:

1. Diep D, Mittal N, Sangha H, Farag J. Cryoneurolysis for non-cancer knee pain: A scoping review. *Interventional Pain Medicine.* 2023;2:100247. doi:10.1016/j.inpm.2023.100247.

2. Radnovich R, Scott D, Patel AT, et al. Cryoneurolysis to treat the pain and symptoms of knee osteoarthritis: A multicenter, randomized, double-blind, sham-controlled trial. *Osteoarthritis Cartilage.* 2017;25:1247-56. doi:10.1016/j.joca.2017.03.006.

3. Urban JA, Dolesh K, Martin E. Preoperative cryoneurolysis for total knee arthroplasty to reduce pain, opioid consumption, and length of stay. *Arthroplasty Today.* 2021;10:87-92. doi:10.1016/j.artd.2021.06.008.

Shear wave elastography in musculoskeletal injuries

45

Why this topic is important

Shear wave elastography (SWE) is an innovative ultrasound-based imaging modality that measures tissue stiffness by tracking the propagation speed of acoustic waves. Its ability to provide quantitative stiffness data has revolutionized musculoskeletal (MSK) medicine, offering insights into the pathophysiology of soft tissue conditions. With applications spanning tendon, ligament, muscle, and nerve pathologies, SWE is emerging as a valuable diagnostic tool in MSK imaging.

Despite its potential, SWE adoption in clinical practice has been limited due to challenges in standardization, interpretation, and integration into existing workflows. This review by Chowdhary et al. (2024) synthesizes recent findings on SWE's diagnostic utility, underscoring its role in improving the assessment and management of MSK injuries.

Objectives of this update

- Summarize the diagnostic applications of SWE in various MSK conditions.

- Highlight SWE's reliability, sensitivity, and specificity compared to traditional imaging modalities.

- Discuss the limitations and future directions for SWE in MSK medicine.

What is new

- Recent studies demonstrate SWE's diagnostic accuracy in conditions like Achilles tendinopathy, median mononeuropathy, and plantar fasciitis.

- Advances in SWE technology have improved interobserver reliability and accessibility in outpatient settings.

- A lack of consensus on SWE standardization continues to limit its widespread clinical use.

Overview of shear wave elastography

- **Principles of operation:**
  - SWE generates and measures the speed of shear waves as they travel through tissue, producing a color-coded map and quantitative stiffness values (measured in m/s).
  - Applications include liver fibrosis assessment and tumor characterization in breast, thyroid, and prostate tissues.

- **Advantages over traditional imaging:**
  - Superior spatial resolution compared to MRI for certain MSK structures.
  - Ability to detect subtle mechanical changes in tissues, offering diagnostic and prognostic value.

Applications in musculoskeletal injuries

- **Tendinopathies:**
  - **Achilles tendinopathy:** SWE identifies increased stiffness in symptomatic tendons compared to healthy controls, aiding in early diagnosis.
  - **Rotator cuff tears:** Studies show SWE can distinguish between partial and full-thickness tears by measuring supraspinatus and infraspinatus stiffness.

- **Neuropathies:**
  - **Median mononeuropathy (carpal tunnel syndrome):** SWE effectively measures increased stiffness in the median nerve, correlating with symptom severity.
  - **Ulnar neuropathy:** SWE assists in diagnosing entrapment at the elbow, particularly when clinical findings are inconclusive.

- **Ligament injuries:**
  - **Anterior cruciate ligament (ACL) reconstruction:** SWE monitors graft integrity and stiffness during rehabilitation, providing functional insights not captured by MRI alone.

- **Plantar fasciitis:**
  - SWE reveals increased stiffness in the plantar fascia, particularly in chronic cases, aiding in differential diagnosis from other causes of heel pain.

Diagnostic reliability and reproducibility

- **Interobserver and intraobserver reliability:**
  - Studies report high reproducibility for SWE in static MSK structures (e.g., tendons, ligaments).
  - Dynamic structures (e.g., muscles during contraction) show variability, emphasizing the need for standardized protocols.

- **Comparative performance:**
  - SWE has shown comparable or superior sensitivity and specificity to traditional ultrasound and MRI in various MSK conditions.

Challenges and limitations

- **Standardization issues:**
  - Variability in equipment, operator technique, and tissue heterogeneity complicate the interpretation of SWE findings.
  - Consensus guidelines are needed to define thresholds for clinical decision-making.

- **Tissue-specific challenges:**
  - MSK tissues, unlike organs, are subject to dynamic stresses, influencing SWE measurements.
  - Overlying soft tissue and bony structures can interfere with signal acquisition.

Clinical implications

- **Improving early diagnosis:**
  - SWE offers non-invasive, point-of-care diagnostic insights, reducing reliance on more expensive and less accessible imaging modalities like MRI.

- **Guiding treatment strategies:**
  - By quantifying tissue stiffness, SWE informs personalized rehabilitation plans and tracks treatment efficacy.

- **Expanding clinical utility:**
  - Integrating SWE into routine MSK assessments could enhance diagnostic accuracy for complex or ambiguous cases.

Key takeaways

☑ SWE is a valuable tool for diagnosing MSK injuries, particularly tendinopathies and neuropathies.

☑ Its quantitative stiffness measurements complement traditional imaging, offering unique diagnostic and prognostic insights.

☑ Standardization and clinical integration are critical for SWE to achieve widespread adoption.

☑ Future research should focus on refining SWE protocols and exploring its role in personalized medicine.

Additional recommended reading:

1. Chowdhary K, Raum G, Visco C. Diagnostic utility of shear wave elastography in musculoskeletal injuries: *A narrative review. PM&R.* 2024;16:384-397.

2. Davis LC, Baessler B, Rana RS. Applications of elastography in musculoskeletal imaging. *Radiographics.* 2019;39:1478-1495.

3. Lee YH, Kim YH, Seo M, et al. Use of shear wave elastography in assessing tendinopathy: A meta-analysis. *Clin Orthop Relat Res.* 2022;480:679-691.

Cancer Pain

Predictors and consequences of cancer-related and non-cancer-related pain in oncology

46

Why this topic is important

Pain is one of the most debilitating symptoms in cancer patients, affecting nearly 70% of individuals during their disease course. Understanding the distinctions between cancer-related pain and non-cancer-related pain is critical for tailoring interventions to improve quality of life, emotional well-being, and functional outcomes.

This update summarizes findings from Shah et al. (2023) on the predictors and consequences of pain in oncology, emphasizing survival implications, symptom burden, and the role of psychosocial and biological mediators. The study also explores inflammatory pathways as potential links between pain and survival.

Objectives of this update

- Differentiate cancer-related and non-cancer-related pain in terms of predictors, consequences, and survival outcomes.

- Examine psychological and behavioral factors associated with pain.

- Highlight the role of cytokines in mediating the relationship between pain and survival.

What is new

- Cancer-related pain was independently associated with poorer survival outcomes after adjusting for sociodemographic, disease-specific, and psychological factors.

- Non-cancer-related pain, though burdensome, did not significantly impact survival.

- Psychological symptoms like depression and fatigue were more pronounced in patients reporting cancer-related pain.

Pain prevalence and classification

- Among 779 patients with cancer:

  - 46.5% reported cancer-related pain (e.g., from tumor invasion or treatment).

  - 53.5% reported non-cancer-related pain (e.g., musculoskeletal conditions).

- Cancer-related pain was linked to higher depressive symptoms and fatigue levels but did not significantly affect sleep duration compared to non-cancer-related pain.

Predictors of pain intensity and interference

- Education level: Lower educational attainment was associated with higher pain interference, reflecting potential gaps in health literacy and access to care.

- Cancer type: Hepatocellular carcinoma and cholangiocarcinoma were associated with the highest pain interference, possibly due to advanced-stage disease.

Pain and survival outcomes

- Kaplan-Meier analysis revealed significantly shorter median survival for cancer-related pain (26 months) compared to non-cancer-related pain (48 months).

- After controlling for covariates, cancer-related pain remained a significant predictor of poorer survival (HR = 0.646), while non-cancer-related pain did not impact survival (HR = 1.022).

Psychosocial and behavioral impacts

- Both pain types predicted higher depressive symptoms and fatigue levels.

- Affective pain descriptors (e.g., "stabbing" or "miserable") were associated with greater psychological distress and fatigue, further amplifying symptom burden.

Cytokines and inflammation

- Despite hypothesized links between pain, inflammation, and survival, circulating cytokines (e.g., IL-10, TNF-α) did not significantly mediate the relationship between pain type and survival.

Clinical implications

Tailored pain management

- **Holistic assessment**: Evaluate both cancer-related and non-cancer-related pain comprehensively to address physical and psychological dimensions.

- **Psychological screening**: Integrate tools like the CES-D to identify depression early, which may compound pain-related distress.

- **Education initiatives**: Address gaps in pain literacy, particularly in patients with lower educational attainment.

Implications for treatment strategies

- **Targeted therapies**: Focus on multimodal approaches combining pharmacologic, interventional, and psychosocial strategies for cancer-related pain.

- **Minimize opioid reliance**: For non-cancer-related pain, prioritize alternatives to chronic opioid therapy to avoid unnecessary dependence.

- **Inflammation-focused research**: Investigate alternative biomarkers or mechanisms beyond cytokines to elucidate pain and survival connections.

Key takeaways

☑ Cancer-related pain predicts poorer survival, emphasizing the need for proactive management and tailored care.

☑ Depression and fatigue are heightened in patients with cancer-related pain, necessitating integrated mental health interventions.

☑ Non-cancer-related pain, while not directly linked to survival, significantly affects quality of life and should not be overlooked.

☑ Further research is needed to explore the inflammatory and psychosocial underpinnings of pain in oncology.

Additional recommended reading:

1. Shah K, Geller DA, Tohme S, et al. Predictors and consequences of cancer and non-cancer-related pain in those diagnosed with primary and metastatic cancers. *Curr Oncol.* 2023;30:8826-8840.

2. Zylla D, Steele G, Gupta P. A systematic review of the impact of pain on overall survival in patients with cancer. *Support Care Cancer.* 2017;25:1687-1698.

3. Hølen JC, Lydersen S, Klepstad P, et al. The Brief Pain Inventory: Pain's interference with functions is different in cancer pain compared with non-cancer chronic pain. *Clin J Pain.* 2008;24:219-225.

Use of opioids for adults with cancer pain

47

Why this topic is important

Cancer pain is a prevalent and debilitating condition affecting over half of patients undergoing treatment and up to two-thirds of those with advanced disease. Despite the central role of opioids in cancer pain management, their use remains fraught with challenges, including concerns over misuse, stigma, and access barriers. These issues are further complicated by limited evidence to guide opioid selection, titration, and management of side effects.

The American Society of Clinical Oncology (ASCO) convened an expert panel to address these challenges and provide evidence-based recommendations for optimizing opioid use in cancer care. This update synthesizes key findings from their 2022 guidelines, offering practical strategies to improve analgesia while minimizing risks.

Objectives of this update

- Outline evidence-based criteria for offering opioids to adults with cancer pain.

- Review best practices for opioid initiation, titration, and management of breakthrough pain.

- Provide recommendations to prevent and manage opioid-related adverse effects.

What is new

- Clear guidance on initiating opioids with immediate-release formulations and titrating to patient-specific goals.

- Emphasis on managing adverse effects proactively, including opioid-induced constipation and neurotoxicity.

- Recommendations for tailoring opioid selection in patients with renal or hepatic impairment.

Criteria for opioid use

- **Indications for initiation:**

  - Opioids should be offered to patients with moderate-to-severe pain related to cancer or its treatment, provided no contraindications exist.

  - Before prescribing, clinicians should establish goals for pain relief and functional outcomes and address concerns about opioids with patients and caregivers.

- **Pain assessment:**

  - Identify pain mechanisms (e.g., nociceptive vs. neuropathic) and review prior responses to non-opioid analgesics.

  - Consider risk factors for misuse using validated tools such as the Opioid Risk Tool.

Opioid initiation and titration

- **Starting dose:**

  - Initiate opioids at the lowest effective dose using immediate-release formulations, titrating based on patient response.

  - Begin with an approximate daily morphine milligram equivalent (MME) of 30 mg.

- **Titration principles:**

  - Adjust doses by 25-50% based on pain intensity and breakthrough medication usage.

  - Regularly reassess efficacy, side effects, and patient goals, especially during the first weeks of therapy.

- **Breakthrough pain management:**

  - Prescribe immediate-release opioids at 5-20% of the daily MME for breakthrough pain.

  - Evidence for a specific short-acting opioid remains insufficient, though sublingual fentanyl shows promise.

Opioid selection and special populations

- **Preferred opioids:**

  - Morphine remains the gold standard for most cancer pain scenarios.

  - Methadone may be preferred for neuropathic pain or renal impairment but requires expertise in prescribing.

- **Renal and hepatic impairment:**

  - Methadone is safe in renal failure, while morphine and codeine should be avoided due to the risk of metabolite accumulation.

  - In hepatic impairment, dose reductions and close monitoring are essential.

- **Substance use disorder:**

  - For patients with a substance use disorder, clinicians should collaborate with a palliative care, pain, and/or substance use disorder specialist to determine the optimal approach to pain management.

Managing opioid-related adverse effects

- **Constipation:**

  - Initiate prophylactic bowel regimens with stimulant laxatives like senna.

  - Consider peripherally acting mu-opioid receptor antagonists (e.g., methylnaltrexone) for refractory cases.

- **Nausea and vomiting:**

  - Manage with metoclopramide or prochlor-perazine; tolerance typically develops within a few days.

- **Neurotoxicity:**

  - Monitor for signs such as myoclonus or confusion, particularly with rapid dose escalation.

  - Rotate to alternative opioids or reduce doses as needed.

- **Sedation and respiratory depression:**
  - Educate patients on expected transient sedation during dose initiation or escalation.
  - Consider psychostimulants for persistent sedation or naloxone for emergency use in high-risk cases.

Access barriers and patient communication

- **Regulatory challenges:**
  - Misinterpretation of opioid guidelines, reimbursement issues, and supply shortages hinder access.
  - Clinicians must advocate for patients and navigate these barriers to ensure timely pain relief.
- **Stigma and education:**
  - Patients often fear addiction or feel guilt about opioid use.
  - Clear communication about the role of opioids in cancer care and safe use practices is essential.

Clinical implications

- **Comprehensive approach:**
  - Combine opioids with non-opioid analgesics and non-pharmacologic therapies to optimize outcomes.
- **Individualized care:**
  - Tailor opioid selection and dosing to the patient's clinical profile, comorbidities, and goals of care.
- **Proactive management:**
  - Prevent and address adverse effects early to maintain adherence and improve quality of life.

Future directions

- Research to evaluate the comparative efficacy of different opioids in cancer pain subtypes.
- Development of precision medicine approaches, including pharmacogenetic testing for opioid selection.
- Advocacy for policy changes to reduce barriers to opioid access.

Key takeaways

- ☑ Opioids remain essential for managing moderate-to-severe cancer pain when used judiciously.
- ☑ Initiate therapy with immediate-release formulations and adjust doses based on patient needs.
- ☑ Proactively address common side effects, including constipation and sedation, to improve adherence.
- ☑ Tailor opioid selection in special populations, such as those with renal or hepatic impairment.

Additional recommended reading:

1. Paice JA, Bohlke K, Barton D, et al. Use of opioids for adults with pain from cancer or cancer treatment: ASCO guideline. *J Clin Oncol.* 2022;41(4):914-930.

2. Mercadante S, Porzio G. Opioid treatment in cancer pain: Moving forward. *Cancers.* 2020;12(152).

3. Wiffen PJ, Wee B, Moore RA. Opioids for cancer pain: An overview of Cochrane reviews. *Cochrane Database Syst Rev.* 2017;(7):CD012592.

Opioid analgesics for nociceptive cancer pain

48

Why this topic is important

Cancer pain remains one of the most burdensome symptoms, impacting up to 75% of patients at various stages of their disease. Effective pain control is a cornerstone of oncology care, aiming to improve quality of life and functionality. Opioid analgesics are considered the mainstay for managing moderate to severe nociceptive cancer pain. However, questions about efficacy, side effects, and long-term outcomes persist.

This review by Shaheed et al. (2023) synthesizes the current evidence on the role of opioids in managing nociceptive cancer pain, addressing gaps in research, evaluating their comparative effectiveness, and discussing adjunctive strategies to mitigate adverse effects.

Objectives of this update

- Explore the efficacy and safety of various opioids for nociceptive cancer pain.

- Highlight alternatives and adjunctive treatments to optimize opioid therapy.

- Review challenges and future directions in the management of nociceptive cancer pain.

What is new

- Recent findings suggest NSAIDs may offer equivalent efficacy to opioids for moderate to severe nociceptive cancer pain in specific contexts.

- Oral tapentadol has emerged as a potential alternative to traditional opioids for chronic malignant pain.

- Strategies to mitigate opioid-induced toxicities, particularly gastrointestinal effects, are receiving greater attention.

The role of opioids in nociceptive cancer pain

- **Mechanisms and indications**

  - Opioids target mu-opioid receptors, modulating nociceptive pathways to provide analgesia.

  - They remain the first-line option for background cancer pain and breakthrough pain unresponsive to non-opioid therapies.

- **Comparative effectiveness**

  - Morphine, traditionally the gold standard, shows similar efficacy to hydromorphone, oxycodone, and fentanyl, with no one agent consistently superior.

  - Tapentadol demonstrates promising results for chronic malignant pain but lacks robust comparative studies against established opioids.

Alternatives and adjunctive strategies

- **Non-opioid analgesics**

  - NSAIDs: Aspirin, diclofenac, and piroxicam have shown comparable pain relief to opioids in some studies, particularly for somatic and bone pain.

  - Acetaminophen, often used in combination with opioids, has limited evidence supporting its independent effectiveness in cancer pain.

- **Adjuvants**

  - Antidepressants: Amitriptyline and duloxetine may enhance pain relief and address concurrent depression, though the evidence is mixed.

  - Anticonvulsants: Pregabalin and gabapentin show limited efficacy for nociceptive cancer pain compared to neuropathic pain.

- **Combination therapies**

  - Opioid-sparing approaches using NSAIDs or antidepressants can reduce required opioid doses, potentially lowering the risk of adverse effects.

Safety considerations and toxicities

- **Common adverse effects**

  - Gastrointestinal toxicities, including constipation and nausea, are prevalent and impact patient compliance.

  - CNS effects, such as sedation and cognitive impairment, may further limit use in vulnerable populations.

- **Strategies to mitigate adverse effects**

  - Prophylactic use of laxatives for opioid-induced constipation is widely recommended.

  - Emerging therapies like peripheral mu-opioid receptor antagonists (e.g., naloxegol) offer targeted relief from constipation without compromising analgesia.

Clinical implications

- **Personalized opioid therapy**

  - The choice of opioid should be guided by patient-specific factors such as pharmacokinetics, comorbidities, and access to medications.

  - Rotating opioids may be beneficial in cases of intolerance or inadequate pain control.

- **Integrating non-opioid options**

  - NSAIDs should be considered, particularly for patients with contraindications to opioids or as part of multimodal therapy.

  - Adjuvants targeting specific pain mechanisms can optimize overall pain management.

- **Managing breakthrough pain**

  - Rapid-onset opioids like sublingual or intranasal fentanyl provide effective control of acute pain episodes but require careful titration to balance efficacy with side effects.

Future directions

- **Refining guidelines:**
  - ○ Standardized recommendations for integrating opioids with adjuvant therapies and alternatives are needed.

- **Research gaps:**
  - ○ More placebo-controlled trials are required to validate the efficacy of opioids and adjunctive treatments in diverse patient populations.

- **Mitigating toxicities:**
  - ○ Innovative drug delivery systems and new formulations targeting opioid-related side effects will be critical for improving patient outcomes.

Key takeaways

- ☑ Opioids remain a cornerstone for nociceptive cancer pain but require careful management to balance efficacy with side effects.

- ☑ NSAIDs and adjuvants, such as antidepressants, provide valuable alternatives and complement opioid therapy.

- ☑ Comprehensive, patient-specific approaches integrating pharmacologic and non-pharmacologic strategies optimize pain relief and quality of life.

Additional recommended reading:

1. Shaheed CA, Hayes C, Maher CG, et al. Opioid analgesics for nociceptive cancer pain: A comprehensive review. *CA Cancer J Clin*. 2024;74:286-313.

2. Mercadante S, Porzio G. Opioid dose titration for cancer pain: A systematic and practical approach. *J Pain Symptom Manage*. 2022;64(5):e319-e328.

3. Fallon M, Hanks G, Cherny N, et al. Guidelines on the management of cancer pain in adults. *Ann Oncol*. 2018;29(Suppl 4):iv166-iv191.

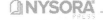

Neuropathic pain in cancer: Diagnosis and management

49

Why this topic is important

Neuropathic cancer pain (NCP) affects 30-40% of cancer patients, profoundly impairing their quality of life. It arises from nerve compression, tumor infiltration, or the toxic effects of chemotherapy and radiation. NCP often coexists with nociceptive and inflammatory pain, creating a complex mixed-pain syndrome.

Despite its prevalence and severity, NCP remains underdiagnosed and undertreated. A systematic and mechanistic approach is essential for tailoring treatment to the underlying pain etiology. Recent advancements in diagnostic tools and multimodal treatments offer significant opportunities to improve outcomes for cancer patients suffering from NCP. This review by Mulvey et al. (2024) summarizes the current guidelines regarding neuropathic cancer pain.

Objectives of this update

- Review the mechanisms and diagnostic approaches for NCP.

- Explore pharmacological and interventional strategies for managing NCP.

- Highlight gaps in current clinical practices and emerging solutions.

What is new

- Standardized screening tools, including the Leeds Assessment of Neuropathic Symptoms and Signs (LANSS) and painDETECT, improve diagnostic accuracy.

- Advances in targeted treatments, including ziconotide and novel NMDA receptor antagonists, offer promise for refractory cases.

- Enhanced understanding of mixed-pain syndromes emphasizes the need for multimodal interventions.

Mechanisms and diagnostic tools

- **Pathophysiology:**

  - NCP results from nerve damage caused by tumors or cancer treatments, leading to central and peripheral sensitization.

  - Mechanisms include direct nerve injury, abnormal ion channel activity, and inflammation.

- **Diagnostic approaches:**

  - Standardized tools like DN4 (Douleur Neuropathique en 4 questions) and LANSS help differentiate neuropathic from nociceptive pain.

  - Quantitative sensory testing (QST) is emerging for phenotyping patients and tailoring treatments.

Pharmacological management

- **Opioids:**

  - While opioids remain a cornerstone for cancer pain, their efficacy in pure NCP is limited. High doses may be required, increasing the risk of side effects.

  - Methadone, with its NMDA receptor antagonism, shows particular promise in NCP management.

- **Adjuvant therapies:**

  - Anticonvulsants (e.g., gabapentin, pregabalin) and antidepressants (e.g., amitriptyline, duloxetine) are first-line agents for NCP.

  - Evidence supports their combination with opioids to enhance analgesia and reduce opioid consumption.

- **Emerging agents:**

  - Ziconotide, an N-type calcium channel blocker, provides significant pain relief but has a narrow therapeutic window.

  - Research into cannabinoids and NMDA receptor antagonists is ongoing, with mixed results.

Interventional approaches

- **Intrathecal drug delivery:**

  - Intrathecal administration of opioids and adjuvants offers targeted relief, particularly in refractory NCP cases.

  - Advances in pump technology and catheter placement have improved safety and efficacy.

- **Nerve blocks and neurolysis:**

  - Techniques such as radiofrequency and cryoablation target specific pain pathways, providing durable relief.

- **Ablation and radiotherapy:**

  - Ablative techniques reduce tumor burden and alleviate associated nerve compression.

  - External beam radiotherapy (EBRT) remains a mainstay for bone metastasis-related NCP.

Clinical implications

- **Personalized management:**

  - Tailor treatments are based on the underlying pain mechanisms and patient-specific factors, such as life expectancy and comorbidities.

  - Use multimodal approaches combining pharmacological and interventional therapies for optimal outcomes.

- **Routine screening and assessment:**

  - Implement validated screening tools during routine oncology visits to identify NCP early.

  - Standardize assessments using the International Association for the Study of Pain (IASP) diagnostic algorithm.

- **Access to advanced therapies:**

  - Expand training in interventional techniques and improve access to specialized centers.

Future directions

- Develop high-quality clinical trials to evaluate the long-term efficacy of novel agents and interventions.

- Integrate quantitative sensory testing into routine practice to identify mechanistic subgroups.

- Advance molecular research to discover new analgesic targets, including selective ion channel modulators.

Key takeaways

☑ NCP is a prevalent yet underdiagnosed condition requiring a mechanistic approach to management.

☑ Multimodal strategies combining opioids, adjuvants, and interventional techniques offer the best outcomes.

☑ Emerging diagnostic tools and therapies pave the way for more precise and effective treatments.

☑ Routine screening and personalized care are essential to improving the quality of life for patients with NCP.

Additional recommended reading:

1. Mulvey MR, Paley CA, Schuberth A, et al. Neuropathic pain in cancer: What are the current guidelines? *Curr Treat Options Oncol.* 2024;25:1193-1202.

2. Fallon M, Giusti R, Aielli F, et al. Management of cancer pain in adult patients: ESMO clinical practice guidelines. *Ann Oncol.* 2018;29(Suppl 4):iv166-iv191.

3. Shkodra M, Mulvey M, Fallon M, et al. Application and accuracy of the EAPC/IASP diagnostic algorithm for neuropathic cancer pain. *Pain Rep.* 2024;9(2):e1140.

Predictors of successful opioid response in cancer patients

50

Why this topic is important

Potent opioids remain the cornerstone of cancer pain management, providing critical relief for patients with moderate to severe pain. However, opioid efficacy varies significantly among individuals, influenced by factors such as pain type, comorbidities, and drug metabolism. Despite their essential role, no universal guidelines exist for selecting the most effective opioid for individual patients, often resulting in trial-and-error prescribing.

This comprehensive analysis of data from four randomized controlled trials (RCTs), as reviewed by Imkamp et al. (2024), identifies predictors of opioid response in cancer pain patients, highlighting the complexity of treatment and underscoring the need for personalized approaches.

Objectives of this update

- Identify clinical and pharmacological factors influencing opioid efficacy in cancer pain management.

- Examine short- and medium-term treatment outcomes based on opioid type and patient characteristics.

- Propose future directions for developing predictive models to optimize opioid therapy.

What is new

- **Opioid type and pain characteristics**: Fentanyl, methadone, and mixed pain (nociceptive and neuropathic) are significantly associated with treatment success.

- **Anxiety as a barrier**: Anxiety negatively impacts medium-term opioid response, emphasizing the need for holistic care.

- **Limitations of prediction models**: Current models lack sufficient discriminative power, highlighting the need for novel predictive markers, including genetic factors.

Mechanisms and baseline considerations

- **Pain types:**

  - Nociceptive pain responds well to opioids like morphine and oxycodone.

  - Mixed pain, with both nociceptive and neuropathic components, demonstrates lower response rates.

- **Opioid pharmacology:**

  - Due to their unique receptor profiles, methadone and buprenorphine show variable efficacy depending on pain type and patient characteristics.

  - Fentanyl is associated with suboptimal response in medium-term outcomes compared to morphine.

- **Patient-specific factors:**

  - Male sex and anxiety are negatively associated with medium-term treatment success.

  - Depression correlates with short-term response, indicating possible overlaps between psychological and analgesic benefits.

Treatment outcomes

- **Short-term success (1 week):**

  - Defined as ≥ 50% reduction in pain scores.

  - Predictors: Mixed pain was negatively associated, and fentanyl, methadone, and buprenorphine showed less effectiveness compared to morphine.

- **Medium-term success (4-5 weeks):**

  - Predictors: Male sex, anxiety, and fentanyl (compared to morphine) were negatively associated with response.

  - Predictive models for medium-term outcomes showed poor calibration, reflecting the complexity of pain management.

Implications for opioid selection

- **Morphine as a reference standard:**

  - Despite being the most commonly used opioid, morphine's comparative success rates indicate its continued relevance in treatment protocols.

- **Alternative opioids:**

  - Methadone may be more effective for mixed pain due to its NMDA receptor antagonist properties, although further trials are needed.

  - Buprenorphine's dual agonist-antagonist action may offer advantages in select neuropathic pain populations.

Barriers to optimal treatment

- **Predictive limitations:**

  - Existing models lack strong discriminative power, with AUC values below 0.7.

  - Factors like genetic variability, metabolic profiles, and psychosocial influences remain underexplored.

- **Pain assessment challenges:**

  - Inconsistent pain characterization across studies complicates the generalization of findings.

Clinical implications

- **Personalized opioid therapy:**
  - Selection should be informed by pain type and patient-specific factors, such as comorbid anxiety or depression.
  - Methadone or buprenorphine may be prioritized for patients with mixed pain profiles.

- **Integrated care models:**
  - Multidisciplinary approaches addressing both physical and psychological dimensions of pain are essential.
  - Early identification and management of anxiety and depression can enhance treatment outcomes.

- **Role of genetic markers:**
  - Genetic factors such as CYP2D6 enzyme activity and opioid receptor polymorphisms warrant further investigation to refine opioid selection.

Key takeaways

☑ Potent opioids remain essential for managing cancer pain, but treatment response varies widely based on pain type and opioid pharmacology.

☑ Morphine demonstrates consistent efficacy, while methadone shows promise for mixed pain.

☑ Anxiety and male sex are barriers to medium-term treatment success, highlighting the need for integrated psychosocial interventions.

☑ Predictive models are currently limited but hold potential for transforming personalized cancer pain management.

☑ Recent studies suggest potential conflicts of interest in some opioid prescribing guidelines, advising caution in their interpretation.

Additional recommended reading:

1. Imkamp MS, Theunissen M, van Kuijk SM, et al. Finding predictors for successful opioid response in cancer patients: An analysis of data from four randomized controlled trials. *Pain Pract.* 2024;24:101-108.

2. Wiffen PJ, Wee B, Moore RA, et al. Opioids for cancer pain - An overview of Cochrane reviews. *Cochrane Database Syst Rev.* 2017;(7):CD012592.

3. Mercadante S, Porzio G. Opioid treatment in cancer pain: Moving forward. *Cancers.* 2020;12:152.

Optimizing opioid dose titration for cancer pain

51

Why this topic is important

Cancer-related pain is a significant public health issue, affecting approximately 45% of cancer patients, with moderate-to-severe pain reported in many cases. Despite opioids being the cornerstone of pain management, the process of opioid dose titration remains complex, requiring careful balancing between achieving effective analgesia and minimizing adverse effects.

The ongoing opioid crisis further complicates this landscape, as healthcare providers must manage concerns of opioid misuse while ensuring adequate treatment of cancer pain. This update synthesizes findings from Mercadante (2024) and other recent studies, providing evidence-based recommendations to guide clinicians in the effective titration of opioids in patients with cancer pain.

Objectives of this update

- Outline evidence-based strategies for initiating and titrating opioids in cancer pain management.

- Highlight approaches tailored to opioid-naive and opioid-tolerant patients.

- Discuss the use of parenteral and extended-release opioid formulations for acute and long-term pain relief.

What is new

- **Updated guidelines**: Immediate-release formulations remain the preferred starting point for titration, but extended-release formulations offer comparable outcomes when combined with as-needed dosing.

- **Tailored approaches**: Differentiating strategies for opioid-naive versus opioid-tolerant patients optimizes safety and efficacy.

- **Parenteral opioids**: Rapid titration protocols using intravenous opioids provide a valuable tool for managing cancer pain emergencies.

Opioid-naive patients

- **Initiation and titration:**

  - Immediate-release morphine is commonly used, starting with low doses of 15-30 mg/day oral morphine equivalents (OME).

  - Dose increments of 25%-50% are recommended every 24 hours based on response.

  - Alternative agents like methadone (6-9 mg/day) show efficacy, particularly in cases of inadequate response to traditional opioids.

- **Effectiveness:**

  - Studies indicate rapid analgesia within 24-48 hours in most patients using immediate-release opioids.

  - Adverse effects such as nausea and sedation are transient and manageable in the majority of cases.

Opioid-tolerant patients

- **Challenges:**

  - Patients on long-term opioids often require higher starting doses to overcome tolerance.

  - Dose increments are dictated by prior opioid exposure, typically ranging from 30%-50%.

- **Titration protocols:**

  - Both immediate-release and sustained-release formulations are effective, with comparable times to stable pain relief (2-3 days).

  - Parenteral administration is recommended for patients with severe, refractory pain or gastrointestinal issues.

Opioid formulations and their roles

Immediate-release opioids

- Preferred for rapid titration due to shorter onset and duration of action.

- Commonly used as the initial step to determine effective dosing.

Extended-release opioids

- Provide prolonged pain relief with fewer doses per day.

- Best suited for patients with stable pain once titration is complete.

- Effective when combined with rescue doses of immediate-release opioids during titration.

Transdermal opioids

- Reserved for patients unable to tolerate oral or parenteral routes.

- Slower onset limits utility in rapid titration scenarios but effective for maintenance therapy.

Parenteral opioids

- Critical for managing cancer pain emergencies.

- Intravenous morphine or fentanyl achieves significant pain relief within minutes.

- Conversion to oral dosing should follow stabilization of pain control using established equianalgesic ratios.

Clinical implications

- **Personalized titration:**

  - Tailor dosing strategies to patient-specific factors, including pain intensity, opioid tolerance, and comorbid conditions.

  - Use flexible titration protocols that allow for rapid adjustments based on patient response.

- **Monitoring and safety:**

  - Assess pain intensity, functional outcomes, and side effects regularly using validated tools like the Visual Analog Scale (VAS).

  - Implement strategies to mitigate common side effects, such as constipation and nausea.

- **Opioid rotation:**

  - Switching between opioids may improve response to analgesics in cases where pain control or side effects are suboptimal, ensuring individualized care.

- **Role of specialist care:**

  - Refer complex cases to palliative care specialists for advanced pain management, including parenteral opioid titration.

Key takeaways

- ☑ Opioid dose titration is essential for achieving effective cancer pain relief while minimizing adverse effects.

- ☑ Immediate-release opioids remain the gold standard for initiation, with extended-release formulations suited for maintenance.

- ☑ Tailored approaches for opioid-naive and tolerant patients optimize outcomes and enhance safety.

- ☑ Parenteral titration offers a rapid solution for cancer pain emergencies and should be integrated into specialized care settings.

- ☑ Opioid rotation is a valuable strategy to improve analgesic response and should be considered when traditional titration fails to achieve adequate relief.

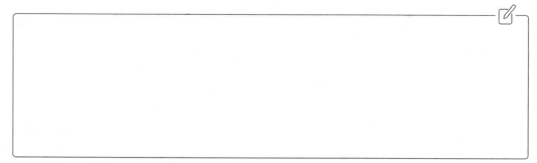

Additional recommended reading:

1. Mercadante S. Opioid dose titration for cancer pain. *Eur J Pain.* 2024;28:359—368.

2. Paice JA, et al. Use of opioids for adults with pain from cancer or cancer treatment: ASCO guideline. *J Clin Oncol.* 2023;41:914-930.

3. Klepstad P, et al. Immediate- or sustained-release morphine for dose finding during start of morphine in cancer patients. *Pain.* 2003;101:193-198.

Pain management in cervical cancer

52

Why this topic is important

Cervical cancer (CC) remains one of the most significant contributors to cancer-related morbidity and mortality globally, particularly in low- and middle-income countries. Pain is a predominant and debilitating symptom in CC, affecting up to 86% of patients with advanced disease. This pain stems from a complex interplay of tumor invasion, adverse effects of treatments like chemotherapy and radiotherapy, and procedural discomfort.

Managing pain in CC is essential for preserving patients' quality of life, yet gaps persist in delivering adequate, evidence-based care. Recent advances emphasize a multidisciplinary approach, combining pharmacological, interventional, and integrative therapies to address the diverse pain mechanisms in this population. This review by Aguiar-Rosas et al. (2024) synthesizes current evidence and recommendations regarding CC pain management.

Objectives of this update

- Outline evidence-based recommendations for managing pain in cervical cancer.

- Highlight advances in pharmacological and interventional treatments, including superior hypogastric plexus (SHP) neurolysis and integrative therapies.

- Discuss the role of a personalized and holistic approach in optimizing pain relief and improving outcomes.

What is new

- **Updated pharmacological guidelines**: Recommendations tailored to pain type (nociceptive, neuropathic, or mixed) and patient-specific considerations, such as renal or hepatic impairment.

- **Enhanced interventional strategies**: Advances in superior hypogastric plexus and impar ganglion neurolysis offer significant pain relief in pelvic and perineal cancer pain.

- **Integrative therapies**: Techniques like mindfulness meditation, acupuncture, and aromatherapy have demonstrated efficacy in alleviating anxiety and enhancing pain relief.

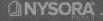

Pain mechanisms and prevalence

- **Tumor-related pain**: Direct invasion of visceral and somatic structures, nerve compression, or bone metastasis leads to nociceptive and neuropathic pain.

- **Treatment-related pain**: Chemotherapy-induced peripheral neuropathy (CIPN) occurs in 30-68% of patients, while radiotherapy may result in radiation-induced plexitis and enteritis.

- **Procedure-related pain**: Placement of nephrostomy tubes or catheters can cause localized pain and discomfort.

Pain remains prevalent across disease stages:

- 59% of patients with locally advanced CC report moderate to severe pain.

- Up to 33% of cancer survivors continue to experience chronic pain.

Pharmacological treatment

The World Health Organization's (WHO) analgesic ladder remains foundational but requires adaptations for CC-specific needs.

Mild pain

- **NSAIDs**: Useful for inflammation but limited by risks of gastrointestinal and renal toxicity, particularly in patients with impaired renal function.

- **Acetaminophen**: Effective for mild nociceptive pain; limit to 3 grams/day to avoid hepatotoxicity.

Moderate to severe pain

- **Opioids**: Morphine is the first-line therapy for visceral or somatic pain. Alternative opioids like fentanyl or buprenorphine are preferred for renal impairment.

- **Neuropathic pain adjuvants:**

  - **Gabapentinoids**: Gabapentin (1200-3600 mg/day) and pregabalin (300-600 mg/day) alleviate neuropathic pain.

  - **Serotonin and norepinephrine reuptake inhibitors**: Duloxetine and venlafaxine are effective for CIPN.

  - **Ketamine infusions**: Beneficial for refractory mixed pain syndromes.

Challenges and optimization

- Tailor therapy to pain type and patient-specific factors, such as organ function and comorbidities.

- Incorporate prophylactic treatments for opioid-induced nausea and constipation.

Interventional pain management

For patients unresponsive to pharmacological treatments, interventional procedures offer targeted pain relief.

- **Superior hypogastric plexus (SHP) neurolysis**

  - Blocks pelvic visceral pain, including pain from tumor invasion.

  - Studies demonstrate up to 70% reduction in baseline pain scores, with sustained relief for months.

  - Transdiscal and transvascular approaches provide similar efficacy.

- **Impar ganglion block**

  - Targets perineal and genital pain, frequently seen in CC.

  - Demonstrates a 70% reduction in pain in clinical studies.

- **Advanced technologies**

  - Pulsed radiofrequency combined with SHP neurolysis enhances pain control without increasing adverse effects.

  - Neurostimulation, including spinal cord and dorsal root ganglion stimulation, shows promise in refractory pelvic cancer pain.

Integrative therapies

Non-pharmacological approaches complement medical and interventional treatments, addressing psychological and emotional dimensions of pain.

- **Mindfulness meditation**: Reduces pain via non-opioidergic pathways, targeting brain regions like the orbitofrontal cortex.

- **Acupuncture**: Minimally invasive and effective for neuropathic and nociceptive pain, with minimal side effects.

- **Aromatherapy and reflexology**: Proven to alleviate anxiety and pain during treatments like brachytherapy.

When integrated into multimodal pain management plans, these therapies improve quality of life and patient satisfaction.

Clinical implications

- **Comprehensive assessment**: Evaluate pain type, intensity, and patient-specific factors using tools like the Visual Analog Scale (VAS) and McGill Pain Questionnaire.

- **Tailored interventions:** Align treatment strategies with pain mechanisms, disease stage, and patient preferences.

- **Multidisciplinary approach**: Combine pharmacological, interventional, and integrative therapies for optimal pain control.

Key takeaways

- ☑ Pain in cervical cancer is multifactorial, requiring personalized, multimodal management strategies.

- ☑ Pharmacological treatments remain the cornerstone, with adjuvants addressing neuropathic and mixed pain.

- ☑ Interventional therapies like SHP and impar ganglion neurolysis are essential for refractory cases.

- ☑ Integrative therapies enhance overall outcomes by addressing the emotional and psychological dimensions of pain.

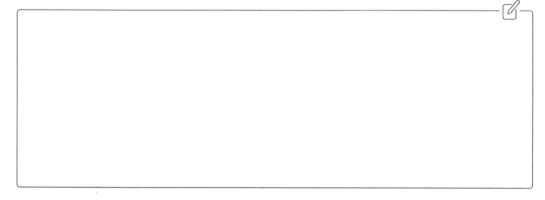

Additional recommended reading:

1. Aguiar-Rosas S, Plancarte-Sanchez R, Hernandez-Porras BC, et al. Pain management in cervical cancer. *Front Oncol.* 2024;14:1371779.

2. Yoon SY, Oh J. Neuropathic cancer pain: prevalence, pathophysiology, and management. *Korean J Intern Med.* 2018;33:1058-69.

3. Mercadante S, Klepstad P, Kurita GP, et al. Sympathetic blocks for visceral cancer pain management: A systematic review and EAPC recommendations. *Crit Rev Oncol Hematol.* 2015;96:577-83.

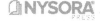

Pharmacologic management of cancer-related pain in pregnant patients

53

Why this topic is important

Cancer during pregnancy is a rare but growing challenge, affecting approximately 1 in 1000 pregnancies in the U.S. Managing cancer-related pain in this population requires balancing the need for effective analgesia with minimizing risks to both the mother and fetus. Despite being integral to comprehensive care, pain management for pregnant cancer patients is understudied and often undertreated due to concerns over teratogenicity and altered pharmacokinetics during pregnancy.

This update synthesizes the latest evidence provided by Zerfas et al. (2023) to guide clinicians in providing safe, effective pain relief for pregnant patients, emphasizing individualized therapy based on pain mechanisms and gestational considerations.

Objectives of this update

- Understand the challenges of managing cancer-related pain during pregnancy.

- Explore the pharmacologic options for nociceptive, neuropathic, and nociplastic pain in pregnant patients.

- Highlight safety profiles and potential risks associated with commonly used analgesics.

What is new

- **Improved safety data**: Expanded evidence supports acetaminophen and buprenorphine as primary options for nociceptive pain during pregnancy.

- **Guidelines for adjunct therapies**: The use of duloxetine and gabapentin for neuropathic and nociplastic pain is gaining traction, though caution is required.

- **Emerging protocols**: Novel low-dose buprenorphine initiation strategies mitigate opioid withdrawal risks while ensuring pain control.

Mechanisms and types of cancer-related pain

- **Nociceptive pain:**

  ○ Results from somatic or visceral tissue damage, often due to tumor burden or metastases.

  ○ Common treatments: Acetaminophen, NSAIDs (limited to early pregnancy), corticosteroids, and opioids.

- **Neuropathic pain:**

  ○ Caused by nerve injury from tumors, chemotherapy, or radiation, presenting as burning, sharp, or shooting pain.

  ○ Preferred agents: Duloxetine and gabapentin.

- **Nociplastic pain:**

  ○ Central sensitization leads to widespread pain unrelated to identifiable tissue damage.

  ○ Effective treatments include duloxetine and gabapentin.

Pharmacologic options

- **Nociceptive pain management:**

  ○ **Acetaminophen:**

    · First-line treatment due to its mild teratogenic risk.

    · May impact neurodevelopment with excessive use; thus, use the lowest effective doses.

  ○ **NSAIDs:**

    · Useful for inflammatory pain but limited to the first 20 weeks due to risks of fetal ductus arteriosus closure and renal dysfunction.

  ○ **Corticosteroids:**

    · Effective for bone and inflammatory pain, with dexamethasone preferred for its minimal fluid retention effects. Short courses are advised.

- ○ **Opioids:**

    · Reserved for moderate-to-severe pain. Buprenorphine is preferred due to its partial agonist profile, reducing risks of respiratory depression and neonatal opioid withdrawal syndrome (NOWS).

- **Neuropathic pain management:**

  ○ **Duloxetine:**

    · First-line agent, especially for patients with comorbid anxiety or depression. Slight risk of postpartum hemorrhage warrants careful monitoring.

  ○ **Gabapentin:**

    · Effective for neuropathic symptoms, though associated with preterm birth and neonatal intensive care admissions with prolonged use in late pregnancy.

  ○ **Pregabalin:**

    · Limited safety data; use gabapentin preferentially due to greater evidence.

  ○ **Avoidance:**

    · Venlafaxine and tricyclic antidepressants (TCAs) carry higher maternal and fetal risks and are not recommended as first-line options.

- **Nociplastic pain management:**

  ○ Duloxetine and gabapentin remain the mainstays of treatment.

  ○ Cyclobenzaprine may be considered cautiously in early trimesters, as anticholinergic effects and risks of ductal closure in late pregnancy are concerns.

Safety considerations

- **Maternal risks:**

  - Opioids: Constipation, sedation, and potential for respiratory depression.

  - Corticosteroids: Hyperglycemia and increased gestational diabetes risk.

  - NSAIDs: Increased risk of bleeding and prolonged labor.

- **Fetal risks:**

  - Acetaminophen: Possible neuro-developmental effects.

  - NSAIDs: Renal dysfunction and premature ductus arteriosus closure with late use.

  - Opioids: Potential for low birth weight, neonatal respiratory depression, and withdrawal.

- **Mitigating risks:**

  - Use the lowest effective doses of medications for the shortest duration.

  - Prioritize medications with established safety profiles, such as acetaminophen and buprenorphine.

Clinical implications

- **Personalized care:**

  - Tailor treatment plans based on the type and mechanism of pain, balancing analgesia and safety.

  - Multidisciplinary collaboration with obstetricians, oncologists, and pain specialists is critical.

- **Close monitoring:**

  - Conduct regular fetal assessments for potential adverse effects of medications.

- **Access to advanced therapies:**

  - Expand the use of interventional procedures, such as nerve blocks and intrathecal delivery, for refractory cases.

Key takeaways

- ☑ Nociceptive pain should be managed with acetaminophen and short-term corticosteroids, with buprenorphine favored for severe cases.

- ☑ Duloxetine and gabapentin are effective for neuropathic and nociplastic pain, but late pregnancy use requires caution.

- ☑ Careful monitoring and a multidisciplinary approach are essential for optimizing outcomes.

Additional recommended reading:

1. Zerfas I, McGinn R, Smith MA. Pharmacologic management of cancer-related pain in pregnant patients. *Drugs*. 2023;83:1067-1076.

2. Bruera E, Paice JA. Cancer-related pain management: safe and effective use of opioids. *ASCO Educ Book*. 2015:e593-599.

3. Haywood A, Good P, Khan S, et al. Corticosteroids for cancer-related pain: A comprehensive review. *Cochrane Database Syst Rev*. 2015;(4):CD010756.

Cancer pain management in inpatient specialized palliative care settings

54

Why this topic is important

Cancer pain remains a major concern in oncology, affecting nearly 55% of patients with advanced disease. Despite advancements in analgesic strategies, undertreatment persists, impacting patients' quality of life, psychological well-being, and ability to engage in daily activities. Specialized palliative care (SPC) teams play a critical role in addressing refractory cancer pain through comprehensive, patient-centered approaches.

A recent study by Tagami et al. (2024) highlights the time-sensitive nature of pain management in inpatient SPC, focusing on personalized pain goals, patient-reported outcomes (PROs), and multidisciplinary strategies. This study provides critical insights into how SPC interventions can enhance pain relief, improve patient satisfaction, and minimize adverse events.

Objectives of this update

- Explore the effectiveness of SPC interventions in achieving cancer pain management (CPM) goals.

- Discuss strategies for implementing patient-reported outcome measures (PROMs) in pain management.

- Provide actionable recommendations for reducing pain-related interference with activities of daily living (ADLs) and sleep.

What is new

- **Rapid relief timeline**: SPC achieved CPM in a median of 3 days, with over 94% of patients reaching their pain goals within 1 week.

- **PROM integration**: Assessment tools such as the Brief Pain Inventory (BPI) demonstrated significant improvements in pain intensity and interference with ADLs.

- **Refined opioid strategies**: Adjustments to morphine equivalent daily doses (MEDD) facilitated tailored pain relief while minimizing rescue medication use.

Cancer pain management: Clinical insights

Pathophysiology and challenges

Cancer pain is multifactorial, involving somatic, visceral, and neuropathic components. Tumor invasion, metastasis, and treatment-related complications exacerbate this complexity. Pain intensity and response vary widely, influenced by cancer type, location, and comorbidities.

Role of SPC

SPC offers a multidisciplinary approach, incorporating medical, psychological, and rehabilitative therapies. This tailored strategy addresses the dynamic needs of patients with advanced cancer, particularly those with refractory pain.

Rapid achievement of CPM

- **Population characteristics:**
  - A total of 355 patients with 438 episodes of cancer pain were included.
  - The mean patient age was 62.9 years, with lung and gastrointestinal cancers being the most common primary sites.
  - Mixed pain types (nociceptive and neuropathic) were predominant, requiring diverse treatment modalities.
- **Pain relief outcomes:**
  - **Success rates**: CPM was achieved in 87.9% of cases, with a median time of 3 days.
  - **Pain intensity reduction:**
    - Worst pain intensity improved from 6.9 to 4.0 (mean reduction of 2.9 points on a numerical rating scale).
    - Average pain intensity decreased from 4.4 to 2.1.

- **Interference with daily life:**
  - General activity impairment decreased significantly (mean reduction: 3.0 points).
  - Sleep interference improved by 2.8 points on average, enhancing overall well-being.
- **PROMs and patient satisfaction:**
  - Over 81% of patients reported satisfaction with their pain management.
  - Personalized pain goals (PPGs) were achieved in 88.6% of cases.

Multimodal approaches in SPC

Pharmacological interventions

- **Regular opioid use:**
  - The majority (78%) of patients were prescribed opioids, with oxycodone being the most common.
  - Opioid doses were adjusted to a median MEDD of 45 mg/day by the end of the observation period.
- **Adjuvant therapies:**
  - Gabapentinoids (pregabalin, gabapentin) were used in 19.8% of cases to address neuropathic pain.
  - Corticosteroids and antidepressants provided additional pain modulation and mood stabilization.
- **Rescue medications:**
  - The frequency of rescue medication use decreased significantly, reflecting improved baseline pain control.

Non-pharmacological strategies

- **Psycho-oncology support:**
  - Psychological interventions addressed fear, anxiety, and depression, enhancing patient resilience.
- **Rehabilitation and mobility aids:**
  - Physical therapy improves functional capacity, reducing pain-related disability.

Clinical implications

- **PROM integration:**
  - Tools like the BPI enable personalized care by monitoring pain intensity, ADL interference, and sleep quality.
  - Real-time feedback fosters shared decision-making between patients and providers.

- **Tailored opioid regimens:**
  - Balancing efficacy with safety is crucial, particularly in managing higher MEDD thresholds.

- **Comprehensive SPC models:**
  - Daily team-based interventions ensure rapid pain relief while addressing holistic patient needs.

Key takeaways

- ☑ Inpatient SPC achieves cancer pain relief rapidly and effectively, with a median timeline of 3 days.

- ☑ PROMs are essential for evaluating patient satisfaction and tailoring individualized care plans.

- ☑ Multimodal approaches, combining pharmacological and non-pharmacological therapies, optimize outcomes and enhance quality of life.

- ☑ Future directions should explore expanding SPC access and refining PROM-based assessments in outpatient and home care settings.

Additional recommended reading:

1. Tagami K, Chiu S, Kosugi K, et al. Cancer pain management in patients receiving inpatient specialized palliative care. *J Pain Symptom Manage.* 2024;67:27-38.

2. Hui D, Bruera E. A personalized approach to assessing and managing pain in patients with cancer. *J Clin Oncol.* 2014;32:1640-1646.

3. Mercadante S, Gebbia V, David F, et al. Does pain intensity predict a poor opioid response in cancer patients? *Eur J Cancer.* 2011;47:713-717.

Multimodal locoregional procedures for cancer pain management

55

Why this topic is important

Cancer pain is one of the most distressing symptoms for patients, especially in advanced stages of disease, affecting up to 80% of those with progressive cancer. Despite global efforts to improve analgesic approaches, nearly 30-50% of patients remain undertreated, enduring unnecessary suffering and diminished quality of life. While pharmacological options, including opioids, remain the cornerstone of cancer pain management, locoregional interventions provide a critical alternative for refractory pain.

This review by Iezzi et al. (2022) explores the expanding role of minimally invasive locoregional procedures such as percutaneous neurolysis, vertebral augmentation, and transarterial embolization (TAE). These techniques enhance pain control, improve functionality, and reduce systemic side effects associated with conventional analgesics.

Objectives of this update

- Highlight the most effective locoregional procedures for managing cancer pain.

- Discuss their mechanisms, safety profiles, and applications.

- Provide practical recommendations for integrating these techniques into multidisciplinary care models.

What is new

- **Innovative neurolysis approaches**: Techniques such as cryoablation and radiofrequency neurolysis offer pain relief and reduce procedural discomfort.

- **Combination therapies**: Augmenting locoregional interventions with systemic treatments maximizes therapeutic benefits.

- **Advances in augmentation techniques**: New implant-based technologies improve structural support in metastatic bone disease.

Locoregional interventions for cancer pain management

Percutaneous neurolysis

Technique and indications

Percutaneous neurolysis involves disrupting pain pathways through chemical or thermal ablation. Chemical agents like phenol and ethanol induce Wallerian degeneration, while radiofrequency and cryoablation use thermal energy for nerve destruction. This method is particularly suited for advanced cancer patients with localized, opioid-refractory pain and a life expectancy of 6-12 months.

Innovations in neurolysis

- **Radiofrequency ablation (RFA):** Provides precise, durable denervation. Studies report pain relief in over 70% of patients.

- **Cryoablation**: Superior imaging visibility of ablation zones and lower intraprocedural discomfort make cryoablation an attractive option.

Vertebral augmentation

Technique and applications

- **Vertebroplasty**: Injection of bone cement to stabilize vertebral fractures caused by metastasis.

- **Balloon kyphoplasty**: Adds a cavity-creating step to restore vertebral height before cement injection.

- **Implant-based technologies**: New materials like PEEK cages provide enhanced biomechanical support.

Efficacy

Vertebral augmentation alleviates pain in 60-85% of patients, with minimal complications like asymptomatic cement leakage.

Transarterial embolization (TAE)

Mechanism and benefits

TAE reduces tumor vascularity, alleviating pain caused by pressure on the periosteal and surrounding tissues. It also aids in controlling tumor progression, especially in spinal metastases.

Clinical outcomes

- Pain relief success rates: 50-97%.

- Median duration of symptom relief: ~8 months.

- Enhanced outcomes when combined with other therapies, such as vertebroplasty or external beam radiation therapy (EBRT).

Radiation therapy

Techniques and innovations

- **External beam radiotherapy (EBRT):**

  - Mainstay for uncomplicated bone metastases.

  - Single-fraction protocols (e.g., 8 Gy) improve pain control while minimizing patient burden.

- **Stereotactic body radiation therapy (SBRT):**

  - Delivers high doses with precision, sparing adjacent healthy tissues.

  - Offers durable pain relief in up to 80% of patients.

- **Interventional radiotherapy (IRT):**

  - Combines brachytherapy with percutaneous procedures for metastatic lesions unresponsive to conventional treatments.

Outcomes

- EBRT and SBRT significantly alleviate pain in 50-80% of cases, with complete pain relief in one-third of patients.

- IRT improves local tumor control and reduces analgesic requirements.

Clinical implications

- **Patient selection:**

  - Locoregional techniques are ideal for patients with refractory cancer pain or contraindications to systemic therapies.

  - Multidisciplinary evaluation is critical to align treatment with patient goals and prognosis.

- **Combination strategies:**

  - Pairing locoregional approaches with systemic therapies enhances overall pain control and functional outcomes.

- **Resource optimization:**

  - Expanding access to minimally invasive technologies requires investment in clinician training and procedural infrastructure.

Key takeaways

☑ Locoregional interventions like neurolysis, vertebral augmentation, and TAE are pivotal for managing cancer pain that is unresponsive to systemic therapies.

☑ Advancements in cryoablation, implant technologies, and SBRT have improved the precision and durability of pain relief.

☑ Multidisciplinary collaboration ensures comprehensive care tailored to the individual needs of cancer patients.

Additional recommended reading:

1. Iezzi R, Kovács G, Dimov V, et al. Multimodal locoregional procedures for cancer pain management: A literature review. *Br J Radiol.* 2022;96:e20220236.

2. Christo PJ, Mazloomdoost D. Interventional pain treatments for cancer pain. *Ann N Y Acad Sci.* 2008;1138:299-328.

3. Moynagh MR, Kurup AN, Callstrom MR. Thermal ablation of bone metastases. *Semin Intervent Radiol.* 2018;35:299-308.

Epidural analgesia for intractable cancer pain

56

Why this topic is important

Cancer-related pain affects a significant proportion of patients, especially those with advanced or metastatic disease. Up to 66% of individuals with terminal cancer experience severe pain, with 10-20% reporting intractable pain unresponsive to systemic therapies. Effective management of this pain is crucial for improving quality of life, yet achieving relief remains challenging due to treatment side effects, variability in pain mechanisms, and limitations of conventional analgesics. Cancer pain is commonly managed using intrathecal pumps or neurolytic blocks. Recently, epidural analgesia has emerged as a key interventional approach, offering localized, potent pain control for patients with severe or refractory symptoms.

This systematic review by Hsieh et al. (2023) evaluates the efficacy and safety of epidural analgesia in managing cancer pain, providing a comprehensive analysis of its role in clinical practice.

Objectives of this update

- Assess the effectiveness of epidural analgesia in reducing intractable cancer pain.

- Evaluate the comparative safety and outcomes of epidural versus systemic opioid administration.

- Explore the role of adjuvants, injection techniques, and delivery methods in optimizing epidural analgesia.

What is new

- Evidence indicates that coadministration of epidural opioids with local anesthetics or adjuvants significantly enhances pain relief.

- Continuous infusion has no clear advantage over intermittent bolus administration, though higher catheter placement may reduce dose requirements.

- Emerging strategies for adjuvants such as clonidine, ketamine, and dexamethasone demonstrate promise for refractory cases.

Mechanisms of action and advantages

Epidural analgesia provides targeted delivery of medications directly to the dorsal spinal cord, bypassing the blood-brain barrier and first-pass metabolism. This results in enhanced analgesia with lower systemic drug exposure, reducing the risk of side effects compared to systemic administration.

Pain relief and efficacy

- **Epidural opioids:**
  - Morphine and sufentanil are commonly used epidural opioids. Studies consistently show significant reductions in pain scores when administered epidurally.
  - Compared to systemic opioids, epidural administration achieves similar analgesia but with reduced systemic side effects in some studies.

- **Coadministration with local anesthetics:**
  - Combining opioids with agents like bupivacaine enhances efficacy by producing a synergistic effect.
  - One RCT demonstrated that sufentanil combined with bupivacaine provided superior pain relief compared to sufentanil alone.

- **Adjuvants:**
  - Clonidine: Enhances analgesia, particularly for neuropathic pain.
  - Ketamine and neostigmine: Improve pain relief duration and reduce opioid requirements.
  - Dexamethasone: Provides additional anti-inflammatory benefits.

Delivery methods and techniques

- **Intermittent bolus versus continuous infusion:**
  - There are no significant differences in pain control between these methods.
  - Continuous infusion may require higher dose escalation over time, raising concerns about long-term use.

- **Injection levels:**
  - Higher-level epidural injections (e.g., cervical or thoracic) are associated with faster and longer-lasting pain relief due to reduced drug requirements.

Comparative outcomes

- **Neuropathic vs. nociceptive pain:**
  - Epidural analgesia is more effective for somatic/nociceptive pain compared to neuropathic pain.
  - Patients with neuropathic pain may benefit from adjuvants such as clonidine or ketamine.

- **Quality of life improvements:**
  - Limited data on quality of life outcomes; some studies report better symptom control and reduced hospitalization for pain management.

- **Reduction in systemic opioid use:**
  - Several studies report decreased oral and systemic opioid consumption following epidural analgesia.

Safety and complications

- **Adverse events:**

    - Common side effects: Nausea, constipation, urinary retention, and catheter-related issues.

    - Serious complications: Rare but include epidural hematoma and infection requiring surgical intervention.

- **Risk mitigation:**

    - Adherence to strict aseptic techniques and careful patient monitoring minimizes complications.

Clinical implications

- **Tailored approach:**

    - Patient selection should consider pain mechanisms (nociceptive vs. neuropathic) and overall clinical condition.

    - Coadministration of opioids with local anesthetics or adjuvants enhances outcomes, particularly for refractory pain.

- **Role in cancer care:**

    - Epidural analgesia is particularly valuable for terminal-stage patients or those with limited life expectancy, offering immediate and effective pain relief.

- **Integration into multimodal therapy:**

    - Combining epidural analgesia with systemic treatments and non-pharmacologic interventions may optimize pain management.

Key takeaways

☑ Epidural analgesia is an effective option for intractable cancer pain, especially for somatic/nociceptive pain.

☑ Combining opioids with local anesthetics or adjuvants enhances analgesia while reducing opioid requirements.

☑ While complications are rare, adherence to best practices and rigorous patient monitoring are essential for safety.

Additional recommended reading:

1. Hsieh Y-L, Chen H-Y, Lin C-R, Wang C-F. Efficacy of epidural analgesia for intractable cancer pain: A systematic review. *Pain Pract.* 2023;23(8):956-969.

2. Mercadante S, Porzio G. Neuraxial analgesia in cancer pain management: Evidence-based recommendations. *J Pain Res.* 2017;10:1423-1431.

3. Bruel BM, Burton AW. Interventional techniques for cancer pain management. *Pain Med.* 2016;17:2404-2421.

Intrathecal drug delivery in cancer-related pain

57

Why this topic is important

Cancer-related pain is a debilitating and common symptom affecting patients in advanced stages of the disease. Despite advancements in systemic opioid therapy, many patients continue to experience inadequate relief or intolerable side effects, underscoring the need for alternative strategies.

Intrathecal drug delivery (IDD) is a targeted intervention that offers precise pain relief by administering analgesics directly into the intrathecal space, reducing systemic exposure and its associated toxicity. A systematic review and meta-analysis by Perruchoud et al. (2021) synthesized decades of evidence to evaluate IDD's efficacy and safety for cancer pain management, providing critical insights for clinicians and researchers.

Objectives of this update

- Review IDD's short-, mid-, and long-term efficacy for cancer pain.

- Highlight its impact on systemic opioid use and associated complications.

- Discuss clinical implications for integrating IDD into cancer pain management pathways.

What is new

- IDD consistently reduces pain scores by over 4 points on a 0-10 scale in the short and mid-term and by 3.3 points over 6 months, maintaining effectiveness despite disease progression.

- Patients experience a dramatic reduction in systemic opioid consumption, averaging over 50%, minimizing opioid-related adverse effects.

- Infection rates remain low (~3%) across studies, with comparable risks between external and implanted IDD systems.

Efficacy of IDD

- **Pain relief**

  - Short-term (4-5 weeks): A meta-analysis of 13 studies showed an average pain reduction of 4.34 points.

  - Mid-term (6-12 weeks): Ten studies reported a similar reduction of 4.3 points.

  - Long-term (> 6 months): Pain scores de-creased by 3.3 points.

- **Durability**

  - Pain relief was sustained even in patients with advanced or metastatic cancers, suggesting the intervention's resilience against disease progression.

Reduction in systemic opioid use

- Patients who transitioned to IDD experienced a weighted mean opioid reduction of 308.24 mg/day in oral morphine equivalents (OME).

- In studies focusing on implanted pumps, opioid use decreased even more dramatically, with an average reduction of 487.23 mg/day.

Safety profile

- Infection rates:

  - Implanted pumps: 2.8%.

  - External pumps: 2.9%.

- Most complications, including infections, catheter malfunctions, and cerebrospinal fluid leaks, were manageable.

Clinical implications

- **Patient selection**

  - IDD is recommended for patients with refractory cancer pain who are unresponsive to systemic treatments or those experiencing significant opioid-related side effects.

- **Device selection**

  - Both external and implanted pumps offer comparable pain relief. However, patient preferences, life expectancy, and healthcare resource availability should guide the choice.

- **Multimodal approach**

  - Combining IDD with systemic therapies, psychological support, and palliative care improves overall quality of life.

- **Resource considerations**

  - Training clinicians in IDD techniques and expanding access to devices are crucial to addressing inequities in advanced pain management options.

Key takeaways

- ☑ IDD significantly reduces cancer pain, providing durable relief across disease stages.

- ☑ Substantial reductions in systemic opioid use lower the risk of adverse effects and improve patient tolerance.

- ☑ Infection rates remain low, supporting the intervention's safety in both implanted and external systems.

- ☑ Incorporating IDD into cancer care pathways requires careful patient selection and multidisciplinary collaboration.

Additional recommended reading:

1. Perruchoud C, Dupoiron D, Papi B, et al. Management of cancer-related pain with intrathecal drug delivery: A systematic review and meta-analysis of clinical studies. *Neuromodulation*. 2021;26(8):1142-1152.

2. Smith TJ, Staats PS, Deer T, et al. Randomized clinical trial of an implantable drug delivery system compared with comprehensive medical management for refractory cancer pain: Impact on pain, drug-related toxicity, and survival. *J Clin Oncol*. 2002;20:4040-4049.

3. Mercadante S, Intravaia G, Villari P, et al. Intrathecal treatment in cancer patients unresponsive to multiple trials of systemic opioids. *Clin J Pain*. 2007;23:793-798.

Efficacy and safety of intrathecal infusion devices for cancer pain

58

Why this topic is important

Cancer-related pain, particularly in advanced stages, often becomes refractory to conventional analgesics. Intrathecal infusion therapy (IIT) is a vital intervention for managing moderate to severe cancer pain, offering direct delivery of analgesics to the cerebrospinal fluid for superior efficacy and reduced systemic side effects.

This review by Díaz-Rodríguez et al. (2024) compares two types of intrathecal infusion devices: partially externalized devices (PEDs) and totally implanted devices (TIDs). Understanding the differences in their efficacy, safety, and suitability is crucial for optimizing patient care and resource allocation in oncology.

Objectives of this update

- Compare the effectiveness of PEDs and TIDs in managing cancer pain.
- Evaluate the safety profiles and complication rates of both devices.
- Provide guidance on device selection based on patient characteristics and life expectancy.

What is new

- PEDs are effective for short-term pain relief but carry higher risks of catheter-related complications.
- TIDs demonstrate greater long-term stability, with fewer infections and reduced hospital readmissions.
- Enhanced insights into functional improvements and episodic pain control provide a nuanced perspective on device selection.

Device mechanisms and usage

- **Partially Externalized Devices (PEDs):**

  - Designed for patients with a life expectancy of under three months.

  - Simpler surgical procedure with reduced implantation time and lower cost.

  - Higher risk of bacterial colonization and catheter dislocation due to the externalized port.

- **Totally Implanted Devices (TIDs):**

  - Indicated for patients with longer life expectancies.

  - A completely internalized system reduces infection risks and minimizes maintenance needs.

  - More complex implantation procedure with higher initial costs.

Pain control outcomes

- **Overall efficacy:**

  - Both PEDs and TIDs achieve significant pain relief, with an average reduction of 4.8 points on the Visual Analog Scale (VAS) at one month.

  - No significant differences in pain reduction between devices at three and six months.

- **Onset of analgesia:**

  - PEDs provide faster pain relief, with 68.4% of patients reporting improvement within 24 hours compared to 47.1% in the TID group.

- **Episodic and nocturnal pain:**

  - Both devices effectively reduce nocturnal pain incidence from 50% to 4.3% in six months.

  - Episodic pain remains challenging, with 53.8% of patients still reporting episodes at six months.

Functional and safety outcomes

- **Functional improvement:**

  - TIDs are associated with better functional outcomes, with fewer bedridden patients (5.6% vs. 22% for PEDs).

  - The Karnofsky Performance Scale (KPS) scores were higher in the TID group before implantation (61.63 vs. 42.22 for PEDs).

- **Complications:**

  - PEDs have a higher overall complication rate (43.3% vs. 25% for TIDs).

  - Common complications include catheter migration and needle dysfunction, with infections more frequent in PEDs (5% vs. 0%).

- **Hospital admissions:**

  - TID-related complications often necessitate hospital readmissions and additional surgeries, increasing healthcare resource utilization.

Clinical implications

- **Device selection:**

  - PEDs are preferable for patients with limited life expectancy due to their cost-effectiveness and rapid pain relief.

  - TIDs are better suited for patients requiring long-term pain control and those with higher functional capacity.

- **Episodic pain management:**

  - The persistent nature of episodic pain highlights the need for adjunctive therapies alongside intrathecal infusion.

- **Risk mitigation:**

  - Stringent aseptic techniques and close monitoring are critical to reducing infection risks, particularly for PEDs.

  - Regular follow-up visits and proactive management of catheter-related issues enhance outcomes for both device types.

Key takeaways

☑ Both PEDs and TIDs provide effective pain relief for moderate to severe cancer pain, with nuanced differences in safety and practicality.

☑ PEDs offer rapid pain relief for short-term needs but are associated with higher infection and complication rates.

☑ TIDs provide greater long-term stability and improved functionality, though they require more complex implantation procedures.

☑ Personalized device selection based on patient characteristics and life expectancy is crucial for optimizing outcomes.

Additional recommended reading:

1. Díaz-Rodríguez D, Fontán-Atalaya IM, Peralta-Espinosa E, et al. Differences in efficacy and safety between intrathecal infusion devices in cancer pain. *Pain Pract.* 2024;24:42-51.

2. Smith TJ, Staats PS, Deer T, et al. An implantable drug delivery system (IDDS) for refractory cancer pain provides sustained pain control. *Ann Oncol.* 2005;16:825-33.

3. Stearns LM, Perruchoud C, Spencer R, et al. Intrathecal drug delivery systems for cancer pain: An analysis of a prospective, multicenter product surveillance registry. *Anesth Analg.* 2020;130:289-97.

Cancer-related pain management in suitable intrathecal therapy candidates

59

Why this topic is important

Cancer pain remains one of the most challenging symptoms in oncology care, particularly in advanced stages, where pain affects up to 80% of patients. Intrathecal therapy (IT) offers significant pain relief by delivering medications directly into the cerebrospinal fluid, enhancing efficacy while minimizing systemic side effects. IT is often underutilized despite its benefits due to a lack of standardized protocols, variable referral practices, and misconceptions about its risk-benefit profile.

The Spanish Multidisciplinary Expert Consensus outlined by Pérez et al. (2023) provides actionable recommendations for optimizing IT use in cancer pain management. By addressing patient selection, care pathways, and healthcare coordination, these guidelines aim to expand access to IT and improve outcomes for patients with refractory cancer pain.

Objectives of this update

- Review best practices for patient selection and referral to intrathecal therapy.

- Highlight care protocols and quality indicators for IT implementation.

- Identify barriers and propose solutions for integrating IT into cancer pain care pathways.

What is new

- Consensus recommendations prioritize timely referrals (< 48 hours for urgent cases).

- Emphasis on comprehensive patient evaluation, including functional and psychosocial assessments.

- Clear guidelines for post-implantation follow-up, including personalized monitoring and patient education.

Patient selection criteria

- **Eligibility**

  ◦ Suitable for patients with refractory cancer pain who are unresponsive to conventional treatments or intolerant to systemic therapies.

  ◦ IT can be implemented at any stage of the disease, not limited to end-of-life care.

- **Comprehensive assessment**

  ◦ Functional status, life expectancy, comorbidities, and psychosocial factors are key determinants of IT candidacy.

  ◦ Psychological evaluations should identify potential barriers to adherence and emotional readiness.

Protocols for care

- **Referral pathways**

  ◦ Early referral to pain units ensures timely access to IT, with urgent cases evaluated within 48 hours and preferential cases within a week.

  ◦ Standardized referral criteria reduce delays caused by variability in primary care practices.

- **Multidisciplinary approach**

  ◦ Effective coordination among oncology, pain management, and palliative care teams is essential.

  ◦ Nursing professionals play a critical role in patient education and post-discharge support.

Intrathecal therapy implementation

- **Pharmacologic considerations**

  ◦ Medications include opioids (e.g., morphine, hydromorphone), local anesthetics (e.g., bupivacaine), and adjuvants (e.g., ziconotide, clonidine).

  ◦ Direct delivery to the spinal cord allows for lower doses and reduced systemic side effects.

  ◦ Drug selection and dosing are tailored to the patient's pain profile and comorbidities.

  ◦ Monitoring for drug interactions and response ensures safety and efficacy.

- **Post-implantation follow-up**

  ◦ Monitoring pain intensity, functional outcomes, and adverse events is essential.

  ◦ Address complications promptly with facilitated healthcare access, such as direct contact lines or telemedicine.

  ◦ Adjust medication dosages based on changes in pain or functional status.

  ◦ Multidisciplinary coordination enhances safety and optimizes treatment outcomes.

- **Patient education**

  ◦ Provide comprehensive instruction on device care, recognizing complications, and adhering to follow-up protocols.

  ◦ Supplement verbal explanations with written materials detailing the therapy plan and troubleshooting steps.

  ◦ Deliver education during hospital discharge tailored to the patient's literacy and learning preferences.

  ◦ Empower patients and caregivers with contact information for medical assistance.

- **Multidisciplinary care coordination**

  ◦ Involve pain specialists, oncologists, nurses, and other providers for holistic care.

  ◦ Foster regular communication among team members to address pain's physical, psychological, and social aspects.

  ◦ Use structured protocols for referrals, device implantation, and follow-up to streamline care delivery.

These strategies collectively enhance the effectiveness and safety of intrathecal therapy, improving patient outcomes and quality of life.

Barriers and proposed solutions

- **Healthcare professional training**

  - Limited availability of qualified specialists is a significant barrier.

  - Continuous training programs in IT techniques and patient communication are recommended.

- **Referral delays**

  - Standardizing referral pathways and educating primary care providers can reduce delays.

  - Establishing dedicated pain management centers improves accessibility.

- **Patient misconceptions**

  - Addressing fears about surgical risks and clarifying the benefits of IT through educational campaigns can enhance acceptance.

Clinical implications

- **Early intervention**

  - IT should be considered proactively for patients with escalating pain or poor tolerance to systemic treatments.

- **Comprehensive care models**

  - Integration of psychological and social support into IT care pathways improves patient outcomes.

- **Quality metrics**

  - Key indicators include patient satisfaction, reduced hospitalizations, and fewer device-related complications.

Key takeaways

☑ IT is an effective, underutilized option for managing refractory cancer pain, suitable across all disease stages.

☑ Multidisciplinary coordination, early referrals, and patient-centered care pathways are critical for successful IT implementation.

☑ Addressing barriers, including training gaps and patient misconceptions, can expand access to this life-changing therapy.

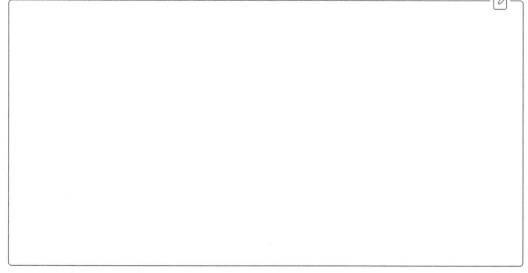

Additional recommended reading:

1. Pérez C, Quintanar T, García C, et al. Cancer-related pain management in suitable intrathecal therapy candidates: A Spanish multidisciplinary expert consensus. *Curr Oncol.* 2023;30:7303-7314.

2. Deer TR, Hayek SM, Grider JS, et al. The Polyanalgesic Consensus Conference (PACC)®: Updates on Clinical Pharmacology and Comorbidity Management in Intrathecal Drug Delivery for Cancer Pain. *Neuromodulation.* Published online September 20, 2024.

3. Bruel BM, Burton AW. Intrathecal therapy for cancer-related pain. *Pain Med.* 2016;17:2404-2421.

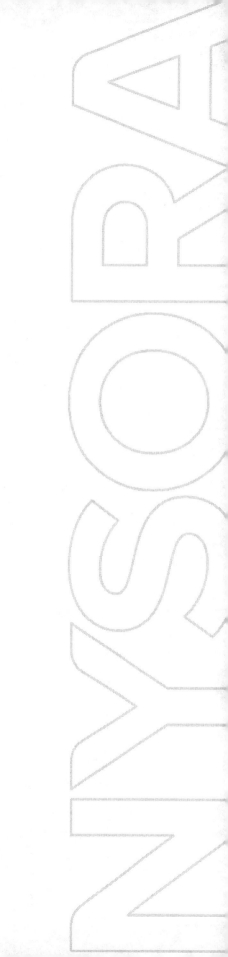

Controversies in intrathecal drug delivery for cancer pain

60

Why this topic is important

Intrathecal drug delivery (IDD) has been a cornerstone for managing refractory cancer pain, offering effective analgesia while minimizing systemic side effects. However, controversies persist in its implementation, particularly concerning catheter tip positioning, trialing protocols, and drug selection. These uncertainties limit IDD's optimization and broader adoption, especially in patients with complex pain syndromes.

Brogan et al.'s review (2022) provides a detailed exploration of these challenges, emphasizing evidence-based guidance and identifying areas for future research. This update distills these insights to aid clinicians in refining their approach to IDD.

Objectives of this update

- Discuss controversies surrounding catheter tip positioning and its impact on drug delivery efficacy.

- Evaluate the necessity of trialing protocols in cancer pain management.

- Highlight advances and challenges in using intrathecal agents like ziconotide and local anesthetics.

What is new

- **Catheter positioning:** Evidence suggests that placing the catheter near the pain dermatome optimizes drug efficacy. However, dorsal vs. ventral placement shows no clinical superiority.

- **Trialing:** Data challenge the necessity of pre-implantation trials, particularly in patients with limited life expectancy.

- **Ziconotide use:** While effective, its implementation is constrained by a narrow therapeutic window and high cost.

Intrathecal catheter tip positioning

- **Receptor targeting:**

  ◦ Mu opioid receptors (MOR) and N-type calcium channels are concentrated in the dorsal horn. Positioning the catheter near the pain-affected dermatome enhances drug action.

- **Cerebrospinal fluid (CSF) dynamics:**

  ◦ Contrary to earlier assumptions of uniform drug distribution via CSF, studies indicate that intrathecal drugs primarily disperse through local diffusion and pulsatile flow, reinforcing the importance of precise catheter placement.

- **Dorsal vs. ventral placement:**

  ◦ There is no clinical advantage for dorsal placement compared to ventral, although theoretical benefits for dorsal placement exist based on nociceptive pathway anatomy.

Trialing in cancer pain

- **Purpose and utility:**

  ◦ Trials aim to predict long-term efficacy, determine drug tolerability, and guide dose selection. However, trialing often delays definitive therapy and imposes additional risks, such as infection and procedural complications.

- **Evidence limitations:**

  ◦ Retrospective studies in non-cancer populations have shown a limited correlation between trial success and long-term outcomes. Similar evidence in cancer pain is scarce, with one manufacturer database reporting only 21.6% of cancer patients undergoing trials.

- **Practical considerations:**

  ◦ Trialing adds logistical challenges, particularly in patients with advanced cancer requiring rapid symptom control. Current guidelines suggest making trials optional based on patient and clinician discretion.

Advances in intrathecal drug delivery

- **Ziconotide:**

  ◦ As a non-opioid, N-type calcium channel blocker, ziconotide offers analgesia without risks of tolerance or respiratory depression.

  ◦ Its adoption is limited by a high incidence of neurological side effects and the need for slow titration, making it less suitable for patients with short life expectancy.

  ◦ Multimodal regimens combining ziconotide with low-dose opioids are emerging as a way to balance efficacy and side effect profiles.

- **Local anesthetics:**

  ◦ Bupivacaine, often combined with opioids, reduces the required opioid dose and enhances analgesic efficacy. Emerging agents like ropivacaine show promise but require further study.

- **Combination therapies:**

  ◦ Combining ziconotide with opioids or local anesthetics can achieve synergistic effects, although concerns about drug stability in admixtures persist. Recent evidence indicates that such combinations significantly reduce systemic opioid requirements, addressing concerns about opioid-related side effects.

Controversies in intrathecal drug delivery for cancer pain

Clinical implications

- **Personalized catheter positioning:**
  - Consider the pain's dermatomal distribution and drug properties (e.g., lipophilicity) when deciding on catheter placement.

- **Rethinking trialing protocols:**
  - Avoid mandatory trials for patients with advanced cancer unless clinically justified. Focus on rapid initiation of definitive therapy.

- **Expanding access to ziconotide:**
  - Streamline protocols to improve tolerability, such as slow titration and early recognition of side effects.

- **Optimizing combination therapies:**
  - Leverage multimodal strategies to enhance efficacy and minimize side effects, particularly in complex pain syndromes.

Key takeaways

☑ Precise catheter positioning is crucial for optimizing IDD efficacy, with dorsal placement offering theoretical but unproven benefits.

☑ Trialing protocols should be flexible and patient-centered, avoiding unnecessary delays in treatment.

☑ Ziconotide represents a valuable option for refractory cancer pain but requires careful management to mitigate side effects.

☑ Multimodal approaches combining opioids, local anesthetics, and ziconotide can enhance pain relief and reduce systemic toxicity. Such strategies are especially beneficial in reducing disparities in access and improving outcomes across diverse patient populations.

Additional recommended reading:

1. Brogan SE, Sindt JE, Odell DW, et al. Controversies in intrathecal drug delivery for cancer pain. *Reg Anesth Pain Med.* 2023;48:319-325.

2. Perruchoud C, Dupoiron D, Papi B, et al. Management of cancer-related pain with intrathecal drug delivery: A systematic review and meta-analysis of clinical studies. *Neuromodulation.* 2022;26(8):1142-1152.

3. Deer TR, Pope JE, Hayek SM, et al. The Polyanalgesic Consensus Conference (PACC): Recommendations for intrathecal drug infusion systems. *Neuromodulation.* 2017;20(2):96-132.

Pharmacology & Transitional Pain

Pharmacodynamic effects of co-administered cannabinoids and opioids in pain management

61

Why this topic is important

Chronic pain management increasingly incorporates multimodal strategies to address its complex pathophysiology. While opioids remain a mainstay, their long-term use is limited by risks of dependency, tolerance, and adverse effects. Cannabinoids, particularly Δ9-tetrahydrocannabinol (THC) and cannabidiol (CBD), have gained attention for their analgesic and adjunctive properties. However, their pharmacodynamic interactions with opioids pose challenges and opportunities for optimizing pain relief while minimizing harm. This update reviews findings from a scoping review by Guy et al. (2024) exploring these interactions, shedding light on their clinical implications.

Objectives of this update

- Assess the evidence on the analgesic effects of combined cannabinoids and opioids.

- Identify non-analgesic pharmacodynamic effects, including cognitive, respiratory, and cardiovascular outcomes.

- Provide insights into the clinical integration of this co-administration strategy.

What is new

- **Modest opioid-sparing effects**: Co-administered cannabinoids, particularly THC, demonstrated potential to enhance opioid analgesia, though results were inconsistent across studies.

- **Additive risks**: Combined use increases the likelihood of cognitive impairment, respiratory depression, and cardiovascular effects, particularly at higher THC doses.

- **Context-dependent outcomes**: Cannabinoid-opioid interactions were influenced by dosing regimens, routes of administration, and patient populations, highlighting the need for tailored use.

Analgesic effects

The review analyzed 16 human experimental studies, including chronic non-cancer pain (CNCP), cancer pain, and healthy volunteers exposed to nociceptive stimuli.

- **Chronic non-cancer pain (CNCP)**
  - Studies involving CNCP patients on stable opioid regimens showed mixed results. Inhaled THC reduced daily pain scores by 27% on the Visual Analog Scale (VAS).
  - Oral THC or THC-CBD preparations yielded variable results, with some studies failing to demonstrate significant pain reduction compared to placebo.

- **Cancer pain**
  - Pain improvements with oral THC-CBD combinations were inconsistent, with notable efficacy only at low doses. Higher doses did not outperform placebo.
  - Opioid consumption remained stable with cannabinoid use in some trials, suggesting potential opioid-sparing effects.

- **Experimental nociception in healthy adults**
  - Co-administration of inhaled THC and low-dose opioids increased pain thresholds and tolerance in cold-press tests, mimicking the effect of higher opioid doses.
  - However, other studies found no additive analgesic benefits when combining cannabinoids with opioids under experimental conditions.

Non-analgesic effects

- **Psychiatric and cognitive outcomes**
  - Co-administration often potentiated THC's euphoric and sedative effects, with participants reporting heightened feelings of "high" and arousal.
  - Cognitive effects included confusion and impaired memory, particularly with oral THC-CBD combinations in cancer patients.

- **Respiratory effects**
  - THC did not significantly alter the respiratory rate or oxygen saturation in CNCP patients on opioids. However, in healthy adults, IV THC reduced compensatory hyperventilation in response to hypercarbia, indicating additive respiratory depression when combined with opioids.

- **Cardiovascular effects**
  - Cannabinoids increased heart rate and reduced blood pressure through dose-dependent mechanisms. Reflex tachycardia was noted with IV THC in opioid-naïve participants.
  - Long-term use of THC-CBD combinations in chronic pain patients showed a gradual normalization of cardiovascular parameters.

- **Neuromuscular effects**
  - Increased dizziness, gait disturbances, and muscle weakness were common, especially during acute exposure. These side effects were attenuated with prolonged cannabinoid use.

- **Gastrointestinal effects**
  - Cannabinoid use frequently exacerbated nausea, vomiting, and dry mouth but had inconsistent effects on appetite.

Clinical implications

- **Potential analgesic synergy**
  - While evidence of opioid-sparing effects exists, these benefits were inconsistent across studies and settings. More robust trials are needed to confirm whether cannabinoids enhance opioid analgesia.

- **Safety concerns**
  - Cognitive impairment, respiratory de-pression, and cardiovascular instability are significant risks when co-administering these agents, particularly at higher doses.
  - Patient selection and careful dose titration are critical to minimize adverse effects.

- **Dose titration:**

  - For opioids, titration should be guided by pain relief and side effect profiles. Common agents like morphine and hydromorphone allow incremental dose adjustments to achieve optimal analgesia.

  - Cannabinoid dosing, such as THC and CBD preparations, requires a stepwise titration approach, with weekly adjustments based on therapeutic response and tolerability. Individual variability in cannabinoid metabolism underscores the need for personalized titration strategies.

- **Patient selection:**

  - Patients with chronic non-cancer pain (CNCP) or cancer pain (CCP) benefit most from combination therapy, particularly those with stable opioid regimens.

  - Careful evaluation is essential to exclude patients with psychiatric instability or contraindications to cannabinoid therapy.

  - Subgroups, such as cannabis-naïve patients, require cautious introduction to minimize adverse effects while assessing their baseline response to opioid-cannabinoid combinations.

- **Applicability to clinical practice**

  - Current evidence supports cautious co-administration of cannabinoids and opioids in patients with inadequate pain relief from monotherapy.

  - Multimodal approaches integrating non-pharmacologic strategies may optimize outcomes and reduce reliance on these agents.

Limitations

- **Study design:** Most available data come from retrospective or observational studies, limiting the ability to establish causal relationships between dose titration strategies and clinical outcomes.

- **Heterogeneity in dosing protocols:** Variability in opioid and cannabinoid titration protocols across studies complicates the generalization of findings to clinical practice.

- **Patient selection bias:** Studies often included patients with stable opioid regimens or excluded those with psychiatric comorbidities, limiting applicability to broader patient populations with more complex clinical profiles.

- **Lack of long-term data:** Evidence on the prolonged use of cannabinoid-opioid combinations and their impact on pain control, tolerance, and side effects is limited, underscoring the need for longer follow-up periods.

- **Cannabinoid variability:** Differences in THC:CBD ratios, formulations, and administration routes introduce variability in therapeutic responses, making it difficult to standardize recommendations.

- **Confounding factors:** Patient-specific factors, such as prior cannabinoid exposure, metabolic differences, and concurrent medications, may confound the observed effects of combination therapy.

Key takeaways

☑ Combined cannabinoids and opioids showed modest and inconsistent analgesic benefits, with potential opioid-sparing effects in select scenarios.

☑ Co-administration significantly increases risks of cognitive impairment, dizziness, and additive respiratory depression, particularly at high doses.

☑ Thorough patient assessment, gradual dose titration, and vigilant monitoring are essential when incorporating this approach into pain management.

☑ Robust, large-scale clinical trials are needed to fully support safety and efficacy conclusions.

Additional recommended reading:

1. Guy D, Wootten JC, Wong M, et al. Pharmacodynamic effects following co-administration of cannabinoids and opioids: A scoping review of human experimental studies. *Pain Med.* 2024;25(7):423-433.

2. Abrams DI, Couey P, Shade SB, et al. Cannabinoid-opioid interaction in chronic pain. *Clin Pharmacol Ther.* 2011;90(6):844-851.

3. Noori A, Miroshnychenko A, Shergill Y, et al. Opioid-sparing effects of medical cannabis or cannabinoids for chronic pain: a systematic review and meta-analysis of randomised and observational studies. *BMJ Open.* 2021;11(7):e047717.

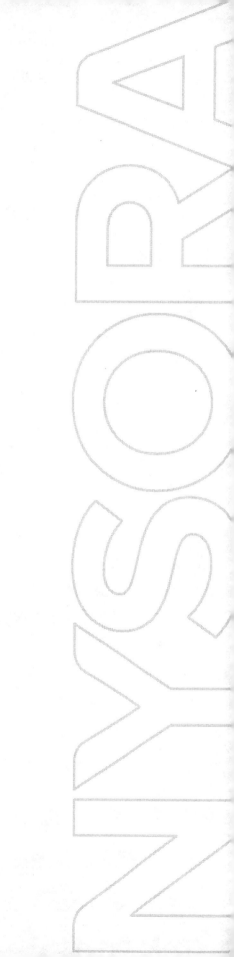

Opioid tapering in patients with chronic non-cancer pain

62

Why this topic is important

Chronic non-cancer pain (CNCP) is a prevalent condition often treated with long-term opioid therapy (LTOT). While opioids can provide short-term relief, prolonged use is associated with risks like dependency, overdose, and reduced quality of life. Efforts to taper opioids in CNCP patients have gained traction as part of deprescribing initiatives. However, understanding individual tapering patterns and factors influencing success remains critical to minimizing adverse outcomes such as withdrawal symptoms and unmanaged pain. This study by Jung et al. (2024) offers key insights into opioid tapering trajectories in patients with CNCP.

Objectives of this update

- Identify common opioid tapering trajectories among patients with CNCP.

- Examine patient-level factors associated with different tapering outcomes.

- Discuss implications for individualized tapering strategies and clinical practice.

What is new

- **Six tapering trajectories**: Groups ranged from low-dose completed tapers to high-dose noncompleted attempts, with medium-dose gradual tapers showing the highest success rates.

- **Predictors of tapering success**: Sociodemographic factors, absence of mental health comorbidities, and lower opioid doses were associated with higher tapering success.

- **Challenges in high-dose tapering**: No patients on high opioid doses completed tapering, underscoring the complexity of managing this population.

Study design

A retrospective cohort study by Jung et al. (2024) analyzed primary care data from 464 practices in Australia. It included 3,369 patients aged ≥ 19 years who initiated opioid tapering after at least six months of stable LTOT for CNCP. Tapering trajectories were tracked over 12 months.

Tapering definition

Tapering was defined as a ≥ 10% reduction in average daily oral morphine equivalents (OME) during the first 90 days post-baseline. An OME of approximately 0 mg marked completion over a rolling 90-day period.

Methods

- **Group-based trajectory modeling**: Identified distinct tapering patterns.

- **Multinomial logistic regression**: Assessed demographic, clinical, and medication-related factors influencing taper trajectories.

Key findings

Tapering trajectories

Six distinct opioid tapering trajectories emerged:

- **Low-dose completed taper** (12.9%): Patients reduced doses successfully from low starting levels (< 50 mg OME).

- **Medium-dose faster taper** (12.2%): Completed taper quickly from medium doses (50-100 mg OME).

- **Medium-dose gradual taper** (6.5%): Completed taper slowly from medium doses.

- **Low-dose noncompleted taper** (21.3%): Failed taper attempts from low doses.

- **Medium-dose noncompleted taper** (30.4%): Failed taper attempts from medium doses.

- **High-dose noncompleted taper** (16.7%): Failed taper attempts from high doses (> 100 mg OME).

Notably, no trajectory involved completed tapering from high doses.

Characteristics influencing trajectories

- **Completed tapers**

  - Patients completing gradual tapers from medium doses were more likely to reside in areas with higher socioeconomic status.

  - A lower prevalence of sleep disorders was observed in this group compared to those failing medium-dose tapers.

- **Noncompleted tapers**

  - High-dose noncompleted tapers were associated with higher rates of strong opioid use (e.g., oxycodone, morphine) and long-acting formulations.

  - Patients with high-dose noncompleted trajectories were also more likely to have concurrent depression or anxiety.

- **Faster versus gradual tapers**

  - Faster medium-dose tapers were more common than gradual tapers, although both achieved completion at similar rates.

Discussion of findings

- **Challenges of tapering high doses**

  - High-dose patients demonstrated significant challenges in achieving tapering goals, with dose levels often rebounding to near baseline.

  - The failure to identify completed high-dose tapering trajectories underscores the complexity of managing this population.

- **Socioeconomic and health disparities**

  - Patients from higher socioeconomic areas were more likely to complete gradual tapers, likely due to better access to healthcare resources and support.

- Comorbidities such as depression, anxiety, and sleep disorders increased the risk of taper failure.

- **Role of medication characteristics**

  - The use of strong or long-acting opioids correlated with tapering challenges, potentially due to higher dependency and withdrawal severity.

  - Adjusting opioid type or formulation could influence tapering success.

- **Clinical implications for tapering strategies**

  - Gradual tapering was associated with better outcomes, aligning with guidelines recommending slow reductions to minimize withdrawal and pain exacerbation.

  - Tailored approaches, including psychological and social support, are critical for high-risk groups.

Clinical implications

- **Personalized tapering plans**

  - Incorporate patient-specific factors like dose level, opioid formulation, comorbidities, and socioeconomic status into tapering strategies.

  - Gradual tapering should be prioritized, especially for patients on medium or high doses.

- **Support for high-risk patients**

  - Patients with depression, anxiety, or sleep disorders require additional psychological and pharmacological support to improve tapering outcomes.

- **Careful selection of opioids**

  - Transitioning to less potent or short-acting opioids may facilitate tapering, particularly in patients struggling with long-acting formulations.

- **Enhanced clinician-patient collaboration**

  - Open communication, shared decision-making, and regular follow-ups are vital to building trust and ensuring adherence to tapering protocols.

Limitations

- **Retrospective design**: The study's observational nature limits its ability to establish causal relationships between tapering trajectories and outcomes.

- **Data gaps**: Reliance on prescribing data needs to capture actual medication consumption or over-the-counter analgesic use, potentially underestimating concurrent therapies.

- **Incomplete referral data**: Information on whether patients accessed referred services (e.g., mental health or physiotherapy) is unavailable, which could influence tapering success.

- **Trajectory classification**: Group-based trajectory modeling forces all patients into predefined trajectories that may not reflect individual tapering patterns optimally.

- **High-dose tapers**: No completed tapering trajectories were identified for patients on high opioid doses, limiting insights into strategies for this challenging subgroup.

- **Generalizability**: The study was conducted in Australian primary care settings, and its findings may not apply to other healthcare systems with differing prescribing practices.

Key takeaways

☑ Six opioid tapering trajectories were identified, with completed tapers more common in low and medium-dose groups.

☑ High-dose tapering remains particularly challenging, with no completed trajectories observed in this cohort.

☑ Sociodemographic factors, comorbidities, and opioid characteristics strongly influence tapering outcomes.

☑ Gradual tapering, combined with tailored support, can improve the likelihood of successful opioid reduction in CNCP patients.

Additional recommended reading:

1. Jung M, Xia T, Ilomäki J, et al. Trajectories of prescription opioid tapering in patients with chronic non-cancer pain: A retrospective cohort study. *Pain Med.* 2024;25(4):263–274. doi:10.1093/pm/pnae002.

2. Dowell D, Ragan KR, Jones CM, et al. CDC clinical practice guideline for prescribing opioids for pain-United States, 2022. *MMWR Recomm Rep.* 2022;71(3):1-95.

3. Glare P, Ashton-James C, Nicholas M. Deprescribing long-term opioid therapy in patients with chronic pain. *Intern Med J.* 2020;50(10):1185-1191.

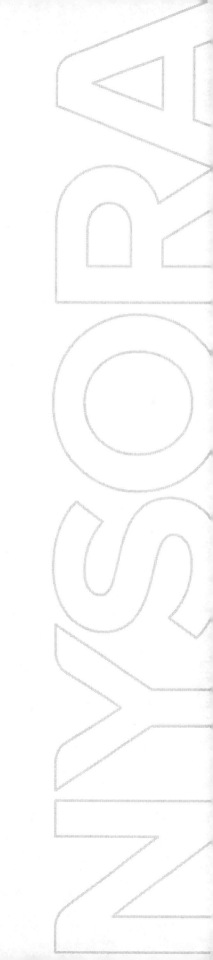

Long-term postoperative opioid use in orthopedic patients

63

Why this topic is important

Orthopedic surgeries, while often essential for restoring function, are associated with significant postoperative pain. Opioid analgesics remain a cornerstone for managing acute pain, but their use can unintentionally transition to long-term dependency, posing challenges such as tolerance, hyperalgesia, and addiction. Identifying the prevalence and predictors of prolonged opioid use is vital to refine perioperative pain management strategies, prevent long-term opioid use, and guide tapering interventions for affected patients. This study by Melis et al. (2024) investigated the long-term postoperative opioid use in orthopedic patients.

Objectives of this update

- Provide insights into the prevalence of long-term opioid use after orthopedic surgery.

- Identify risk factors associated with prolonged opioid use.

- Highlight the importance of patient education and perioperative strategies to mitigate risks.

What is new

- **High prevalence**: Approximately 12.5% of orthopedic surgery patients continued opioid use six months postoperatively.

- **Preoperative predictors**: Pre-surgical opioid use was the strongest predictor of prolonged postoperative dependency.

- **Variation by procedure**: Spine and knee surgeries were associated with the highest rates of persistent use, highlighting the need for procedure-specific interventions.

Prevalence of long-term opioid use

A 2023 prospective cohort study by Melis et al. investigated long-term opioid use in 607 patients who underwent orthopedic surgery. Key findings include:

- **Overall prevalence:**
  - 12.5% of patients reported opioid use six months post-surgery, equating to approximately one in eight patients.
  - Among these, 3.3% represented new long-term opioid users, having no prior opioid exposure before surgery.

- **By body region:**
  - Spine surgery patients exhibited the highest prevalence (28.8%), followed by knee (16.7%), upper extremity (14.3%), foot/ankle (8.1%), and hip surgeries (3.6%).

- **Opioid dosage:**
  - The median daily opioid dose at six months was 29.9 mg morphine equivalents, with a wide interquartile range (10.0-76.1 mg/day).

Risk factors for long-term opioid use

- **Preoperative opioid use:**
  - The strongest predictor of prolonged opioid use. Patients already using opioids preoperatively are significantly more likely to continue postoperatively.

- **Surgical site:**
  - Spine and knee surgeries were associated with the highest likelihood of long-term opioid use. This highlights the need for targeted strategies in these high-risk groups.

- **Pain at discharge:**
  - Higher rest pain scores at discharge showed a trend toward predicting prolonged use but did not reach statistical significance.

- **Demographics:**
  - Neither age nor gender significantly predicted long-term opioid use in this study, contrasting with some prior research.

Patient experiences and tapering willingness

Among the 76 long-term opioid users:

- **Pain and functional impairment:**
  - Mean pain scores were 4.1 at rest and 5.1 during motion, with 52.6% of patients reporting their pain as "unacceptable."
  - High levels of pain catastrophizing and disability were evident, with a mean Pain Disability Index score of 33 (on a 0-70 scale).

- **Willingness to taper:**
  - Encouragingly, 88.2% expressed a desire to reduce or discontinue opioid use.
  - Nearly half (47.8%) preferred professional support for tapering, emphasizing the need for structured interventions.

- **Targeting high-risk groups:**

  - Patients undergoing spine or knee surgeries and those using opioids preoperatively require tailored perioperative pain plans to minimize reliance on opioids.

- **Enhanced perioperative strategies:**

  - Comprehensive pain management plans, including multimodal analgesia, may reduce the need for prolonged opioid use.

  - Early recognition and management of postoperative pain and psychological factors, such as catastrophizing, can prevent the transition to chronic opioid dependence.

- **Education and support:**

  - Educating both patients and healthcare providers about the risks of prolonged opioid use and the benefits of alternative pain management strategies is critical.

  - Structured tapering programs, led by multidisciplinary teams, can aid patients in discontinuing opioids safely and effectively.

- **Prescription practices:**

  - Reevaluating standardized opioid prescriptions, especially for minor or moderate surgeries, is crucial. Evidence suggests that excessive opioid prescribing does not improve pain control but increases the risk of dependency.

Key takeaways

☑ Long-term opioid use affects 12.5% of patients after orthopedic surgery, with spine and knee procedures posing the highest risk.

☑ Preoperative opioid use is the strongest predictor of prolonged postoperative dependence.

☑ Most long-term opioid users wish to discontinue their medication, highlighting the importance of accessible tapering support.

☑ Comprehensive perioperative strategies, including patient education, multimodal analgesia, and early intervention, are essential to prevent long-term opioid use.

Additional recommended reading:

1. Melis EJ, Vriezekolk JE, van der Laan JCC, et al. Long-term postoperative opioid use in orthopedic patients. *Eur J Pain.* 2024;28(5):797-805. doi:10.1002/ejp.2219.

2. Goesling J, Moser SE, Zaidi B, et al. Trends and predictors of opioid use after total knee and total hip arthroplasty. *Pain.* 2016;157:1259-1265. doi:10.1097/j.pain.0000000000000516.

3. Simoni AH, Nikolajsen L, Olesen AE, et al. The association between initial opioid type and long-term opioid use after hip fracture surgery in elderly opioid-naive patients. *Scand J Pain.* 2020;20:755-764. doi:10.1515/sjpain-2019-0170.

Persistent opioid use following traumatic injury

64

Why this topic is important

Traumatic injuries frequently result in acute and chronic pain, with opioids serving as a primary treatment option. However, the transition to long-term opioid use is a growing concern, posing risks such as dependency, misuse, and adverse health outcomes. Understanding the prevalence and predictors of persistent opioid use after traumatic injuries, synthesized by Mauck et al. (2024), is essential to improve pain management strategies and reduce the risks associated with chronic opioid therapy.

Objectives of this update

- Assess the incidence of new persistent opioid use following common traumatic injuries.

- Identify injury-specific and patient-related risk factors contributing to prolonged opioid use.

- Highlight clinical implications for opioid stewardship and pain management after trauma.

What is new

- **High incidence in orthopedic trauma**: One in five patients with long bone fractures transitioned to chronic opioid use.

- **Risk factors**: Preoperative opioid use, injury severity, and comorbid mental health conditions were strongly associated with prolonged use.

- **Opioid-sparing strategies needed**: The findings highlight the urgency of alternative pain management approaches post-trauma.

Incidence of persistent opioid use

A large retrospective cohort study analyzed national insurance claims data from 2001 to 2020, encompassing over 173,000 patients aged 18-65 hospitalized for trauma or surgery. Persistent opioid use was defined as receiving at least one opioid prescription 90-180 days post-injury in patients who were opioid-naïve before hospitalization. Key findings include:

- **Prevalence by trauma type:**
  - **Orthopedic trauma (long bone fractures)**: 20% of patients transitioned to persistent opioid use, the highest among all groups.
  - **Motor vehicle collisions**: Persistent use occurred in 16% of patients.
  - **Burn injuries**: Persistent use was seen in 12% of patients, regardless of whether tissue grafting was required.
- **Comparison with surgical cohorts:**
  - Non-traumatic surgeries showed lower rates of persistent opioid use: 13% for ventral hernia repair (major surgery) and 9% for laparoscopic cholecystectomy (minor surgery).
- **Length of hospital stay:**
  - Patients hospitalized for more than 24 hours had significantly higher rates of persistent opioid use across all trauma types except for burn injuries requiring grafts.

Risk factors for persistent opioid use

- **Trauma-related factors:**
  - **Injury severity:** Orthopedic trauma was associated with the highest risk, reflecting the intense pain and limited alternative treatments for such injuries.
  - **Mechanism of injury:** Motor vehicle collisions and burns also carried notable risks, likely due to prolonged recovery times and post-traumatic complications.

- **Patient characteristics:**
  - **Age**: Advancing age correlated with higher rates of persistent opioid use across trauma types.
  - **Gender**: Women undergoing orthopedic surgery or non-trauma surgeries were more likely to develop persistent opioid use than men.

- **Comorbidities:**
  - Chronic pain conditions (e.g., back and joint pain) and mental health disorders, including anxiety and mood disorders, increased the likelihood of long-term opioid use.
  - Benzodiazepine use, often indicative of coexisting mental health conditions, was another risk factor.

Patterns of opioid prescribing

- **Type of opioids:**
  - Nearly all patients with persistent opioid use (95.9%) were prescribed short-acting opioids, such as hydrocodone (49%), oxycodone (20%), and tramadol (12%).
  - Long-acting opioids were rarely used (3.4%), reflecting prescribing trends aimed at minimizing dependency risks.

- **Daily morphine milligram equivalents (MMEs):**
  - The highest daily opioid doses were seen in orthopedic trauma patients (71 MMEs), followed by burn injuries (67 MMEs) and motor vehicle collisions (64 MMEs).
  - Patients with hospital stays exceeding 24 hours consistently received higher MMEs across all groups.

Clinical implications

- **Opioid stewardship in trauma care:**
  - High rates of persistent opioid use among trauma patients underscore the need for tailored pain management strategies that prioritize alternatives like regional anesthesia, physical therapy, and non-opioid analgesics.
  - Trauma care teams must adopt standardized prescribing practices to limit unnecessary opioid exposure during recovery.

- **Screening for risk factors:**
  - Identifying patients at high risk for persistent use-such as those with preexisting mental health conditions or chronic pain-can inform targeted interventions.

- Addressing mental health comorbidities and offering multidisciplinary support can reduce reliance on opioids post-trauma.

- **Policy and education:**
  - Enhanced provider education on opioid prescribing and robust monitoring systems can ensure adherence to evidence-based guidelines.
  - Policymakers should focus on expanding access to non-opioid pain management options for trauma patients.

Key takeaways

☑ One in five patients hospitalized for orthopedic trauma develops persistent opioid use, with significant rates also observed after motor vehicle collisions (16%) and burn injuries (12%).

☑ Risk factors for long-term opioid use include severe injuries, longer hospital stays, advancing age, female gender, and comorbid chronic pain or mental health conditions.

☑ Short-acting opioids remain the most commonly prescribed, but efforts are needed to reduce dependency through multimodal and non-opioid analgesia.

☑ Comprehensive opioid stewardship programs and early interventions for high-risk patients can improve outcomes and minimize long-term risks.

Additional recommended reading:

1. Mauck MC, Zhao Y, Goetzinger AM, et al. Incidence of persistent opioid use following traumatic injury. *Reg Anesth Pain Med.* 2024;49:79-86. doi:10.1136/rapm-2022-103662.

2. Brummett CM, Waljee JF, Goesling J, et al. New persistent opioid use after minor and major surgical procedures in US adults. *JAMA Surg.* 2017;152:e170504. doi:10.1001/jamasurg.2017.0504.

3. Rosenbloom BN, McCartney CJL, Canzian S, et al. Predictors of prescription opioid use after traumatic musculoskeletal injury: A prospective study. *J Pain.* 2017;18:956-963. doi:10.1016/j.jpain.2017.04.004.

Transitional pain services and postoperative opioid trajectories

65

Why this topic is important

Chronic opioid use after surgery poses significant risks, including dependency, overdose, and reduced quality of life. Addressing these challenges requires effective perioperative pain management strategies. Transitional pain services (TPS) provide multidisciplinary care, bridging acute postoperative pain management with long-term recovery. This update reviews findings from a retrospective cohort study by Ladha et al. (2024) evaluating TPS's role in reducing opioid use after major surgery.

Objectives of this update

- Assess the impact of TPS on postoperative opioid use trajectories.

- Highlight the mechanisms through which TPS facilitates opioid dose reduction.

- Explore implications for implementing TPS in diverse healthcare settings.

What is new

- **Accelerated opioid tapering**: TPS patients achieved significantly faster reductions in opioid doses compared to standard care.

- **Benefits for high-risk patients**: TPS effectively managed patients requiring higher opioid doses immediately post-surgery, minimizing risks of chronic use.

- **Multimodal approach**: Psychological support and multimodal analgesia were integral to TPS success, emphasizing comprehensive care.

Postoperative opioid use and the role of TPS

Background

A significant proportion of surgical patients experience persistent pain and continue using opioids months after discharge. Studies estimate that preoperative opioid use, severe postoperative pain, and lack of follow-up care contribute to this transition. TPS, first implemented at Toronto General Hospital, involves chronic pain specialists, psychologists, and physiotherapists who manage high-risk patients through multimodal analgesia and psychological support.

Study findings

The study compared opioid use in 209 patients enrolled in TPS to a matched cohort of surgical patients receiving standard care at other academic hospitals in Ontario. Key outcomes included reductions in daily opioid doses measured in morphine milligram equivalents (MME).

- **Opioid dose trajectories:**
  - TPS patients achieved a mean monthly reduction of 3.53 MME, significantly faster than the control group's reduction of 1.1 MME per month.
  - The difference-in-difference analysis showed a 2.5 MME monthly advantage for TPS patients.

- **Baseline and early postoperative use:**
  - TPS patients required higher doses immediately post-surgery (mean 46.5 MME) compared to controls (12.7 MME).
  - Despite the higher initial use, TPS patients reached baseline levels faster than controls.

- **Stratified analysis:**
  - Patients without prior opioid prescriptions showed similar trends, highlighting TPS's effectiveness for opioid-naïve individuals.

Mechanisms driving TPS effectiveness

- **Multimodal analgesia:**
  - Combining pharmacologic (e.g., nerve blocks, non-opioid analgesics) and non-pharmacologic (e.g., physical therapy, psychological interventions) methods minimizes opioid reliance.

- **Psychological support:**
  - Acceptance and commitment therapy (ACT) and counseling address anxiety, catastrophizing, and maladaptive behaviors that exacerbate pain perception.

- **Patient education:**
  - TPS emphasizes opioid tapering, pain coping strategies, and realistic expectations for recovery, empowering patients to engage actively in their pain management.

- **Tailored interventions:**
  - Regular follow-ups and individualized care plans adapt to each patient's progress, addressing unique challenges in recovery.

Clinical implications

- **Faster opioid weaning:**
  - TPS reduces opioid use more rapidly than standard care, benefiting high-risk patients who might otherwise transition to chronic opioid dependency.

- **Addressing high postoperative doses:**
  - By intervening early in patients requiring higher opioid doses post-surgery, TPS can mitigate risks associated with prolonged use.

- **Adoption in diverse settings:**
  - While this study involved high-acuity academic centers, scaling TPS to community hospitals requires adapting resource-intensive elements like psychological care.

- **Cost-effectiveness:**
  - Reducing persistent opioid use and associated complications may offset the upfront costs of implementing TPS programs, highlighting their potential value in broader healthcare systems.

Key takeaways

☑ Transitional pain services significantly accelerate opioid dose reduction after surgery, particularly in high-risk patients.

☑ Multimodal strategies, psychological support, and patient education underpin TPS's effectiveness.

☑ Scaling TPS to diverse settings requires addressing resource and infrastructure barriers, but its benefits may justify these investments.

Additional recommended reading:

1. Ladha KS, Vachhani K, Gabriel G, et al. Impact of a Transitional Pain Service on postoperative opioid trajectories: A retrospective cohort study. *Reg Anesth Pain Med.* 2024;49:650-655. doi:10.1136/rapm-2023-104709.

2. Clarke H, Azargive S, Montbriand J, et al. Opioid weaning and pain management in postsurgical patients at the Toronto General Hospital Transitional Pain Service. *Can J Pain.* 2018;2:236-247. doi:10.1080/24740527.2018.1501669.

3. Vetter TR, Kain ZN. Role of the perioperative surgical home in optimizing the perioperative use of opioids. *Anesth Analg.* 2017;125:1653-1657. doi:10.1213/ANE.0000000000002280.

Low-dose naltrexone for centralized pain conditions

66

Why this topic is important

Centralized pain syndromes, including fibromyalgia, complex regional pain syndrome (CRPS), and diabetic neuropathy, are challenging to manage due to their multifactorial pathophysiology and limited treatment options. Traditional therapies, such as antidepressants and anticonvulsants, often yield suboptimal results or cause significant side effects. Low-dose naltrexone (LDN), an opioid receptor antagonist with immunomodulatory properties, has emerged as a novel therapeutic option. This update synthesizes findings by Rupp et al. (2023) on LDN's efficacy and safety in managing centralized pain syndromes.

Objectives of this update

- Evaluate the evidence for LDN's effectiveness in reducing pain and improving functional outcomes in centralized pain syndromes.

- Review its mechanisms of action and safety profile.

- Discuss clinical implications for integrating LDN into chronic pain management.

What is new

- **Neuropathic pain relief**: Significant reductions in pain and disability were observed in fibromyalgia, CRPS, and diabetic neuropathy, with responder rates exceeding 30% in several studies.

- **Immunomodulatory benefits**: LDN's ability to inhibit glial activation and reduce inflammatory cytokines was linked to clinical improvements.

- **Favorable safety profile**: LDN was well-tolerated, with minimal side effects compared to traditional therapies.

Mechanisms of action

At low doses (1-4.5 mg), naltrexone exerts a paradoxical effect, shifting from opioid receptor antagonism to modulating toll-like receptor 4 (TLR4) on microglial cells. This action suppresses the production of pro-inflammatory cytokines and neuropeptides implicated in central sensitization. By disrupting the inflammatory cascade, LDN reduces hyperalgesia and allodynia, hallmarks of centralized pain syndromes.

Key findings

Fibromyalgia

- **Pain reduction:**

  ○ A pilot trial demonstrated a 32.5% reduction in overall symptom severity with LDN compared to 2.3% with placebo over 8 weeks. Patients also reported improvements in fatigue, stress, and gastrointestinal symptoms.

  ○ A larger follow-up study reported a 28.8% pain reduction in LDN-treated patients versus 18.0% in the placebo group over 12 weeks.

- **Inflammatory modulation:**

  ○ LDN was associated with reduced pro-inflammatory cytokine levels, correlating with clinical improvements.

Complex regional pain syndrome (CRPS)

- **Case reports:**

  ○ A series of case reports documented significant pain relief with LDN (3.0-4.5 mg/day), with patients experiencing a reduction in Numeric Rating Scale (NRS) scores from 10/10 to 3/10 within weeks.

  ○ In one case, a patient with CRPS refractory to conventional treatments regained ambulation and reported complete pain resolution after 16 months of LDN.

- **Mechanistic insights:**

  ○ Histopathological analyses revealed microglial activation in CRPS patients, supporting LDN's mechanism of targeting glial-mediated inflammation.

Diabetic neuropathy

1. **RCT findings:**

  ○ A randomized trial compared LDN (2-4 mg) to amitriptyline in patients with painful diabetic neuropathy. Both treatments significantly reduced pain, but LDN exhibited a superior safety profile.

  ○ Case studies highlighted rapid pain reduction, with some patients reporting Visual Analog Scale (VAS) scores decreasing from 9/10 to 0.5/10 after 2 weeks of treatment.

Safety and tolerability

- **Common side effects:**

  ○ Mild and transient side effects such as vivid dreams, nausea, and headaches were reported.

  ○ Severe adverse events were rare, with most patients tolerating the medication well after dose adjustments.

- **Contraindications and considerations:**

  ○ Caution is required when prescribing LDN to patients concurrently using opioid agonists, as competitive receptor antagonism can reduce opioid efficacy.

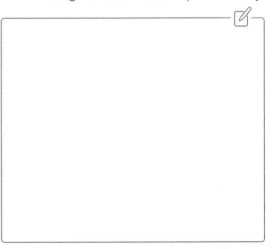

Limitations

- **Study design**: Evidence is limited by small sample sizes, observational designs, and few randomized controlled trials (RCTs).

- **Patient selection**: Lack of standardized inclusion criteria and data on patient-specific factors introduces heterogeneity.

- **Dosing variability**: Inconsistent protocols for starting doses and titration complicate efficacy assessment.

- **Long-Term data**: Limited research on the safety, durability of pain relief, and quality-of-life improvements beyond 12-16 weeks.

- **Mechanistic gaps**: Theoretical mechanisms, such as glial modulation, lack direct clinical correlation.

- **Reporting bias**: Publication bias may overstate efficacy due to the prominence of positive case reports.

Clinical implications

- **Expanding treatment options:**
  - LDN offers a novel mechanism of action distinct from traditional neuropathic pain medications, making it a valuable addition for patients with refractory pain.

- **Tailored dosing:**
  - While 4.5 mg/day is the most commonly studied dose, evidence supports efficacy at doses as low as 1 mg, enabling flexibility based on patient response and tolerability.

- **Integrative approach:**
  - Combining LDN with physical therapy and cognitive-behavioral interventions may maximize benefits for patients with centralized pain.

- **Implementation challenges**
  - Variability in dosing regimens, insurance coverage, and the need for specialized training to monitor and manage side effects present barriers to implementation.

Key takeaways

- ☑ LDN demonstrates significant efficacy in reducing pain and associated symptoms in fibromyalgia, CRPS, and diabetic neuropathy.

- ☑ Its immunomodulatory effects target central sensitization, addressing an underlying mechanism of centralized pain.

- ☑ The favorable safety profile and minimal side effects make LDN a promising option for chronic pain management.

- ☑ Further large-scale, randomized trials are necessary to standardize dosing regimens and establish long-term outcomes.

Additional recommended reading:

1. Rupp A, Young E, Chadwick AL. Low-dose naltrexone's utility for non-cancer centralized pain conditions: A scoping review. *Pain Med.* 2023;24(11):1270-1281. doi:10.1093/pm/pnad074.

2. Younger J, Mackey S. Fibromyalgia symptoms are reduced by low-dose naltrexone: A pilot study. *Pain Med.* 2009;10(4):663-672. doi:10.1111/j.1526-4637.2009.00613.x.

3. Srinivasan A, Dutta P, Hota D. Efficacy and safety of low-dose naltrexone in painful diabetic neuropathy: A randomized, double-blind, active-control, crossover trial. *J Diabetes.* 2021;13(10):770-778. doi:10.1111/1753-0407.13202.

Duloxetine for managing central post-stroke pain

67

Why this topic is important

Central post-stroke pain (CPSP) is a challenging neuropathic condition affecting 1-12% of stroke survivors. Characterized by persistent pain localized to areas corresponding to brain lesions, CPSP significantly impairs quality of life. Current treatment options, including tricyclic antidepressants and anticonvulsants, are often limited by suboptimal efficacy and side effects. Duloxetine, a serotonin-norepinephrine reuptake inhibitor (SNRI), has shown promise in managing other neuropathic pain conditions, making it a potential therapeutic option for CPSP. This update evaluates findings from a randomized trial by Manesh et al. (2023) assessing duloxetine's efficacy and safety for this debilitating condition.

Objectives of this update

- Examine the efficacy of duloxetine in reducing pain intensity in CPSP patients.

- Highlight secondary benefits on pain-related disability and patient-reported outcomes.

- Discuss the safety and tolerability of duloxetine in the context of CPSP management.

What is new

- **Superior pain relief:** Duloxetine significantly reduced pain intensity compared to placebo, with 80.5% of patients achieving meaningful improvement.

- **Improved disability:** Pain-related disability scores and patient-reported outcomes, such as quality of life, were notably enhanced with duloxetine treatment.

- **Tolerable side effects:** While mild side effects like dizziness and nausea occurred, no serious adverse events were reported.

Study design

This single-center, double-blind, randomized controlled trial was conducted at a tertiary care institute in India. Eighty-two patients meeting the inclusion criteria for CPSP were randomized into duloxetine (30-60 mg/day) or placebo groups for four weeks. Participants were aged ≥ 18 years, with unilateral brain lesions confirmed by imaging and moderate-to-severe pain (≥ 4 on the Numeric Rating Scale [NRS]).

Outcomes

- **Primary outcome:** Change in pain intensity measured by NRS from baseline to four weeks.
- **Secondary outcomes:** Changes in pain severity (Short-form McGill Pain Questionnaire-2 [SFMPQ-2]), pain-related disability (Pain Disability Index [PDI]), and global improvement (Patient Global Impression of Change [PGIC]).

Key findings

- **Pain reduction**
  - Duloxetine significantly reduced pain compared to placebo. Mean NRS scores decreased from 6.5 to 3.0 in the duloxetine group versus 6.4 to 4.4 in the placebo group.
  - The duloxetine group's responder rate (≥ 2-point NRS reduction) was significantly higher (80.5%) than the placebo group's (43.9%).

- **Pain-related disability**
  - PDI scores improved significantly in the duloxetine group, dropping from 43.0 to 24.18, compared to 42.1 to 30.1 in the placebo group.
  - Improvements spanned multiple life domains, including family responsibilities, recreation, and self-care.

- **Global improvement**
  - PGIC scores, reflecting patients' perception of overall improvement, were significantly higher in the duloxetine group (5.2) than placebo (3.9).

- **Safety and tolerability**
  - Common side effects included dizziness (17.1%), somnolence (14.6%), and nausea (14.6%), occurring more frequently in the duloxetine group.
  - One patient discontinued due to vomiting. No serious adverse events were reported.

Mechanisms of action

Duloxetine modulates serotonin and nore-pinephrine levels, affecting pain processing at multiple levels of the central nervous system, including the thalamus and descending inhibitory pathways. Additional mechanisms, such as blocking late sodium channel currents implicated in painful channelopathies, may also contribute to its analgesic effects.

Clinical implications

- **Efficacy in CPSP**
  - Duloxetine offers a meaningful reduction in pain and associated disability, positioning it as an effective option for managing moderate-to-severe CPSP.
  - High responder rates suggest potential benefits in patients unresponsive to traditional treatments.

- **Safety considerations**
  - Duloxetine's tolerability aligns with its established profile in neuropathic pain management. Monitoring for common side effects can enhance adherence and patient satisfaction.

- **Integration into practice**
  - Duloxetine may serve as a first-line or adjunctive treatment for CPSP, complementing rehabilitation strategies.

- **Future research**
  - Long-term studies are needed to evaluate sustained benefits and identify predictors of response.

Key takeaways

☑ Duloxetine significantly reduces pain intensity and disability in CPSP patients, with a high responder rate (80.5%) compared to placebo.

☑ Secondary benefits include improved patient-reported outcomes and quality of life, as measured by PGIC scores.

☑ While generally well-tolerated, typical side effects like dizziness and nausea should be managed proactively.

☑ Duloxetine's unique dual action on serotonin and norepinephrine pathways offers distinct advantages in CPSP management.

Additional recommended reading:

1. Manesh B, Singh VK, Pathak A, et al. Efficacy of duloxetine in patients with central post-stroke pain: A randomized double-blind placebo-controlled trial. *Pain Med.* 2023;24(6):610-617. doi:10.1093/pm/pnac182.

2. Vranken JH, Hollmann MW, van der Vegt MH, et al. Duloxetine in patients with central neuropathic pain caused by spinal cord injury or stroke: A randomized, double-blind, placebo-controlled trial. *Pain.* 2011;152(2):267-273. doi:10.1016/j.pain.2010.09.005.

3. Klit H, Finnerup NB, Jensen TS. Central post-stroke pain: Clinical characteristics, pathophysiology, and management. *Lancet Neurol.* 2009;8(9):857-868. doi:10.1016/S1474-4422(09)70176-0.

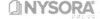

Soticlestat as adjunctive therapy for complex regional pain syndrome

68

Why this topic is important

Complex regional pain syndrome (CRPS) is a debilitating condition characterized by chronic pain, autonomic dysfunction, and sensory abnormalities. Despite an interdisciplinary treatment approach, managing CRPS effectively remains challenging. Soticlestat, a novel cholesterol 24-hydroxylase inhibitor, has shown potential in targeting central sensitization, a key pathophysiological mechanism in CRPS. This study by Ratcliffe et al. (2023) explores the efficacy and safety of soticlestat as an adjunctive therapy in CRPS, offering insights into its potential role in improving patient outcomes.

Objectives of this update

- Evaluate the efficacy of soticlestat in reducing pain intensity and improving functional outcomes in CRPS patients.

- Discuss the safety profile and tolerability of soticlestat in this patient population.

- Highlight key findings and limitations of this pilot study.

What is new

- **Limited efficacy**: Soticlestat did not significantly reduce pain intensity or improve functional outcomes compared to placebo.

- **Targeted mechanisms**: The drug effectively reduced 24-hydroxycholesterol levels, though this pharmacodynamic action did not translate into clinical benefits in chronic CRPS.

- **Safety considerations**: Soticlestat was generally safe, though one severe psychiatric event highlights the need for close monitoring.

Study design

This phase 2a randomized, double-blind, placebo-controlled trial by Ratcliffe et al. (2023) was conducted at two sites in the UK. Twenty-four adults with chronic CRPS (symptoms persisting ≥ 6 months) were randomized 2:1 to receive soticlestat or placebo for 15 weeks, followed by a 14-week open-label extension. Soticlestat was titrated from 100 mg twice daily to 300 mg during maintenance.

Participants

Inclusion criteria required CRPS diagnosis based on Budapest Criteria, moderate-to-severe pain (≥ 4 on an 11-point Numeric Pain Scale [NPS]), and prior failure of standard therapies. Patients with unstable medical conditions or recent ketamine use were excluded.

Outcome measures

- **Primary outcome**: Change in mean 24-hour NPS pain intensity score from baseline to week 15.
- **Secondary outcomes:**
  - Percentage of responders achieving ≥ 30% reduction in NPS score.
  - Changes in quality of life using the PROMIS-29 questionnaire.
  - Patient Global Impression of Change (PGIC) scores.
  - CRPS Severity Score (CSS).
- **Safety endpoints**: Adverse events, lab results, and vital signs.

Key findings

- **Pain intensity**
  - Soticlestat showed a mean change in 24-hour NPS score of -0.75 compared to -0.41 in the placebo group, yielding a non-significant placebo-adjusted difference of -0.34.
- **Responder rates**
  - At week 15, 26.7% of soticlestat patients and 22.2% of placebo patients achieved ≥ 30% pain reduction, indicating no statistically significant difference.

- **Quality of life**
  - Improvements in PROMIS-29 domains, such as physical function and participation in social roles, were observed but were comparable between the soticlestat and placebo groups.
- **Safety profile**
  - Most treatment-emergent adverse events (TEAEs) were mild or moderate, with dizziness, headache, and nausea being the most common.
  - One participant discontinued due to severe depression and suicidal ideation, considered related to soticlestat.

Discussion of findings

- **Efficacy limitations**
  - Soticlestat did not significantly reduce pain intensity or improve responder rates compared to placebo.
  - The small sample size, high baseline variability, and advanced CRPS duration in the soticlestat group may have confounded results.
- **Mechanistic insights**
  - Soticlestat targets central sensitization by modulating NMDA receptor activity. While it lowered plasma 24-hydroxycholesterol levels, this pharmacodynamic effect did not translate into significant clinical benefits in this trial.
- **Safety considerations**
  - The overall safety profile was consistent with previous studies. However, the severe psychiatric event emphasizes the need for careful monitoring in future trials.
- **Potential in early-stage CRPS**
  - Given the pathophysiological emphasis on neurogenic inflammation early in CRPS, soticlestat may hold greater promise for newly diagnosed patients.

Clinical implications

- **Limited current applicability**
  - Soticlestat is not currently recommended for chronic CRPS management due to insufficient evidence of efficacy in this study.

- **Patient selection**
  - Future research should prioritize patients with early-stage CRPS, where soticlestat's mechanisms may better align with active disease processes.

- **Need for larger trials**
  - Adequately powered studies with diverse CRPS populations are necessary to validate these findings and refine patient selection criteria.

Key takeaways

- ☑ During this pilot study, Soticlestat did not significantly reduce pain or improve clinical outcomes in chronic CRPS patients.

- ☑ While generally safe, one severe psychiatric event highlights the need for close monitoring.

- ☑ Further research is needed to explore its potential role in early-stage CRPS and other neuropathic pain conditions.

Additional recommended reading:

1. Ratcliffe S, Arkilo D, Asgharnejad M, et al. The efficacy and safety of soticlestat as adjunctive therapy in adults with complex regional pain syndrome: A randomized controlled study. *Pain Med.* 2023;24(7):872-880. doi:10.1093/pm/pnac198.

2. Harden RN, Oaklander AL, Burton AW, et al. Complex regional pain syndrome: Practical diagnostic and treatment guidelines, 5th edition. *Pain Med.* 2022;23(Suppl 1):S1-S53. doi:10.1093/pm/pnab228.

3. Zhao J, Wang Y, Wang D. The effect of ketamine infusion in the treatment of complex regional pain syndrome: A systematic review and meta-analysis. *Curr Pain Headache Rep.* 2018;22(2):12. doi:10.1007/s11916-018-0666-5.

Analgesic properties of anti-osteoporotic drugs

69

Why this topic is important

Osteoporosis, characterized by diminished bone density and increased fracture risk, affects a significant portion of the aging population. Pain is a frequent and debilitating symptom in osteoporotic patients, often linked to fractures and structural changes in bone. Beyond fracture prevention, emerging evidence suggests that some anti-osteoporotic drugs may possess inherent analgesic properties, offering dual benefits of bone health improvement and pain reduction. Understanding these properties can guide therapeutic choices, improve quality of life, and reduce reliance on traditional analgesics. This review by Pickering et al. (2024) synthesizes the latest evidence on the analgesic effects of anti-osteoporotic drugs.

Objectives of this update

- Examine the evidence for pain relief associated with anti-osteoporotic medications.

- Review mechanisms underlying the analgesic effects of these drugs.

- Provide clinical insights into optimizing treatment strategies for osteoporosis with concurrent pain management.

What is new

- **Pain reduction**: Bisphosphonates and teriparatide demonstrated significant analgesic effects in osteoporotic patients with vertebral fractures.

- **Mechanistic insights**: Pain relief correlated with reduced inflammatory cytokines and osteoclast activity, linking bone health improvements to neuropathic pain modulation.

- **Clinical relevance**: These findings suggest that drug selection in osteoporosis treatment should consider analgesic properties alongside bone density improvement.

Mechanisms of pain in osteoporosis

Osteoporotic pain arises from peripheral and central sensitization triggered by structural bone damage and inflammation.

- **Peripheral drivers**: Fractures disrupt sensory nerve fibers in bone, leading to local acidosis and activation of pain-inducing ion channels such as acid-sensing ion channels (ASICs) and transient receptor potential vanilloid (TRPV1).

- **Central sensitization**: Chronic pain states involve upregulated neurotransmitters, glial cell activation, and descending pain pathway modulation. These processes sustain pain even after structural healing.

- **Inflammatory factors**: Osteoclast activity and osteocyte signaling contribute to pain via neuropeptide release, including nerve growth factor (NGF) and cytokines like tumor necrosis factor-alpha (TNF-α).

Study scope

A scoping review by Pickering et al. (2023) analyzed 31 studies (12 randomized controlled trials [RCTs], 19 observational studies) focusing on pain as a primary or secondary outcome. Drugs assessed included bisphosphonates, denosumab, selective estrogen receptor modulators (SERMs), anabolic agents (e.g., teriparatide), and newer therapies like romosozumab. Many studies included 100% female participants, focusing on postmenopausal osteoporosis and the effects of drugs like bisphosphonates, raloxifene, and teriparatide, reflecting the condition's link to hormonal changes and fracture risk.

Bisphosphonates

- **Mechanism**: Inhibit osteoclast activity, reducing inflammatory cytokines and preventing osteocyte apoptosis.

- **Clinical findings**:
  - Multiple studies showed significant reductions in back pain scores among patients with vertebral fractures.
  - In an RCT, alendronate and calcitonin significantly reduced pain compared to calcium alone.
  - Zoledronate significantly improved overall symptom scores, including pain and standing pain, at 1 year and maintained significant improvements in overall symptoms and pain at 3 years in patients with clinical fractures.

Denosumab

- **Mechanism**: Inhibits receptor activator of nuclear factor kappa-α ligand (RANKL), directly decreasing osteoclastogenesis and associated inflammatory signaling.

- **Clinical findings**:
  - Improved pain-related quality of life in multiple studies, particularly for patients with vertebral fractures.
  - Observational data suggest pain reduction correlates with decreased bone resorption markers.

Selective estrogen receptor modulators (SERMs)

- **Mechanism**: Modulate estrogen pathways, reducing cytokine production and osteoclast activity.

- **Clinical findings**:
  - Raloxifene significantly reduced skeletal pain and analgesic use in a six-month study.
  - Improvements in sleep quality and physical functioning accompanied pain relief.

Anabolic agents (e.g., teriparatide)

- **Mechanism**: Promote bone formation by stimulating osteoblast activity and increasing bone mass.

- **Clinical findings:**

  - Teriparatide showed consistent reductions in back pain intensity across multiple RCTs.

  - A study comparing teriparatide and bisphosphonates found greater pain reduction with teriparatide over 18 months.

  - Pain relief was particularly significant in patients with new vertebral fractures.

Newer agents (romosozumab)

- **Mechanism:** Targets sclerostin to simultaneously inhibit bone resorption and promote formation.

- **Clinical findings:**

  - Emerging data suggest that romosozumab may alleviate pain by improving bone microarchitecture and reducing local inflammatory signaling.

  - Further research is required to confirm its analgesic properties.

Key takeaways

☑ Anti-osteoporotic drugs provide dual benefits of bone health improvement and pain relief, particularly in patients with vertebral fractures.

☑ Teriparatide, bisphosphonates, and denosumab show the most consistent analgesic effects, with teriparatide excelling in acute fracture-related pain.

☑ Combining mechanistic understanding with patient-specific factors, such as fracture history and pain intensity, can optimize therapeutic choices.

☑ Future research should address gaps in the literature, including standardized pain assessment and dose optimization.

Clinical implications

- **Treatment selection:**

  - Anti-osteoporotic drugs with proven analgesic effects, such as teriparatide and bisphosphonates, should be prioritized for patients with concurrent osteoporosis and significant pain.

  - Denosumab offers a suitable alternative for those unable to tolerate bisphosphonates.

- **Mechanism-based therapy:**

  - Understanding the specific pain pathways affected by each drug can guide tailored therapy. For example, teriparatide is more effective for acute fracture-related pain, while bisphosphonates and denosumab may provide longer-term relief.

- **Adjunctive strategies:**

  - Combining anti-osteoporotic drugs with physical therapy and non-opioid analgesics may enhance outcomes.

  - Addressing central sensitization through psychological and pharmacological interventions can further improve quality of life.

- **Monitoring and follow-up:**

  - Regular assessment of pain and quality-of-life metrics ensures timely adjustments to therapy.

  - Attention to adverse effects, such as gastro-intestinal symptoms or rare complications like jaw osteonecrosis, is essential for patient safety.

Additional recommended reading:

1. Pickering M-E, Javier R-M, Malochet S, et al. Osteoporosis treatment and pain relief: A scoping review. *Eur J Pain.* 2024;28(1):3-20. doi:10.1002/ejp.2156.

2. Sambrook PN, Geusens P, Ribot C, et al. Zoledronic acid efficacy and safety in postmenopausal women with osteoporosis: A randomized trial. *J Bone Miner Res.* 2011;26(1):183-190. doi:10.1002/jbmr.243.

3. Hadji P, Zanchetta JR, Russo L, et al. Teriparatide reduces back pain in postmenopausal women with osteoporosis: An 18-month study. *Bone.* 2012;50(3):579-585. doi:10.1016/j.bone.2011.10.003.

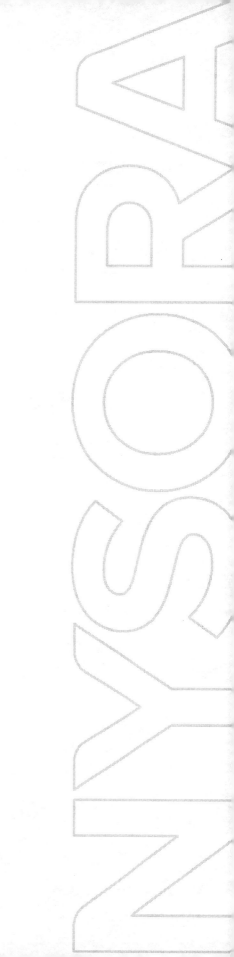

Prescribing patterns in older adults with chronic non-cancer pain

70

Why this topic is important

Chronic non-cancer pain (CNCP) significantly impacts the quality of life in older adults, leading to decreased mobility, increased rates of depression and anxiety, and a heavy societal economic burden. Pain management in this population is challenging due to the coexistence of multiple chronic conditions, high medication use (polypharmacy), and increased susceptibility to adverse drug events. Understanding prescribing patterns in CNCP patients can highlight gaps in care, improve medication safety, and inform clinical decisions to optimize pain management. This study by Goetschi et al. (2024) provides insights into prescribing patterns in older adults with CNCP.

Objectives of this update

- Examine the prevalence of CNCP in older adults with polypharmacy.

- Identify prescribing trends and potentially inappropriate drug combinations in this population.

- Assess patient complexity and implications for optimizing pain management in older adults.

What is new

- **Polypharmacy prevalence**: Older adults with CNCP were prescribed more medications, including higher doses of opioids and co-analgesics, compared to non-CNCP peers.

- **Inappropriate combinations**: High rates of opioid-hypnotic and opioid-gabapentinoid co-prescriptions raise safety concerns.

- **Variations by age:** Patients aged 85+ were more likely to receive paracetamol and lower opioid doses, reflecting tailored prescribing practices.

Prevalence of CNCP in older adults

A four-year study by Goetschi et al. (2024) analyzed data from 20,422 hospital discharges of patients aged 65 and older in Switzerland.

- **Overall prevalence**: CNCP affected 9.7% of older adult inpatients.

- **Prevalence by age group**: Prevalence rose to 11.3% among those aged 85 and older (the "oldest old").

Prescribing trends for CNCP patients

Patients with CNCP exhibited notable differences in medication use compared to their counterparts without CNCP.

- **Analgesic use**

  ◦ CNCP patients were prescribed a median of two analgesics, compared to one in non-CNCP patients.

  ◦ Potent opioids were prescribed to 28.6% of CNCP patients versus 9.6% of non-CNCP patients.

  ◦ Paracetamol was more commonly used in CNCP patients (75.8%) than non-CNCP patients (67.9%).

- **Opioid dosage**

  ◦ CNCP patients were more likely to receive high morphine milligram equivalents (MMEs). Notably, 22.8% received MMEs > 90 mg/day, compared to 7.8% in non-CNCP patients.

- **Co-analgesics**

  ◦ Gabapentinoids were prescribed to 14.1% of CNCP patients versus 5.0% of non-CNCP patients.

  ◦ Tricyclic antidepressants (TCAs) and serotonin-norepinephrine reuptake in-hibitors (SNRIs) were also more common in CNCP patients.

- **Potentially inappropriate combinations**

  ◦ Co-prescription of opioids and hypnotics (e.g., benzodiazepines or Z-drugs) occurred in 24.5% of CNCP patients, raising concerns about increased respiratory depression and mortality risks.

  ◦ Opioid and gabapentinoid combinations were also higher in CNCP patients (8.6% vs. 2.2%), further elevating the risk of sedation and overdose.

Variations in prescribing among the oldest old

Patients aged 85 and older exhibited distinct prescribing trends compared to those aged 65-84:

- **Lower use of potent opioids, NSAIDs, and co-analgesics**: This may reflect concerns about adverse drug events, including gastrointestinal bleeding and renal impairment.

- **Increased paracetamol use**: Paracetamol was prescribed to 78.9% of the oldest old CNCP patients, compared to 74.4% in the younger group.

- **Reduced MMEs**: High-dose opioids (> 90 MME) were prescribed less frequently in the oldest old (18.6% vs. 24.6%).

Patient complexity and comorbidities

Patients with CNCP demonstrated higher complexity and more comorbid conditions than those without CNCP:

- **Polypharmacy**

  ◦ CNCP patients had a median of 11 prescribed medications versus 9 in non-CNCP patients.

- **Comorbidities**

  ◦ CNCP patients were more likely to have inflammatory diseases (15.3% vs. 9.4%), liver failure (9.1% vs. 6.3%), and psychiatric disorders (33.8% vs. 23.5%).

- **Physical and cognitive deficits**

  - CNCP patients exhibited more significant impairments in physical function, with a median deficit index of 0.18 compared to 0.11 in non-CNCP patients.

  - Cognitive deficits were also more pronounced, emphasizing the need for individualized care plans.

Clinical implications

- **Addressing over-reliance on opioids**

  - The high prevalence of opioid prescriptions and excessive dosages in CNCP patients underscores the need for alternative strategies, such as non-pharmacological interventions and multimodal analgesia.

- **Reducing potentially inappropriate com-binations**

  - Co-prescription of opioids with hypnotics or gabapentinoids requires careful review to mitigate risks of respiratory depression and overdose.

- **Optimizing pain management in the oldest patients**

  - For patients aged 85 and older, emphasis on safer analgesics like paracetamol and reducing polypharmacy may prevent adverse outcomes. However, under-treatment of pain in this group should also be avoided.

- **Tailored interventions for complex patients**

  - The elevated comorbid burden and functional deficits in CNCP patients necessitate comprehensive care plans, including regular medication reviews and multidisciplinary support.

Key takeaways

- ☑ CNCP affects nearly 10% of older adults with polypharmacy, rising to 11.3% in the oldest old.

- ☑ CNCP patients are prescribed more analgesics, opioids, and co-analgesics, often in potentially inappropriate combinations.

- ☑ Polypharmacy, comorbidities, and functional impairments are significantly higher in CNCP patients, highlighting their vulnerability.

- ☑ Safer prescribing practices, reduced reliance on high-dose opioids, and regular medication reviews are essential for improving outcomes.

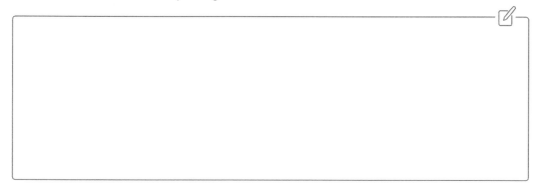

Additional recommended reading:

1. Goetschi AN, Verloo H, Wernli B, et al. Prescribing pattern insights from a longitudinal study of older adult inpatients with polypharmacy and chronic non-cancer pain. *Eur J Pain.* 2024;28:1645-1655. doi:10.1002/ejp.2298.

2. Breivik H, Collett B, Ventafridda V, et al. Survey of chronic pain in Europe: Prevalence, impact on daily life, and treatment. *Eur J Pain.* 2006;10:287-333. doi:10.1016/j.ejpain.2005.06.009.

3. Dowell D, Ragan KR, Jones CM, et al. CDC clinical practice guideline for prescribing opioids for pain-United States, 2022. *MMWR Recomm Rep.* 2022;71(3):1-95. doi:10.15585/mmwr.rr7103a1.

Neuromodulation

A classification and definition framework for neuromodulation for chronic pain

71

Why this topic is important

Neuromodulation, especially implantable electrical modalities, is a cornerstone in managing chronic pain syndromes. The field has grown exponentially, with technologies such as spinal cord stimulation (SCS), deep brain stimulation (DBS), and dorsal root ganglion stimulation revolutionizing patient care. However, this rapid development has led to terminology, classification, and reporting standards inconsistencies. These gaps complicate research, regulatory processes, and clinical practice, ultimately limiting the field's potential to deliver optimal outcomes.

Based on a consensus framework proposed by Sivanesan et al. (2024), this update provides a unified definition and taxonomy for neuromodulation, emphasizing its application in chronic pain management. By standardizing nomenclature and creating a classification system, this framework aims to improve the quality of research, facilitate communication among stakeholders, and guide evidence-based clinical decision-making.

Objectives of this update

- Define neuromodulation in the context of chronic pain.

- Present a classification system for implantable electrical neuromodulation technologies based on their intended use and physical properties.

- Highlight the implications of standardization for research, clinical practice, and policy-making.

What is new

- **Definition clarity**: Neuromodulation is defined as the alteration of nervous system function via direct exogenous application of chemical or physical treatments to neuronal targets.

- **Classification system**: A two-tiered taxonomy based on the anatomical site of modulation and waveform characteristics is introduced, addressing the diversity of emerging modalities.

- **Focus on reproducibility**: Standardized reporting of stimulation parameters (e.g., amplitude, frequency, and electrode configuration) is emphasized to ensure study replicability.

Defining neuromodulation

- Neuromodulation encompasses interventions that modify nervous system activity using direct chemical, electrical, magnetic, or mechanical approaches.

- It excludes treatments that lack a direct, targeted action on named neuronal structures (e.g., general field stimulation).

Classification of electrical neuromodulation

- **Intended use:**

  ○ Central nervous system (e.g., SCS, DBS, motor cortex stimulation).

  ○ Peripheral nervous system (e.g., peripheral nerve stimulation, dorsal root ganglion stimulation).

  ○ Subcutaneous field stimulation targeting peripheral branches.

- **Physical properties:**

  ○ Waveform characteristics (e.g., amplitude, frequency, duty cycle).

  ○ Electrode geometry and configurations (e.g., monopolar, multipolar).

Evolution of spinal cord stimulation

- SCS began in 1967, grounded in Melzack and Wall's gate control theory.

- Advances include miniaturization, MRI compatibility, and the development of high-frequency, burst, and differential target multiplexed waveforms.

- Emerging SCS modalities target structures beyond the dorsal columns, such as visceral and craniofacial pain pathways.

Implications for clinical practice

Enhanced patient selection

- **Precision diagnostics:**

  ○ A detailed understanding of neuromodulatory targets enables better alignment between patient-specific pathology and device selection.

- **Optimized outcomes:**

  ○ Accurate classification improves treatment customization, ensuring appropriate modulation for conditions such as CRPS, PSPS, and diabetic neuropathy.

Reporting and reproducibility

- **Standardized documentation:**

  ○ Clear reporting of stimulation parameters, including amplitude, pulse width, and electrode configuration, ensures reproducibility and cross-study comparability.

- **Framework for meta-analyses:**

  ○ A universal classification system facilitates aggregation of data across studies, enhancing evidence synthesis.

Guiding innovation and policy

- **Technology development:**

  ○ Standardization supports the design of next-generation devices, emphasizing safety and efficacy.

- **Regulatory alignment:**

  ○ Clear definitions assist regulatory bodies in evaluating device claims and streamlining approval processes.

Recommendations

- **Adopt the proposed classification system:**

  ○ Encourage its use across clinical, research, and policy-making domains to ensure consistency and clarity.

- **Invest in education and training:**
  - ◦ Equip clinicians with the knowledge to apply standardized terminology and protocols.

- **Support ongoing refinement:**
  - ◦ Engage stakeholders in iterative updates to the classification framework, reflecting technological and clinical advancements.

Key takeaways

☑ Neuromodulation for chronic pain is defined by its targeted application to specific neuronal structures.

☑ A two-tier classification system based on anatomical targets and physical properties enhances clarity and usability.

☑ Standardization improves research quality, clinical outcomes, and device development.

☑ Alignment with the framework facilitates better communication among researchers, clinicians, payors, and regulatory bodies.

Additional recommended reading:

1. Sivanesan E, North RB, Russo MA, et al. A definition of neuromodulation and classification of implantable electrical modulation for chronic pain. *Neuromodulation*. 2024;27:1-12.

2. Lempka SF, Patil PG. Innovations in spinal cord stimulation for pain. *Curr Opin Biomed Eng*. 2018;8:51-60.

3. Knotkova H, Hamani C, Sivanesan E, et al. Neuromodulation for chronic pain. *Lancet*. 2021;397:2111-2124.

4. Karcz M, Abd-Elsayed A, Chakravarthy K, et al. Pathophysiology of Pain and Mechanisms of Neuromodulation: A Narrative Review (A Neuron Project). *J Pain Res*. 2024;17:3757-3790.

Mitigating complications of neurostimulation

72

Why this topic is important

Neurostimulation therapies, including spinal cord stimulation (SCS), dorsal root ganglion (DRG) stimulation, and peripheral nerve stimulation (PNS), are pivotal in managing chronic pain and movement disorders. While their efficacy is well-documented, complications such as infection, lead migration, hematoma, and neurologic injuries remain significant concerns. These risks necessitate evidence-based strategies to enhance safety and optimize outcomes.

The Neurostimulation Appropriateness Consensus Committee (NACC) has issued updated 2024 guidelines to address these challenges. This update synthesizes new recommendations and expert consensus to assist practitioners in minimizing complications and ensuring durable, successful outcomes.

Objectives of this update

- Highlight key complications associated with neurostimulation therapies.

- Outline evidence-based strategies for mitigating these complications.

- Provide actionable recommendations for integrating safety protocols into clinical practice.

What is new

- **Enhanced anticoagulation management**: Updated recommendations align with contemporary anticoagulation and bleeding risk protocols for neurostimulation procedures.

- **Focus on infection prevention**: Revised guidelines emphasize preoperative and intraoperative measures to mitigate surgical site infections (SSIs).

- **Technology-driven insights**: Incorporation of imaging, advanced neuromonitoring, and antiseptic techniques for improved procedural safety.

Key complications and mitigation strategies

Bleeding risks

Challenges

- Bleeding complications, including epidural hematoma, are rare but potentially catastrophic.

- Risks are heightened in patients on anticoagulants, those with spinal stenosis, or those undergoing lead placement in complex anatomies.

Recommendations

- **Anticoagulant management:**

  - Discontinue anticoagulants based on their pharmacokinetics (e.g., hold warfarin for five days preoperatively).

  - Restart anticoagulants 24 hours post-trial or permanent lead removal.

  - Consult hematologists for high-risk patients.

- **Preoperative imaging**: Review MRI or CT to assess spinal anatomy and plan for lead placement.

- **Education**: Train patients to recognize symptoms of epidural hematoma (e.g., new or worsening neurologic deficits).

Infections

Challenges

- SSIs can lead to device explantation, delayed recovery, and increased healthcare costs.

- Common risk factors include smoking, poorly controlled diabetes, and high-dose opioid use.

Recommendations

- **Preoperative care:**

  - If positive, screen for MSSA/MRSA with nasal swabs and initiate decolonization protocols.

  - Optimize comorbid conditions such as diabetes and smoking cessation.

- **Intraoperative protocols:**

  - Use chlorhexidine-based antiseptics for skin preparation.

  - Implement maximal sterile barriers, including double gloving and cap/mask changes.

- **Postoperative care**: Consider short-term antibiotics for high-risk patients.

Lead migration and integrity

Challenges

- Lead migration or fractures compromise therapeutic efficacy and may necessitate revision surgeries.

Recommendations

- **Secure placement**: Use intraoperative imaging to confirm lead positioning.

- **Anchoring techniques**: Securely anchor leads to prevent displacement.

Neurologic injuries

Challenges

- Risks include spinal cord or nerve root damage during lead placement.

- Injuries are more common in patients with altered spinal anatomy or dense epidural adhesions.

Recommendations

- **Neuromonitoring:**

  - Use sensory and motor evoked potentials during procedures performed under general anesthesia.

  - Ensure patients remain responsive during awake procedures to detect warning symptoms.

- **Training**: Provide regular workshops for physicians to refine lead placement techniques.

Incorporating best practices

Comprehensive planning

- **Patient selection:**

  - Evaluate for modifiable risk factors such as obesity, smoking, and poor glycemic control.

  - Avoid elective procedures in patients with active infections.

- **Multidisciplinary collaboration:** Coordinate with hematologists, infectious disease specialists, and oncologists for complex cases.

Procedural optimization

- **Antibiotic prophylaxis:** Administer weight-based doses of cefazolin (or alternatives for allergies) 60-120 minutes preoperatively.

- **Surgical scrubbing:** Use chlorhexidine for hand and site preparation with a minimum duration of two minutes.

Postoperative monitoring

- **Surveillance:** Monitor patients for early signs of complications such as fever, neurologic changes, or wound discharge.

- **Education:** Teach patients about wound care and signs of device malfunction.

Key takeaways

☑ Neurostimulation procedures are generally safe, but complications such as infection, bleeding, and lead issues require proactive management.

☑ Preoperative preparation, including imaging, anticoagulation assessment, and comorbidity optimization, is essential.

☑ Intraoperative and postoperative protocols must emphasize aseptic techniques, careful lead placement, and patient education.

☑ Collaboration among multidisciplinary teams enhances safety and patient outcomes.

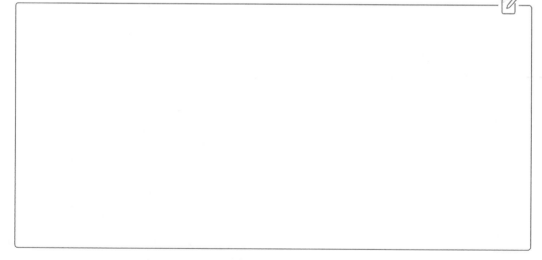

Additional recommended reading:

1. Deer TR, Russo MA, Sayed D, et al. The Neurostimulation Appropriateness Consensus Committee (NACC®): Recommendations for the mitigation of complications of neurostimulation. *Neuromodulation.* 2024;27:977-1007.

2. Hagedorn JM, Strand N, Deer TR, et al. Management of anticoagulation in neurostimulation: A comprehensive review. *Pain Physician.* 2022;25(3):257-269.

3. Provenzano DA, Falowski SM, Pope JE, et al. Infection prevention strategies in neuromodulation: A 10-year update. *Neuromodulation.* 2021;24(8):1254-1264.

Long-term outcomes and salvage strategies in spinal cord stimulation

73

Why this topic is important

Spinal cord stimulation (SCS) has become a cornerstone in managing chronic pain syndromes, such as persistent spinal pain syndrome (PSPS) and complex regional pain syndrome (CRPS). Despite advances in technology, a significant number of patients experience a loss of efficacy (LoE) over time, which can lead to frustration, device explantation, and unmet clinical needs.

The Neurostimulation Appropriateness Consensus Committee (NACC) 2024 recommendations address these challenges, offering evidence-based strategies to enhance long-term therapeutic outcomes and provide effective salvage therapy when initial SCS fails. This update synthesizes key points from the guidelines to aid clinicians in optimizing SCS systems and restoring patient satisfaction.

Objectives of this update

- Explore the phenomenon of LoE in SCS therapy, including potential mechanisms.

- Present evidence-based approaches for programming optimization and salvage strategies.

- Highlight practical considerations for integrating advanced SCS modalities into clinical practice.

What is new

- **Recognition of therapy habituation**: Redefining LoE to include neural and psychological factors contributing to decreased effectiveness.

- **Updated salvage therapies**: New evidence supports transitioning to advanced SCS systems, such as 10 kHz, burst, or dorsal root ganglion (DRG) stimulation.

- **Guidance for device evaluation**: Comprehensive protocols to identify and address mechanical or programming-related causes of therapy failure.safety.

Understanding loss of efficacy (LoE)

- **Neural habituation**: Repetitive stimulation may lead to reduced neural response over time.

- **Psychological factors**: Secondary gain or unmet patient expectations can impact perceived therapy effectiveness.

- **Device-related issues**: Lead migration, impedance changes, or hardware malfunctions may compromise pain relief.

Recommendations for optimizing therapy

Programming adjustments

- **Paresthesia-based tuning**: Reassess lead positioning and stimulation settings to maximize pain coverage.

- **Waveform modifications**: Transition to alternative stimulation patterns, such as burst or high-frequency, for refractory cases.

- **Closed-loop systems**: Utilize real-time feedback mechanisms to maintain stimulation within therapeutic ranges.

Addressing mechanical failures

- **Lead migration:**
  - Confirm with imaging and reposition leads as necessary.

- **Impedance changes:**
  - Investigate high impedance levels for signs of lead fracture or disconnection.

- **Battery issues:**
  - Ensure proper recharging protocols and replace malfunctioning power sources promptly.

Salvage therapy options

High-frequency SCS

- **Evidence**: Proven superior to tonic stimulation for back and leg pain.

- **Applications**: Ideal for patients with LoE due to paresthesia discomfort or inadequate pain coverage.

Burst stimulation

- **Mechanism**: Delivers clustered electrical pulses to reduce habituation and improve analgesia.

- **Benefits**: Effective for patients unresponsive to traditional tonic stimulation.

Dorsal root ganglion (DRG) stimulation

- **Target specificity**: Direct stimulation of the DRG minimizes energy requirements and enhances pain relief for focal conditions like CRPS.

- **Challenges**: Requires precise electrode placement and thorough patient education.

Practical considerations

Patient selection and education

- **Thorough evaluation:**
  - Identify reversible causes of LoE, such as new pain generators or device malfunctions.

- **Setting expectations:**
  - Educate patients about the benefits and limitations of salvage therapies.

Multidisciplinary collaboration

- Engage pain specialists, neurosurgeons, and device representatives to optimize therapy outcomes.

Future directions

- **Personalized neuromodulation:**
  - Incorporate patient-specific factors, such as pain characteristics and anatomical considerations, into device programming.

- **Technological advancements:**
  - Expand access to closed-loop systems and AI-driven optimization tools.

- **Longitudinal research:**
  - Conduct prospective studies to refine salvage strategies and improve durability of outcomes.

Key takeaways

☑ Loss of efficacy in SCS is a multifaceted issue requiring a comprehensive approach to diagnosis and management.

☑ Advanced stimulation modalities, including burst and 10 kHz, provide effective salvage options for refractory cases.

☑ Careful patient evaluation, programming optimization, and device maintenance are critical to long-term success.

☑ Multidisciplinary collaboration enhances therapy outcomes and addresses the complex needs of chronic pain patients.

Additional recommended reading:

1. Deer TR, Russo MA, Grider JS, et al. Recommendations for spinal cord stimulation long-term outcome optimization and salvage therapy. Neuromodulation. 2024;27:951-976.

2. Kumar K, Rizvi S, Bishop S, et al. The phenomenon of tolerance in spinal cord stimulation: A comprehensive review. *Pain Physician.* 2022;25(5):371-383.

3. North RB, Kidd DH, Olin J, et al. Spinal cord stimulation with interleaved pulses: A randomized controlled trial. *Neuromodulation.* 2007;10:349-357.

Factors predicting pain relief after spinal cord stimulation

74

Why this topic is important

Chronic low back pain (CLBP) and radicular leg pain are among the most burdensome conditions globally, significantly affecting patients' quality of life and generating substantial healthcare costs. Spinal cord stimulation (SCS) has emerged as an effective intervention for managing these refractory pain conditions, particularly in persistent spinal pain syndrome (PSPS). However, the success of SCS varies widely, necessitating precise patient selection to optimize outcomes.

This systematic review by Bastiaens et al. (2023) offers valuable insights into predictive factors for achieving clinically meaningful pain relief following SCS. By identifying the characteristics associated with successful outcomes, clinicians can refine patient selection criteria, personalize treatment approaches, and improve long-term efficacy.

Objectives of this update

- Identify key predictive factors for pain relief after SCS in patients with CLBP and/or radicular leg pain.

- Examine the influence of patient demographics, procedural details, and stimulation parameters on treatment outcomes.

- Highlight recommendations for improving patient selection and SCS protocols based on predictive factors.

What is new

- **Predictive factors:**

  - **Back pain relief:** Percutaneous implantation and lower baseline disability scores (Oswestry Disability Index [ODI]) were significant predictors.

  - **Leg pain relief:** Female sex and longer pain duration predicted better outcomes.

  - **General pain relief**: Variable stimulation and percutaneous implantation emerged as key factors.

- **SCS efficacy:** On average, 68% of patients achieved substantial pain relief for leg pain and 63% for back pain at 12 months.

Methods

- **Design**: Systematic review and meta-analysis of 27 studies with 2,220 patients.

- **Inclusion criteria**: Studies reporting ≥ 50% pain relief at 12 or 24 months in CLBP or PSPS patients.

- **Outcomes**: Substantial back, leg, and general pain relief as measured by patient-reported outcomes.

Results

Pain relief outcomes

- **12-month data:**

  - Leg pain relief: 68% of patients achieved ≥ 50% relief.

  - Back pain relief: 63% achieved ≥ 50% relief.

  - General pain relief: 73% achieved ≥ 50% relief.

- **24-month data:**

  - Leg pain relief: Sustained in 63% of patients.

  - Back pain relief: Decreased slightly to 59%.

  - General pain relief: Maintained in 71%.

Predictive factors

- **Back pain relief:**

  - Lower baseline ODI scores indicated higher functional reserve and better outcomes.

  - Percutaneous lead implantation facilitated more targeted stimulation.

- **Leg pain relief:**

  - Female patients showed greater response rates, potentially linked to pain modulation mechanisms.

  - Longer pain duration predicted better outcomes, suggesting chronicity may influence treatment responsiveness.

- **General pain relief:**

  - Variable stimulation (e.g., frequency modulation) enhanced outcomes, likely due to tailored neural engagement.

Implications for clinical practice

Patient selection

- **Screening criteria:**

  - Use ODI scores to assess baseline functional impairment and potential for improvement.

  - Consider pain duration and sex as modifiers for expected outcomes.

- **Tailored approaches:**

  - Incorporate predictive factors into patient selection algorithms to identify the most suitable SCS candidates.

Procedural strategies

- **Implantation technique:**

  - Percutaneous lead placement should be prioritized for its association with improved outcomes.

- **Stimulation optimization:**

  - Employ variable stimulation to enhance efficacy, particularly in general pain management.

Long-term management

- **Monitoring and adjustments:**

  - Regular follow-up is essential to optimize stimulation settings and address emerging patient needs.

- **Multidisciplinary care:**

  - Combining SCS with physical therapy and psychosocial support can amplify benefits.

Recommendations

- **Integrate predictive factors:**
  - ○ Develop structured guidelines incorporating predictive factors like ODI scores, sex, and pain duration into clinical pathways.

- **Enhance data collection:**
  - ○ Establish standardized registries to capture long-term outcomes and refine predictive models.

- **Explore innovative techniques:**
  - ○ Invest in research on novel stimulation modalities (e.g., closed-loop or high-frequency systems) for enhanced efficacy.

Key takeaways

- ☑ SCS is effective for CLBP and radicular leg pain, with 68% of patients achieving significant leg pain relief and 63% experiencing back pain relief at 12 months.

- ☑ Predictive factors, including percutaneous implantation, lower ODI scores, female sex, and longer pain duration, guide patient selection and procedural planning.

- ☑ Optimization of stimulation parameters and comprehensive follow-up are essential for sustained pain relief.

- ☑ Incorporating predictive insights into clinical practice can improve outcomes and enhance the cost-effectiveness of SCS.

Additional recommended reading:

1. Bastiaens F, van de Wijgert IH, Bronkhorst EM, et al. Factors predicting clinically relevant pain relief after spinal cord stimulation for patients with chronic low back and/or leg pain: A systematic review with meta-analysis and meta-regression. *Neuromodulation.* 2024;27:70-82.

2. Taylor RS, Desai MJ, Rigoard P, et al. Predictors of pain relief following spinal cord stimulation: A systematic review. *Pain Pract.* 2014;14:489-505.

3. Eldabe S, Buchser E, Duarte RV. Complications of spinal cord stimulation and the role of assessment tools. *Pain Pract.* 2020;20:25-34.

Differential target multiplexed spinal cord stimulation for intractable low back pain

75

Why this topic is important

Chronic low back pain (CLBP) is a leading cause of disability globally, with a subset of patients ineligible for surgical intervention due to anatomical or medical contraindications. These patients, classified as persistent spinal pain syndrome type 1 (PSPS-T1), often rely on conventional medical management (CMM), which offers limited benefits over time.

Differential Target Multiplexed Spinal Cord Stimulation (DTM SCS) has emerged as a promising treatment alternative, leveraging targeted neural modulation to achieve superior pain relief compared to traditional SCS. This trial by Kallewaard et al. (2024) provides 24-month evidence on the efficacy, safety, and broader benefits of DTM SCS for PSPS-T1 patients, offering critical insights into its role in chronic pain management.

Objectives of this update

- Evaluate the long-term efficacy of DTM SCS compared to CMM in reducing CLBP and improving functional outcomes.

- Explore the impact of DTM SCS on opioid use and quality of life (QoL).

- Provide guidance on integrating DTM SCS into clinical practice for managing PSPS-T1.

What is new

- **Superior long-term outcomes**: DTM SCS achieved > 80% responder rates and > 70% CLBP relief over 24 months.

- **Quality-of-life improvements:** Significant gains in physical and mental functioning, as measured by the EQ-5D-5L and SF-12 indices.

- **Reduced opioid dependency:** DTM SCS patients reduced daily morphine milligram equivalents (MME) by up to 58%.

Methods

- **Design**: Multicenter, randomized controlled trial conducted across four European countries.

- **Participants**: 112 PSPS-T1 patients ineligible for spinal surgery were randomized 1:1 to DTM SCS (n=55) or CMM (n=57).

- **Outcomes measured**: Pain relief (VAS scores), functional disability (ODI), QoL (EQ-5D-5L, SF-12), opioid use, and safety. Follow-up extended to 24 months.

Results

Pain relief

- **Responder rates:**

  - ≥ 50% pain relief was achieved in 80%-85% of DTM SCS patients at all time points compared to < 10% for CMM.

  - Profound responders (≥ 80% pain relief) comprised 65% of the DTM SCS cohort by 24 months.

- **Pain scores:**

  - DTM SCS reduced mean VAS back pain scores from 7.9 cm at baseline to ≤ 2.3 cm (≥ 70% reduction).

  - Leg pain also decreased significantly, with > 5 cm reduction on VAS sustained over 24 months.

Functional and QoL outcomes

- **Oswestry Disability Index (ODI):**

  - ODI scores improved from 49.2 (severe disability) to ≤ 23 (moderate disability) at all time points.

  - Improvements exceeded twice the minimal clinically significant difference (MCID).

- **EQ-5D-5L and SF-12 indices:**

  - QoL indices improved significantly, with EQ-5D-5L gains > 0.3 (triple the MCID).

  - SF-12 physical and mental component scores increased by 11-12 and 6-9 points, respectively, reflecting better overall health and well-being.

Opioid use

- DTM SCS reduced opioid consumption by 38-58% over 24 months, compared to increases in the CMM group.

Safety

- Study-related adverse events (AEs):

  - DTM SCS: AEs occurred in 29.1% of patients, primarily mild to moderate severity.

  - Most common AEs included implant-site pain and infections, with 6.7% requiring surgical intervention.

  - No deaths were reported.

Implications for clinical practice

Candidate selection

- **PSPS-T1 focus:**

  - DTM SCS is a viable option for patients with severe CLBP ineligible for spine surgery, particularly those unresponsive to CMM.

- **Comprehensive evaluation:**

  - Incorporate detailed pain, functional, and QoL assessments to identify appropriate candidates for DTM SCS.

Treatment considerations

- **Superior efficacy:**

  - DTM SCS offers significantly better pain relief and QoL improvements compared to CMM, with long-term benefits.

- **Minimized opioid dependency:**

  - Integration of DTM SCS can reduce reliance on opioid medications, improving safety and patient satisfaction.

Post-procedure management

- **Close monitoring:**
  - ○ Regular follow-up to optimize stimulator settings and address potential complications, such as infections.

- **Patient education:**
  - ○ Set realistic expectations for pain relief and functional improvements to enhance satisfaction and adherence.

Key takeaways

- ☑ DTM SCS achieves > 80% responder rates and sustained pain relief in PSPS-T1 patients over 24 months, outperforming CMM.

- ☑ Patients experience significant functional and QoL improvements, with reductions in opioid use.

- ☑ Safety outcomes are consistent with other SCS studies, affirming DTM SCS as a reliable treatment option.

- ☑ Comprehensive assessment and tailored patient selection are critical for optimizing outcomes.

Additional recommended reading:

1. Kallewaard JW, Billet B, Van Paesschen R, et al. Differential target multiplexed spinal cord stimulation versus conventional medical management: 24-month results. *Eur J Pain*. 2024;28:1745-1761.

2. Deer TR, Krames ES, Mekhail N, et al. Comprehensive chronic pain management with spinal cord stimulation: A review. *Pain Pract*. 2023;23:1187-1201.

3. Patel K, Wilson P, Whitworth J, et al. Comparing neuromodulation approaches for chronic pain: Focus on new technologies. *Pain Med*. 2023;24:860-873.

The duration of carryover effects in spinal cord stimulation

76

Why this topic is important

Spinal cord stimulation (SCS) has been established as an effective therapy for managing chronic neuropathic pain, providing patients with significant relief and improved functionality. However, the phenomenon known as the "carryover effect"-a temporary extension of pain relief after SCS deactivation-remains underexplored. This effect has implications for understanding the underlying mechanisms of SCS, optimizing clinical protocols, and designing robust clinical trials.

The EChO (Examining the Carryover Effect) study by Meier et al. (2024) is the first systematic investigation of this phenomenon. By quantifying the carryover effect and analyzing patient-specific factors, the study advances our understanding of how SCS therapy interacts with neuromodulatory and neuroplastic processes.

Objectives of this update

- Define the carryover effect and its relevance to SCS therapy.

- Examine patient and treatment variables influencing carryover duration.

- Discuss implications for clinical practice, including device programming and trial design.

What is new

- **Quantified carryover effect**: Median duration of 5 hours, with substantial variability between patients.

- **Correlations identified**: Longer carryover durations linked to high-frequency (10 kHz) stimulation, back pain indications, and higher baseline pain scores.

- **Practical applications**: Insights for optimizing intermittent stimulation protocols and designing crossover trials with appropriate washout periods.

Methods

- **Study type**: Open-label, multicenter, investigator-initiated trial.

- **Participants**:

  - 158 adults with SCS implants for chronic neuropathic pain.

  - Included conditions: back pain, radicular pain, CRPS, and peripheral neuropathy.

  - Patients had been on stable SCS therapy for at least 6 months.

- **Procedure**:

  - Patients deactivated their devices at home and recorded pain resurgence using numerical rating scales (NRS).

  - Reactivation occurred upon a pain increase of ≥3 NRS points or the onset of unbearable symptoms.

Results

Carryover duration

- Median duration: 5 hours, with a wide range (0.9-62.8 hours).

- Longest carryover times observed in:

  - **Back pain patients**: Median of 25 hours.

  - **High-frequency stimulation users**: Median of 22.8 hours.

Influential factors

1. **Pain characteristics**:

   - Patients with predominantly spike-like pain experienced longer carryover durations (median: 11.4 hours) than those with constant pain (median: 4.5 hours).

2. **Stimulation paradigms**:

   - High-frequency (10 kHz) stimulation was associated with significantly longer carryover effects than tonic and burst paradigms.

3. **Baseline pain scores**:

   - Higher pain levels at deactivation correlated with extended carryover durations.

4. **Geographic variability**:

   - Patients from certain centers (e.g., Canada) exhibited longer carryover times, potentially due to differences in programming practices and patient demographics.

Implications for clinical practice

Device programming

- **Intermittent stimulation**:

  - Leveraging carryover effects can extend battery life and reduce habituation.

  - Automated on/off cycles should consider individual carryover durations for optimal efficacy.

- **Personalized settings**:

  - Programming should account for patient-specific factors like pain type and baseline scores.

Trial design

- **Crossover studies**:

  - Appropriate washout periods must consider interindividual variability in carryover duration to avoid confounding results.

- **Treatment optimization**:

  - Understanding carryover dynamics allows better evaluation of new stimulation paradigms and settings.

Patient education and management

- Periodic deactivation can be introduced safely, minimizing pain resurgence in patients with longer carryover durations.

- Education on managing temporary pain increases is critical for patient adherence.

Recommendations

- **Consider carryover dynamics in protocols:**
  - Intermittent and cyclic stimulation settings could potentially be tailored to individual patient profiles, but further research is needed to confirm their effectiveness.

- **Enhance data collection efforts:**
  - Future studies could explore neurochemical and neuroplastic correlates of the carryover effect, which could help refine therapeutic strategies.

- **Expand patient stratification approaches:**
  - Baseline pain characteristics and stimulation parameters might be useful in predicting carryover duration, but more evidence is required to support the customization of care based on these factors.

Key takeaways

☑ The carryover effect may extend SCS pain relief post-deactivation, with reported durations ranging from minutes to days.

☑ Longer carryover durations appear associated with high-frequency stimulation and back pain conditions, although more data is needed to generalize these findings.

☑ An improved understanding of this phenomenon could potentially inform device programming, reduce habituation, and refine clinical trial designs.

☑ Patient education and thoughtful integration of carryover dynamics into clinical protocols may help optimize therapy outcomes.

Additional recommended reading:

1. Meier K, de Vos CC, Bordeleau M, et al. Examining the duration of carryover effect in patients treated with spinal cord stimulation: Results from the EChO study. *Neuromodulation*. 2024;27:887-898.

2. Tieppo Francio V, Polston KF, Murphy MT, et al. Management of chronic and neuropathic pain with 10-kHz spinal cord stimulation: A review. *Biomedicines*. 2021;9:732.

3. Wolter T, Winkelmüller M. Continuous versus intermittent spinal cord stimulation: An analysis of clinical efficacy. *Neuromodulation*. 2012;15:13-19.

4. Braun E, Khatri N, Kim B, et al. A Prospective, Randomized Single-Blind Crossover Study Comparing High-Frequency 10,000 Hz and Burst Spinal Cord Stimulation. *Neuromodulation*. 2023;26(5):1023-1029.

Impact of prior lumbar spine surgeries on spinal cord stimulation outcomes

77

Why this topic is important

Chronic low back pain (CLBP) is one of the leading causes of disability worldwide, often necessitating lumbar spine surgeries to alleviate symptoms. However, persistent spinal pain syndrome (PSPS), commonly known as failed back surgery syndrome (FBSS), occurs in 10%-40% of patients following lumbar spine surgery. These individuals frequently experience persistent pain and functional impairment despite surgical interventions.

Spinal cord stimulation (SCS) has emerged as a viable treatment for refractory pain in PSPS patients. While SCS is well-documented as an effective therapy, the influence of prior lumbar surgeries on SCS outcomes remains unclear. This study by Hagedorn et al. (2024) investigates the relationship between the number of prior lumbar spine surgeries and pain relief following SCS implantation. Its findings offer critical insights into optimizing SCS as a treatment strategy for PSPS.

Objectives of this update

- Assess whether the number of prior lumbar spine surgeries impacts pain relief outcomes following SCS implantation.

- Explore the role of device waveforms in influencing outcomes based on surgical history.

- Provide guidance for selecting SCS candidates and tailoring treatment based on prior surgical history.

What is new

This multicenter, retrospective study reveals several key findings:

- **Comparable outcomes across surgeries**: Patients with one prior surgery experienced similar pain relief as those with two or more surgeries.

- **No influence of waveform**: Device waveform (burst-DR, tonic, or 10-kHz) did not significantly impact outcomes relative to prior surgeries.

- **Broad applicability of SCS**: Findings support SCS as an effective option for PSPS, regardless of the number of previous lumbar surgeries.

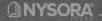

Methods

- **Design**: Multisite, retrospective pooled analysis of 468 patients across five pain centers.

- **Participants:**

  - Inclusion: Patients with PSPS who underwent SCS implantation after at least one lumbar spine surgery.

  - Groups: Patients stratified by one prior surgery (n=268) versus two or more surgeries (n=200).

- **Outcomes measured:**

  - Primary: Mean percentage pain relief 12 months post-implantation.

  - Secondary: Responder rates (≥ 30% and ≥ 50% pain relief thresholds).

Results

Pain relief outcomes

- Mean pain relief was similar between patients with one prior surgery (28.2%) and those with two or more (25.8%).

- No significant association between the number of surgeries (as a categorical or continuous variable) and pain relief (adjusted β-coefficient -1.5).

Responder rates

- **≥ 30% pain relief**: Achieved by 39.9% of patients with one surgery and 37.5% with two or more.

- **≥ 50% pain relief**: Achieved by 25.4% of patients with one surgery and 24.0% with two or more.

Subgroup analysis by waveform

- Waveform type (burst-DR, tonic, or 10-kHz) did not significantly influence pain relief outcomes across surgical histories.

- Pain relief ranged from 26.3% to 33.9%, with no meaningful differences observed.

Implications for clinical practice

Candidate selection

- **Broad applicability:**

  - SCS provides comparable relief for patients with one or multiple prior lumbar surgeries, supporting its use across a broad spectrum of PSPS cases.

  - Past surgical history should not preclude patients from being considered for SCS.

- **Surgical factors and timing:**

  - While surgery count does not predict SCS success, assessing functional impairment, chronicity of pain, and surgical details can guide patient expectations.

Waveform selection

- **Flexibility in waveform use:**

  - No significant differences in outcomes based on device waveform were observed, allowing clinicians to tailor waveform selection to patient-specific needs and preferences.

- **Consider device capabilities:**

  - When choosing a device, focus on other factors such as battery life, patient comfort, and programming options.

Setting realistic expectations

- Only 25% of patients achieved ≥50% pain relief, emphasizing the importance of multidisciplinary pain management.

- Educate patients on realistic goals, including functional improvement and reduced reliance on opioids.

Recommendations

- **Evaluate comprehensively:**

  - Consider SCS for all PSPS patients with persistent pain, regardless of surgical history.

  - Assess psychosocial factors, opioid use, and comorbidities that may influence outcomes.

- **Optimize pre-implantation strategies:**
  - Conduct psychological evaluations and optimize physical therapy to enhance response rates.

- **Post-implantation care:**
  - Monitor pain scores and device functionality closely, making programming adjustments as needed.

Key takeaways

☑ The number of prior lumbar spine surgeries does not significantly influence SCS outcomes, supporting its use in diverse PSPS populations.

☑ SCS provides comparable pain relief and responder rates for patients with varying surgical histories.

☑ Device waveform type does not impact outcomes, allowing for individualized device selection.

☑ Comprehensive preoperative evaluation and realistic patient counseling remain essential for optimizing SCS success.

Additional recommended reading:

1. Hagedorn JM, D'Souza RS, Yadav A, et al. Relationship between number of prior lumbar spine surgeries and outcomes following spinal cord stimulator implantation: A multisite, retrospective pooled analysis. *Pain Pract.* 2024;24:882-890.

2. Kumar K, Taylor RS, Jacques L, et al. Spinal cord stimulation versus conventional medical management for neuropathic pain: A multicentre randomized controlled trial. *Pain.* 2007;132(1-2):179-188.

3. North RB, Kidd DH, Farrokhi F, et al. Spinal cord stimulation versus repeated lumbosacral spine surgery for chronic pain: A randomized, controlled trial. *Neurosurgery.* 2005;56(1):98-107.

Outcomes of single-stage spinal cord stimulation

78

Why this topic is important

Chronic pain is a leading cause of disability, with conditions like persistent spinal pain syndrome (PSPS) and failed back surgery syndrome (FBSS) representing significant therapeutic challenges. Spinal cord stimulation (SCS) is a proven treatment modality for these conditions, typically requiring a two-stage process involving a trial period before permanent implantation. However, the necessity of this trial period has been increasingly debated.

Single-stage SCS (SS-SCS), which bypasses the external trial period and incorporates intraoperative testing, has emerged as a cost-effective alternative. This approach simplifies the procedure, reduces infection risk, and minimizes healthcare burden while maintaining long-term efficacy. The study by De Negri et al. (2023) evaluates real-world outcomes of SS-SCS, providing critical data to guide clinical decision-making.

Objectives of this update

- Evaluate the long-term efficacy of SS-SCS in chronic pain management.

- Compare SS-SCS to traditional two-stage SCS approaches regarding safety, pain relief, and quality of life.

- Assess implications for patient selection and clinical practice.

What is new

- **Sustained pain relief**: SS-SCS delivers a 5-point reduction in pain scores sustained over 12 months.

- **Improved quality of life (QoL)**: Significant enhancements in QoL scores align with population norms.

- **High responder rates**: Over 70% of patients achieve ≥ 50% pain relief, matching outcomes of traditional two-stage SCS.

Methods

- **Design**: Multicenter, observational case series involving 171 chronic pain patients across 18 European centers.

- **Participants**:
  - Patients aged ≥ 18 years diagnosed with PSPS, FBSS, or other chronic pain syndromes.
  - Mean age: 59.4 years; 53.2% female.

- **Intervention**: SS-SCS with intraoperative testing and immediate permanent implantation.

- **Outcomes measured**:
  - Pain intensity (Numerical Rating Scale [NRS]).
  - QoL (EuroQol 5 Dimensions-5L [EQ-5D-5L]).
  - Responder rates (≥ 50% pain reduction).

Results

Pain relief

- **Overall pain**:
  - Baseline NRS: 8.1 (severe pain).
  - Reduction of 5 points to 3.1 at 3 months, sustained at 12 months and the last follow-up (mean: 408 days).
  - By the last follow-up, 50.3% of patients achieved mild pain levels (NRS ≤ 3).

- **Subgroup pain scores**:
  - Low back pain: Reduced by 4.5 points.
  - Leg pain: Reduced by 5.1 points.

Quality of life

- **EQ-5D-5L improvements**:
  - Baseline score: 25.0 (severe impairment).
  - Last follow-up: 70.2 (healthy population norms).

Responder rates

- **≥ 50% pain relief:** 71.3% of patients achieved this, aligning with two-stage SCS outcomes reported in prior studies.

Safety

- **Adverse events:**
  - Infection risk was minimized by avoiding prolonged trial periods.
  - No major complications directly attributed to SS-SCS.

Implications for clinical practice

Rethinking the trial period

- **Clinical value:**
  - The necessity of a trial period for predicting long-term outcomes is increasingly questioned, as SS-SCS outcomes mirror those of traditional two-stage SCS.

- **Cost and efficiency:**
  - SS-SCS reduces procedural costs, healthcare visits, and infection risks, presenting a compelling case for broader adoption.

Patient selection

- **Criteria refinement:**
  - SS-SCS may be preferable for patients with high predicted response likelihood, minimizing delays and resource use.

- **Comorbidities:**
  - Patients with conditions increasing infection risk (e.g., diabetes) are ideal candidates for SS-SCS.

Integration into care pathways

- **Intraoperative testing:**
  - Ensures appropriate lead placement and therapy response without needing a prolonged trial.

- **Enhanced QoL:**
  - Improved QoL metrics emphasize SS-SCS as a transformative therapy for chronic pain patients.

Recommendations

- **Expand SS-SCS adoption:**

  ○ Utilize to meet the criteria for SCS therapy, particularly for patients with comorbidities or logistical constraints.

- **Streamline protocols:**

  ○ Develop standardized protocols for intraoperative testing and immediate implantation.

- **Prioritize patient-centered care:**

  ○ Engage patients in discussions about the benefits and limitations of SS-SCS versus traditional approaches.

Key takeaways

☑ SS-SCS achieves comparable pain relief and QoL improvements to two-stage SCS, with fewer procedural burdens.

☑ Simplifying the SCS process minimizes infection risk and reduces healthcare costs.

☑ Patient selection and intraoperative testing are pivotal for successful outcomes.

☑ SS-SCS represents an innovative, patient-centered approach to managing chronic pain.

Additional recommended reading:

1. De Negri P, Paz-Solis JF, Rigoard P, et al. Real-world outcomes of single-stage spinal cord stimulation in chronic pain patients: A multicenter, European case series. *Interventional Pain Medicine*. 2023;2:100263.

2. Eldabe S, Duarte RV, Gulve A, et al. Does a screening trial for spinal cord stimulation in patients with chronic pain of neuropathic origin have clinical utility and cost-effectiveness? *Pain*. 2020;161(12):2820-2829.

3. North R, Vangeneugden J, Raftopoulos C, et al. Postoperative infections associated with prolonged spinal cord stimulation trial duration. *Neuromodulation*. 2020;23(5):620-625.

Long-term outcomes of closed-loop and open-loop spinal cord stimulation

79

Why this topic is important

Spinal cord stimulation (SCS) is an established therapy for managing chronic, refractory pain. However, traditional open-loop SCS (OL-SCS) systems rely on fixed stimulation outputs that do not adapt to the dynamic environment of the spinal cord, often resulting in inconsistent pain relief. To address these limitations, closed-loop SCS (CL-SCS) systems have been developed, using real-time evoked compound action potentials (ECAPs) to adjust stimulation based on neural feedback.

The EVOKE trial (Mekhail et al., 2023) is a landmark randomized, double-blind clinical study that provides the first long-term comparative evaluation of CL-SCS and OL-SCS systems. The 36-month follow-up data demonstrate the superior efficacy, safety, and durability of CL-SCS, marking a significant advancement in the field of neuromodulation.

Objectives of this update

- Compare the long-term efficacy of CL-SCS versus OL-SCS in chronic pain management.

- Assess holistic outcomes, including function, sleep, and emotional well-being improvements.

- Discuss the implications of neural activation accuracy on clinical outcomes.

What is new

- **Improved pain relief**: At 36 months, 77.6% of CL-SCS patients achieved ≥50% pain reduction, compared to 49.3% of OL-SCS patients.

- **Enhanced holistic outcomes**: CL-SCS patients showed superior improvements in functional, emotional, and sleep domains, with 44.8% classified as holistic treatment responders versus 28.4% in the OL-SCS group.

- **Sustained efficacy**: No explants due to loss of efficacy were observed in the CL-SCS group, emphasizing its long-term reliability.

Methods

- **Design:** Multicenter, double-blind, randomized clinical trial conducted across 13 U.S. sites.

- **Participants:** 113 adults with chronic back and leg pain refractory to conservative therapy, randomized to CL-SCS or OL-SCS.

- **Intervention:** Both groups received the same neuromodulation system with ECAP-guided programming. In the CL-SCS group, feedback loops adjusted stimulation in real time.

Results

Pain relief

- **Primary endpoint:**
  - 77.6% of CL-SCS patients achieved ≥ 50% pain relief at 36 months, compared to 49.3% in the OL-SCS group.
  - 49.3% of CL-SCS patients experienced ≥80% pain relief, compared to 31.3% in the OL-SCS group.

- **Magnitude of improvement:**
  - Mean reduction in pain scores: 69.6% for CL-SCS versus 53.9% for OL-SCS.

Holistic treatment response

- **Composite outcomes:**
  - CL-SCS outperformed OL-SCS across domains, including physical function, sleep quality, emotional well-being, and health-related quality of life.
  - 44.8% of CL-SCS patients achieved holistic responder status (≥ 1 clinically meaningful improvement in all impaired domains), compared to 28.4% of OL-SCS patients.

Neural activation

- **Accuracy:**
  - CL-SCS systems demonstrated threefold greater accuracy in maintaining target ECAP levels compared to OL-SCS systems.
  - Greater neural activation was consistently observed in the CL-SCS group.

Clinical implications

Advancing neuromodulation

- **Adaptive therapy:**
  - CL-SCS provides real-time feedback, optimizing therapy delivery and maintaining consistent neural activation.
  - This adaptability translates into superior long-term outcomes compared to static OL-SCS systems.

- **Holistic benefits:**
  - Beyond pain relief, CL-SCS addresses broader aspects of patient well-being, including physical, emotional, and functional domains.

Durability and safety

- **Explants:**
  - No explants due to loss of efficacy were reported in the CL-SCS group, indicating robust long-term performance.

- **Comparable safety:**
  - Adverse events and explant rates were similar across both groups, with no device-specific complications observed.

Personalized medicine

- **Targeted outcomes:** CL-SCS's real-time adjustment capabilities make it ideal for patients with dynamic pain patterns or those who have failed traditional SCS systems.

Limitations

- CL-SCS requires frequent recharging due to higher energy consumption, though device improvements are anticipated in the near future.

Recommendations

- **Adopt CL-SCS as the standard:**
  - Given its proven efficacy, durability, and holistic benefits, CL-SCS should be considered the first-line SCS therapy for chronic pain.

- **Integrate holistic assessments:**
  - Use multidimensional outcomes to evaluate treatment success, ensuring a patient-centered approach.

- **Optimize programming:**
  - Clinicians should leverage ECAP-guided programming to maximize therapeutic outcomes and minimize variability.

Key takeaways

- ☑ Closed-loop SCS offers superior and sustained pain relief compared to open-loop systems, with 77.6% of patients achieving ≥ 50% pain reduction at 36 months.

- ☑ CL-SCS's holistic benefits include improvements in function, emotional well-being, and sleep quality, reflecting its broader impact on patient health.

- ☑ CL-SCS systems demonstrate greater accuracy and consistency in neural activation, underscoring the value of real-time feedback mechanisms in neuromodulation.

Additional recommended reading:

1. Mekhail NA, Levy RM, Deer TR, et al. ECAP-controlled closed-loop versus open-loop SCS for the treatment of chronic pain: 36-month results of the EVOKE blinded randomized clinical trial. *Reg Anesth Pain Med.* 2024;49:346-354.

2. Hagedorn JM, Karantonis DM, Poree L, et al. Innovations in closed-loop neuromodulation for chronic pain management. *Pain Physician.* 2022;25(3):271-282.

3. Deer TR, Mekhail N, Pope JE, et al. Advances in neuromodulation: real-time feedback in spinal cord stimulation. *Neuromodulation.* 2021;24(5):451-460.

Identifying nonresponders to high-frequency spinal cord stimulation

80

Why this topic is important

Chronic low back pain (CLBP) is among the leading causes of disability worldwide, imposing a significant burden on patients and healthcare systems. Spinal cord stimulation (SCS) has emerged as a promising intervention for patients with refractory chronic pain, offering long-term relief and functional improvement. Despite its growing utilization, approximately 30% of patients fail to achieve meaningful pain relief after SCS implantation.

High-frequency (10 kHz) SCS represents a technological advancement with improved efficacy and reduced side effects compared to traditional low-frequency systems. However, variability in patient response underscores the importance of identifying predictors of treatment success. This study by Francio et al. (2024) investigates clinical, psychological, and demographic factors associated with nonresponse to 10 kHz SCS, providing critical guidance for optimizing patient selection and outcomes.

Objectives of this update

- Identify baseline variables linked to nonresponders in 10 kHz SCS therapy for CLBP.

- Highlight the role of psychological factors, such as pain catastrophizing and kinesiophobia, in influencing outcomes.

- Provide recommendations for preoperative screening and patient optimization.

What is new

This study offers several key findings:

- **Psychological factors matter:** High levels of kinesiophobia and pain catastrophizing were significantly associated with nonresponse to 10 kHz SCS.

- **Baseline disability and pain intensity predict outcomes:** Greater disability and severe pain levels correlated with poorer treatment response.

- **No significant impact from demographic variables:** Age, gender, BMI, and psychiatric illness did not predict nonresponse in this study.

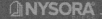

Methods

- **Design:** Retrospective observational study at a single university center.
- **Participants:** 237 patients with CLBP who underwent successful trial stimulation and subsequent implantation of a 10 kHz SCS system.
  - **Responders:** ≥ 50% improvement in pain scores (n=160).
  - **Nonresponders:** < 50% improvement in pain scores (n=77).
- **Outcomes measured:** Baseline demographic, clinical, and psychological variables, including pain intensity (NRS), disability (ODI), pain catastrophizing (PCS), and kinesiophobia (TSK).

Results

Psychological predictors

- **Kinesiophobia (fear of movement):**
  - Nonresponders had significantly higher mean TSK scores (44.8 vs. 38.8 in responders).
  - Clinically relevant kinesiophobia (TSK > 37) was present in 76.5% of nonresponders, compared to 56.5% of responders.
- **Pain catastrophizing:**
  - Nonresponders had higher PCS scores, indicating greater levels of pain-related rumination and helplessness.
  - Clinically relevant pain catastrophizing (PCS > 30) was significantly more frequent in nonresponders (53.8% vs. 36.4%).

Clinical predictors

- **Disability (Oswestry Disability Index):**
  - Nonresponders reported higher baseline disability scores (47.9 vs. 43.6).
  - Severe disability (ODI ≥ 59) increased the likelihood of nonresponse.

- **Pain intensity:**
  - Nonresponders had higher baseline NRS scores (6.3 vs. 5.6).
  - Longer pain duration was associated with poorer outcomes.

Demographic and other variables

- **No significant differences** were observed in age, gender, BMI, history of spinal surgery, opioid use, or psychiatric illness between responders and nonresponders.

Implications for clinical practice

Preoperative screening

- **Psychological evaluation:**
  - Incorporate validated tools like TSK and PCS into routine preoperative assessments to identify high-risk patients.
  - Patients with clinically relevant levels of kinesiophobia (TSK > 37) or pain catastrophizing (PCS > 30) may require targeted interventions before SCS.
- **Functional assessment:**
  - Evaluate baseline disability using ODI to identify patients with severe functional impairment, as this may predict nonresponse.

Patient optimization

- **Address modifiable psychological factors:**
  - Consider prehabilitation programs, including pain neuroscience education and cognitive behavioral therapy, to reduce fear-avoidance behaviors and catastrophizing.
- **Tailor expectations:**
  - Provide realistic counseling on anticipated outcomes, particularly for patients with severe baseline disability or long-standing pain.

Recommendations

- **Screen comprehensively:**
  - Combine psychological, functional, and pain assessments to guide patient selection.

- **Optimize before implantation:**
  - Address modifiable risk factors, such as kinesiophobia and catastrophizing, through multidisciplinary pain management strategies.

- **Develop targeted protocols:**
  - Incorporate findings into standard clinical pathways for SCS to improve long-term success rates.

Key takeaways

☑ High levels of kinesiophobia and pain catastrophizing strongly predict nonresponse to 10 kHz SCS.

☑ Greater baseline disability and pain intensity are associated with poorer outcomes.

☑ Preoperative psychological and functional assessments are essential for optimizing patient selection and enhancing SCS success rates.

☑ Multidisciplinary approaches can mitigate modifiable risk factors, including prehabilitation and pain education.

☑ Findings align with patterns observed in other SCS modalities, highlighting the importance of addressing psychological and clinical predictors across all waveform types.

☑ When interpreting its findings, it is important to consider the study's retrospective design and funding support from the manufacturer of the 10 kHz SCS system.

Additional recommended reading:

1. Francio VT, Alm J, Leavitt L, et al. Variables associated with nonresponders to high-frequency (10 kHz) spinal cord stimulation. *Pain Pract.* 2024;24:584-599.

2. Bendinger T, Plunkett A. Predictors of outcomes in spinal cord stimulation for chronic pain: A systematic review. *Pain Med.* 2016;17(6):1066-1076.

3. Goudman L, Moens M, Billot M, et al. Predicting the response to spinal cord stimulation for chronic pain: Machine-learning insights. *J Pain Res.* 2021;14:489-500.

Intrathecal drug delivery for chronic noncancer pain

81

Why this topic is important

Chronic noncancer pain represents a significant public health challenge, affecting millions of individuals and presenting a major burden on healthcare systems. Intrathecal drug delivery (IDD) offers a targeted therapeutic option for refractory pain, delivering medication directly into the cerebrospinal fluid to optimize pain control while minimizing systemic side effects.

While IDD has been transformative in pain management, its use demands precision in patient selection, drug choice, and procedural technique to ensure safety and efficacy. The 2024 Polyanalgesic Consensus Conference (PACC®) guidelines offer updated evidence-based recommendations for IDD, addressing key aspects such as patient optimization, medication management, trialing strategies, and infection prevention.

Objectives of this update

- Highlight the latest recommendations for IDD in managing chronic noncancer pain.

- Explore best practices for patient selection, trialing, and device management.

- Provide actionable insights into optimizing therapy and minimizing complications.

What is new

- **Emphasis on psychological screening**: Updated recommendations stress psychological evaluations to predict treatment success.

- **Refined trialing techniques**: Evidence supports diverse methods tailored to patient-specific needs and medications.

- **Advanced infection control**: Strategies for infection prevention now incorporate updated perioperative and postoperative protocols.

Key findings and recommendations

Patient optimization for IDD

- **Psychological evaluation:**

  ○ Pain perception and treatment outcomes are influenced by psychological factors such as depression and catastrophizing.

  ○ Preimplant evaluations are essential to identify barriers to success and establish readiness for therapy.

- **Opioid reduction:**

  ○ IDD candidates should aim to reduce or discontinue systemic opioids before implantation, given the risks of opioid-induced hyperalgesia and respiratory depression.

- **Lifestyle modifications:**

  ○ Weight loss, smoking cessation, and improved physical activity are recommended to enhance therapy outcomes.

Trialing strategies

- **Methods of trialing:**

  ○ Single-shot bolus injections, continuous infusions, and staged catheter trials are effective, with no one method superior overall.

  ○ Medication selection (e.g., hydrophilic vs. lipophilic drugs) guides the choice of trialing approach.

- **Ziconotide-specific trialing:**

  ○ This hydrophilic peptide should be trialed intrathecally using small bolus injections due to its restricted dural distribution and neuropsychiatric side effects.

- **Trialing location:**

  ○ While outpatient settings are feasible for bolus trials, inpatient trials are recommended for high-risk patients requiring catheter placement.

Infection prevention

- **Preoperative measures:**

  ○ Screen for MRSA/MSSA and initiate decolonization protocols when necessary.

  ○ Optimize comorbid conditions such as diabetes and ensure proper skin preparation with chlorhexidine.

- **Intraoperative protocols:**

  ○ Limit operating room traffic and use iodine-impregnated drapes to maintain asepsis.

- **Postoperative care:**

  ○ Educate patients on wound management and monitor for early signs of infection, with follow-up within two weeks of implantation.

Medication management

- **On- vs. off-label medication:**

  ○ Off-label use is common but requires strict adherence to sterile compounding guidelines to prevent adverse events.

- **Pharmacokinetics:**

  ○ Hydrophilic drugs like morphine provide broader CSF distribution, while lipophilic drugs such as fentanyl demand precise catheter placement for localized pain.

- **Initial dosing:**

  ○ Start with low doses to minimize side effects and allow upward titration based on patient response.

Intrathecal catheter and pump considerations

- **Catheter placement**

  ○ For optimal pain relief, the catheter should be placed dorsally, and the tip should align with the affected dermatome, provided it is anatomically feasible.

- **Pump implantation**

  ○ While the abdominal wall remains the standard site, alternative placements (e.g., paraspinal, buttocks) are viable for patients with anatomical challenges.

- **Programming and maintenance**

  - Flex dosing and patient-controlled boluses offer flexibility, enhancing pain management while reducing local complications like granuloma formation.

- **Imaging guidance**

  - Consider using ultrasound or fluoroscopy guidance in patients with challenging body habitus to enhance procedural success and minimize risks.

Health Economic Considerations

- **Cost-effectiveness**

  - IDD is cost-effective for well-selected patients, with long-term savings from reduced hospitalizations and medication use offsetting initial high costs.

- **Savings timeline**

  - Cost benefits typically emerge 2-3 years post-implantation, though payer transitions can shift financial responsibilities.

- **Evidence gaps**

  - Economic analyses need stronger data; integrating health economics early in clinical trials could improve evaluations.

- **Evaluation metrics**

  - Key factors include costs of screening, implantation, and maintenance, measured using Quality-Adjusted Life Years (QALYs).

- **Recommendations**

  - Embedding economic assessments in clinical trials aids informed decision-making and policy development.

Clinical implications

- **Improving access:**

  - The PACC® guidelines provide a roadmap to expand the safe and effective use of IDD for chronic pain.

- **Tailored therapy:**

  - Recommendations underscore the importance of personalized approaches, from trialing methods to catheter placement, to optimize outcomes.

- **Safety focus:**

  - Comprehensive infection control and close postoperative monitoring mitigate the risks associated with IDD systems.

Key takeaways

- ☑ IDD offers targeted and effective pain relief for chronic noncancer pain when implemented with evidence-based protocols.

- ☑ Psychological screening, lifestyle optimization, and opioid tapering are critical for selecting ideal candidates.

- ☑ Trialing strategies and medication choices should align with patient needs and anatomical considerations.

- ☑ Infection prevention protocols, precise catheter placement, and tailored dosing enhance safety and efficacy.

Additional recommended reading:

1. Deer TR, Hayek SM, Grider JS, et al. The Polyanalgesic Consensus Conference (PACC®): Intrathecal drug delivery guidance on safety and therapy optimization when treating chronic noncancer pain. *Neuromodulation*. 2024;27:1107-1139.

2. Prabhala T, Johansen A, Grider JS, et al. Advancing patient selection for IDD systems: A review of psychosocial screening tools. *Pain Physician*. 2022;25:467-482.

3. Yaksh TL, Bernards CM. Intrathecal drug delivery: Mechanisms and clinical implications. *Anesth Analg*. 2010;110:123-132.

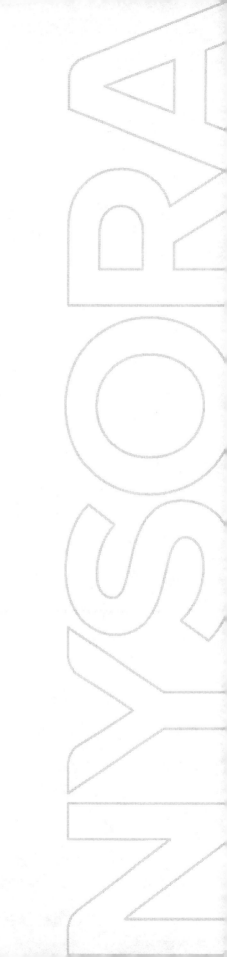

The efficacy of 60-day percutaneous peripheral nerve stimulation after total knee arthroplasty

82

Why this topic is important

Total knee arthroplasty (TKA) is a highly effective surgical intervention for end-stage osteoarthritis and other severe knee joint conditions. However, up to 20% of patients experience persistent postoperative pain beyond the typical healing period, contributing to decreased mobility, functional limitations, and a diminished quality of life. Managing such chronic postoperative pain remains a complex challenge, with existing treatments offering inconsistent efficacy and often relying on opioids, which carry significant risks of dependence and adverse effects.

Percutaneous peripheral nerve stimulation (PNS) has emerged as a promising nonopioid therapy targeting persistent postoperative pain. This intervention may provide meaningful pain relief and functional improvements by stimulating sensory nerves associated with the affected knee. This update examines findings from a randomized, double-blind, placebo-controlled trial by Goree et al. (2024) evaluating the safety and efficacy of a 60-day PNS treatment for chronic postoperative pain after TKA, providing valuable insights for clinicians managing these patients.

Objectives of this update

- Assess the effectiveness of 60-day PNS in reducing pain and improving function after TKA.

- Evaluate the treatment's impact on mobility and quality of life (QoL).

- Highlight the clinical implications of incorporating PNS into postoperative pain management pathways.

What is new

- **Clinically meaningful pain relief**: PNS was associated with ≥ 50% pain relief in 60% of patients compared to 24% in the placebo group during weeks 5-8 of treatment.

- **Improved mobility**: On the 6-minute walk test (6MWT), PNS participants demonstrated a 47% increase in walking distance compared to a 9% decrease in the placebo group.

- **Enhanced quality of life**: Significant improvements in the Western Ontario and McMaster Universities Osteoarthritis Index (WOMAC) scores and Patient Global Impression of Change (PGIC) ratings were observed among PNS recipients.

Methods

- **Study design**: Multicenter, randomized, double-blind, placebo-controlled trial conducted from 2020 to 2023.

- **Participants**: 52 adults with persistent moderate-to-severe pain (≥ 5/10 on the Brief Pain Inventory) following TKA, stratified into PNS (n=28) and placebo (n=24) groups.

- **Intervention**: Ultrasound-guided placement of percutaneous leads targeting femoral and sciatic nerves, delivering charge-balanced stimulation at 100 Hz for eight weeks in the PNS group. Sham devices mimicking active stimulation were used for placebo participants.

Key findings

Pain relief

- **Primary endpoint**: 60% of PNS patients achieved ≥ 50% pain relief during weeks 5-8 compared to 24% in the placebo group.

- **Overall pain reduction**: At the end of treatment (EOT), the mean reduction in pain scores was significantly greater in the PNS group (54%) than in the placebo group (26%).

Functional outcomes

- **Walking ability (6MWT)**:

  - **Baseline**: Both groups demonstrated below-average walking distances compared to matched healthy controls.

  - **At EOT**: PNS patients increased walking distance by 47%, surpassing healthy thresholds, while placebo participants experienced a 9% decline.

- **WOMAC scores**:

- The PNS group reported a 62% improvement in total WOMAC scores at EOT, significantly surpassing the 35% improvement observed in the placebo group.

Quality of life

- **PGIC ratings**:

  - 90% of PNS participants reported improvement (PGIC ≥ 1) at EOT compared to 55% in the placebo group.

  - Holistic responders (patients showing combined pain relief, functional gains, and QoL improvements) constituted 75% of the PNS group versus 35% of the placebo group at EOT.

Clinical implications

Nonopioid pain management

- **Reduced dependence on medications**: Pain relief and functional improvements achieved through PNS may minimize reliance on opioids and their associated risks.

- **Enhanced recovery protocols**: Incorporating PNS into multimodal analgesic strategies can optimize rehabilitation outcomes for patients with refractory postoperative pain.

Personalized patient care

- **Targeted therapy**: PNS provides a minimally invasive, focused approach to managing persistent pain localized to the knee.

- **Selection criteria**: Patients with severe, refractory pain following TKA who do not respond to conventional therapies represent ideal candidates for this intervention.

Broader impact on mobility and function

- **Restoring independence**: By addressing pain and stiffness, PNS facilitates improvements in mobility, enabling patients to return to daily activities.

- **Complementing physical therapy**: The functional benefits of PNS may enhance the efficacy of concurrent rehabilitation programs.

Recommendations

- **Expand PNS access**: Advocate for broader adoption of PNS as a standard nonopioid intervention for chronic postoperative pain.

- **Refine patient selection**: Develop protocols incorporating clinical, functional, and imaging criteria to identify suitable candidates for PNS.

- **Integrate with multimodal care**: Combine PNS with pharmacologic, physical therapy, and psychological interventions for comprehensive pain management.

Key takeaways

☑ Sixty-day percutaneous PNS provides significant pain relief and functional improvements in patients with persistent postoperative pain after TKA.

☑ Improvements in walking ability, WOMAC scores, and PGIC ratings underscore the therapy's broad benefits for QoL and mobility.

☑ PNS offers a promising alternative to opioids, addressing an unmet need in chronic postoperative pain management.

Additional recommended reading:

1. Goree JH, Grant SA, Dickerson DM, et al. Randomized placebo-controlled trial of 60-day percutaneous peripheral nerve stimulation treatment indicates relief of persistent postoperative pain and improved function after knee replacement. *Neuromodulation*. 2024;27:847-861.

2. Ilfeld BM, Gabriel RA, Said ET, et al. Ultrasound-guided percutaneous peripheral nerve stimulation for postoperative pain: A systematic review. *Pain Med*. 2022;23(6):1032-1042.

3. Kroin JS, Buvanendran A, Tuman KJ, et al. Novel approaches to minimizing chronic pain after total knee arthroplasty. *J Arthroplasty*. 2021;36(9):3093-3099.

Pre-implant diagnostic nerve blocks for peripheral nerve stimulation

83

Why this topic is important

Peripheral nerve stimulation (PNS) is a rapidly advancing therapy for managing chronic pain syndromes such as complex regional pain syndrome (CRPS), phantom limb pain, and postsurgical neuropathy. While widely adopted, selecting appropriate candidates for PNS remains a challenge. Pre-implant diagnostic nerve blocks are often utilized to assess potential response to therapy, mimicking practices used for medial branch blocks before radiofrequency ablation.

This study by Hoffmann et al. (2024) comprehensively evaluates the prognostic value of pre-implant nerve blocks in predicting pain relief following PNS implantation. The research challenges conventional practices by analyzing ten years of data across various PNS types and provides actionable insights into optimizing patient selection and procedural workflows.

Objectives of this update

- Determine whether pre-implant diagnostic nerve block outcomes correlate with post-implant PNS efficacy.

- Evaluate differences in short- and long-term pain relief in temporary and permanent PNS.

- Offer clinical guidance on incorporating diagnostic nerve blocks into the PNS workflow.

What is new

- **Key findings:**

  - Pre-implant diagnostic blocks do not predict long-term PNS efficacy for either temporary or permanent implants at six months.

  - Short-term correlations exist, with diagnostic block response associated with pain relief at three months for temporary PNS only.

- **Broader implications:**

  - Diagnostic blocks may delay implantation and increase healthcare costs without clear long-term prognostic value.

  - PNS efficacy may rely on distinct neuromodulatory mechanisms that differ from the localized action of nerve blocks.

Methods

- **Design**: Retrospective, multicenter analysis at Mayo Clinic facilities, including 173 patients treated with PNS from 2014 to 2023.

- **Patient stratification:**

  ○ Temporary PNS (n=112): Short-term percutaneous implants used for 60 days.

  ○ Permanent PNS (n=61): Fully implanted systems with leads targeting specific nerves.

- **Intervention**: Pre-implant nerve blocks using 1-2 mL lidocaine, followed by temporary or permanent PNS based on clinical indications.

- **Outcomes**: Pain relief (percentage reduction) at three and six months post-implant.

Results

Diagnostic block outcomes

- 77.5% of patients underwent pre-implant nerve blocks, reporting a mean pain relief of 70.1% immediately post-block.

PNS efficacy

- **Overall cohort:**

  ○ Mean pain relief at three months: 39.4%.

  ○ Mean pain relief at six months: 32.8%.

- **Temporary PNS:**

  ○ Three-month relief: 37.9% with blocks; 49.8% without blocks.

  ○ Six-month relief: 23.3% with blocks; 45.7% without blocks.

- **Permanent PNS:**

  ○ Three-month relief: 42.4% with blocks; 43.2% without blocks.

  ○ Six-month relief: 44.3% with blocks; 38.8% without blocks.

Correlations with diagnostic blocks

- Pain relief from diagnostic blocks correlated with three-month outcomes in temporary PNS.

- No significant association at six months for either temporary or permanent PNS.

Clinical implications

Revisiting the role of diagnostic blocks

- **Prognostic limitations:**

  ○ The lack of long-term predictive value challenges the routine use of diagnostic blocks for patient selection.

  ○ Patients achieving minimal relief from nerve blocks may still respond to PNS due to its central and peripheral mechanisms.

- **Short-term utility:**

  ○ While diagnostic blocks offer short-term prognostic insights for temporary PNS, their relevance diminishes over time.

- **Cost and risks:**

  ○ Eliminating unnecessary blocks could reduce procedural delays, healthcare costs, and patient exposure to risks (e.g., bleeding, infection).

Optimizing PNS workflows

- **Patient selection:**

  ○ Focus on clinical assessment and imaging to identify target nerves without over-reliance on diagnostic blocks.

- **Device considerations:**

  ○ The choice of temporary vs. permanent PNS should depend on patient-specific factors rather than block outcomes.

Recommendations

- **Limit routine diagnostic blocks:**
  - Reserve nerve blocks for cases where anatomical uncertainty exists or alternative pain generators must be ruled out.

- **Focus on short-term predictors:**
  - Use diagnostic block outcomes to guide expectations for temporary PNS but avoid using them as exclusion criteria.

- **Prioritize multidisciplinary assessment:**
  - Integrate clinical, imaging, and patient-reported outcomes for comprehensive PNS candidate evaluation.

Key takeaways

- ☑ Diagnostic nerve blocks lack long-term prognostic value for PNS efficacy, particularly for permanent implants.

- ☑ Short-term correlations suggest limited utility for predicting three-month outcomes in temporary PNS.

- ☑ Eliminating unnecessary blocks can streamline care, reduce costs, and prevent procedural delays.

- ☑ Comprehensive clinical evaluation remains essential for successful PNS implementation.

Additional recommended reading:

1. Hoffmann CM, Butler CS, Pingree MJ, et al. Is response to a pre-implant diagnostic peripheral nerve block associated with efficacy after peripheral nerve stimulation implantation? A ten-year enterprise-wide analysis. *Neuromodulation.* 2024;27:873-880.

2. Strand N, D'Souza RS, Hagedorn JM, et al. Evidence-based clinical guidelines for implantable peripheral nerve stimulation in chronic pain. *J Pain Res.* 2022;15:2483-2504.

3. Deer TR, Naidu R, Strand N, et al. The bioelectronic implications of peripheral nerve stimulation in chronic pain. *Bioelectron Med.* 2020;6:9.

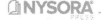

Multifidus dysfunction and restorative neurostimulation

84

Why this topic is important

Chronic low back pain (CLBP) is a prevalent and debilitating condition, affecting an estimated 568 million people globally and leading to significant healthcare costs, functional impairments, and reduced quality of life. Traditional treatment modalities often focus on structural issues, leaving many cases of nonspecific CLBP unresolved.

Emerging research highlights multifidus dysfunction-a functional condition characterized by impaired neuromuscular control and spinal instability-as a critical contributor to CLBP in certain patients. Restorative neurostimulation, a novel approach targeting the lumbar multifidus muscle, offers an innovative solution to address this etiology. This update, based on the article by Francio et al. (2023), reviews the pathophysiological basis, diagnostic strategies, and therapeutic benefits of restorative neurostimulation for CLBP, emphasizing its potential to modify disease progression and improve outcomes.

Objectives of this update

- Outline the pathophysiology of multifidus dysfunction and its contribution to CLBP.

- Discuss diagnostic methods for identifying multifidus dysfunction.

- Evaluate the role of restorative neurostimulation as a treatment modality for CLBP associated with multifidus dysfunction.

What is new

Recent advancements in understanding and managing multifidus dysfunction include:

- **Pathophysiology:** Multifidus dysfunction arises from neuromuscular control loss and arthrogenic muscle inhibition (AMI), resulting in chronic instability and pain.

- **Diagnostic clarity:** Enhanced physical examination techniques (e.g., prone instability test) and imaging methods (e.g., MRI and ultrasound) enable precise identification of dysfunction.

- **Therapeutic innovation:** Restorative neurostimulation uniquely stimulates the lumbar medial branch nerve to restore multifidus muscle function, providing long-term pain relief and functional improvements.

Pathophysiology of multifidus dysfunction

- **Role of the lumbar multifidus muscle:**
  - The multifidus contributes to spinal stability, accounting for over two-thirds of spinal stiffness.
  - Dysfunction leads to reduced spinal stiffness and functional instability, creating an environment for CLBP.
- **Neuromuscular control loss:**
  - Chronic pain alters neuromuscular feedback, resulting in poor movement patterns, muscle atrophy, and cortical reorganization.
- **Arthrogenic muscle inhibition (AMI):**
  - A spinal reflex mechanism that inhibits multifidus activation, perpetuating dysfunction and chronic pain.

Diagnosis of multifidus dysfunction

- **Clinical evaluation:**
  - Key features: Predominantly axial pain with mechanical triggers, worsened by postural challenges or minor movements (e.g., leaning or bending).
  - Physical tests:
    - **Prone instability test**: High interrater reliability ($\kappa = 0.87$) for identifying functional
    - **Aberrant movement patterns**: Indicative of neuromuscular control loss.
- **Imaging:**
  - MRI reveals multifidus atrophy and fat infiltration, while ultrasound assesses dynamic muscle activity.
  - Findings should correlate with clinical presentation, as imaging alone cannot confirm dysfunction.

Restorative neurostimulation

- **Mechanism of action:**
  - Targets the lumbar medial branch nerve, stimulating efferent pathways to elicit repetitive multifidus contractions.
  - Over time, this restores neuromuscular control, improving spinal stability and reducing pain.
- **Indications:**
  - CLBP lasting > 6 months with confirmed multifidus dysfunction.
  - Candidates often have failed conservative therapies but lack surgical indications.
- **Clinical outcomes:**
  - Studies report sustained improvements in pain and disability over 36 months.
  - Additional benefits include reduced opioid dependence and lower healthcare utilization.
- **Comparative advantages:**
  - Unlike traditional neurostimulation (e.g., spinal cord stimulation), restorative neurostimulation addresses muscle dysfunction rather than modulates pain signals.

Implications for clinical practice

Patient selection

- **Identify functional contributors:**

Multifidus dysfunction often coexists with structural issues (e.g., degenerative disc disease) but requires specific diagnostic focus.

- **Multidisciplinary evaluation:**
  - Collaboration with physical therapists and pain specialists ensures comprehensive assessment and tailored treatment planning.

Integrating restorative neurostimulation

- **Timing:**
  - ○ Consider earlier in treatment pathways, particularly for patients with significant neuromuscular control loss and limited response to other modalities.

- **Adjunctive therapies:**
  - ○ Combining restorative neurostimulation with physical therapy, biofeedback, and pain education enhances outcomes.

Recommendations

- **Prioritize functional diagnostics:**
  - ○ Confirm multifidus dysfunction using a combination of clinical tests and imaging, ensuring a functional rather than purely structural focus.

- **Embrace multidisciplinary care:**
  - ○ Collaborative approaches optimize patient selection, address comorbidities, and improve adherence to treatment protocols.

- **Monitor and refine interventions:**
  - ○ Longitudinal follow-up is essential to adjust stimulation parameters and evaluate progress.

Key takeaways

☑ Multifidus dysfunction significantly contributes to nonspecific CLBP, characterized by impaired spinal stability and neuromuscular control loss.

☑ Restorative neurostimulation offers a novel, disease-modifying approach to address this etiology, yielding sustained pain relief and functional improvements.

☑ Comprehensive diagnostic evaluation and multidisciplinary care are critical for optimizing outcomes.

☑ Early intervention with restorative neurostimulation may prevent chronicity, reduce healthcare costs, and enhance the quality of life for CLBP patients.

Additional recommended reading:

1. Francio VT, Westerhaus BD, Carayannopoulos AG, et al. Multifidus dysfunction and restorative neurostimulation: A scoping review. *Pain Med.* 2023;24(12):1341-1354.

2. Gilligan C, Volschenk W, Russo M, et al. Long-term outcomes of restorative neurostimulation for CLBP: Three-year results. *Neuromodulation.* 2023;26(1):87-98.

3. Deckers K, De Smedt K, van Buyten JP, et al. Restorative neurostimulation for chronic low back pain: Clinical results from prospective trials. *Neuromodulation.* 2015;18(6):478-486.

Long-term effectiveness of restorative neurostimulation in multifidus muscle dysfunction

85

Why this topic is important

Chronic low back pain (CLBP) remains a global healthcare challenge, especially in cases involving multifidus muscle dysfunction. Characterized by neuromuscular control deficits, multifidus dysfunction leads to mechanical spinal instability and persistent pain. Conventional treatments often fall short in addressing the underlying pathophysiology, leaving patients with limited options for sustained relief.

Restorative neurostimulation has emerged as a novel intervention targeting this specific dysfunction. By activating the multifidus muscle through the lumbar medial branch nerve, this therapy offers a rehabilitative approach, emphasizing functional recovery rather than mere symptom management. This update reviews the five-year longitudinal outcomes of restorative neurostimulation, investigated by Gilligan et al. (2024), underscoring its safety, durability, and clinical benefits.

Objectives of this update

- Explain the pathophysiology of multifidus dysfunction in CLBP.

- Evaluate the long-term outcomes of restorative neurostimulation based on clinical evidence.

- Highlight implications for integrating this therapy into chronic pain management pathways.

What is new

- **Sustained pain relief**: Significant reductions in pain intensity and disability persisted over five years.

- **Reduced opioid dependence**: Nearly half of opioid users at baseline discontinued use by year five.

Study design

- **Trial type:** Prospective, five-year longitudinal follow-up of the ReActiv8-B pivotal trial.

- **Participants:** 204 adults with refractory mechanical CLBP, confirmed multifidus dysfunction, and no indications for surgery.

- **Intervention:** Restorative neurostimulation targeting the lumbar medial branch nerve to activate multifidus muscles.

Results

Pain and disability

- **Pain intensity (VAS):** Improved from 7.3 cm at baseline to 2.4 cm at five years, with 71.8% achieving ≥ 50% pain reduction.

- **Disability (ODI):** Reduced from 39.1 points (moderate-to-severe disability) to 16.5 points (minimal disability), with 61.1% experiencing ≥ 20-point reductions.

Quality of life

- **EQ-5D-5L index:** Increased from 0.585 to 0.807, nearing population norms, reflecting enhanced health-related QoL.

Opioid use

- Among baseline opioid users, 46% discontinued use, and an additional 23% reduced their dosage.

Safety profile

- Device- or procedure-related adverse events (AEs) were rare, with no lead migrations reported.

- Device durability was validated, with no replacements required due to battery depletion over five years.

Pathophysiology of multifidus dysfunction

- **Role of multifidus muscles:**

  - The multifidus provides segmental spinal stability and protects against perturbations.

  - Dysfunction leads to mechanical instability, repeated microtrauma, and chronic nociceptive input.

- **Mechanisms of dysfunction:**

  - Neuromuscular inhibition following spinal injuries disrupts multifidus activation, perpetuating dysfunction.

Clinical implications

Patient selection

- **Eligibility criteria:**

  - Patients with refractory mechanical CLBP, multifidus dysfunction (positive prone instability test), and no surgical indications.

  - Ideal candidates exhibit pain lasting > 12 months and limited response to conservative therapies.

- **Exclusion criteria:**

  - Structural abnormalities requiring surgical correction or significant psychosocial barriers.

Integration into care pathways

- **Early intervention:**

  - Introducing restorative neurostimulation earlier may prevent progression to chronic disability.

- **Complementary therapies:**

  - Combining neurostimulation with targeted physical therapy optimizes outcomes by reinforcing neuromuscular reeducation.

- **Monitoring and follow-up:**

  - Regular assessments ensure therapy adherence and allow for stimulation parameter adjustments.

Recommendations

- **Adopt restorative neurostimulation for multifidus dysfunction:**

  ○ Its rehabilitative focus aligns with long-term functional recovery goals.

- **Standardize diagnostic protocols:**

  ○ Incorporate tests like prone instability and imaging to confirm multifidus dysfunction before treatment.

- **Expand patient access:**

  ○ Advocate for broader insurance coverage to reduce barriers to this innovative therapy.

- **Leverage real-world evidence:**

  ○ Continued longitudinal studies will refine indications and further validate benefits.

Key takeaways

☑ Restorative neurostimulation provides durable relief for refractory CLBP, targeting the root cause of multifidus dysfunction.

☑ Five-year outcomes demonstrate substantial improvements in pain, disability, and QoL, with reductions in opioid dependence.

☑ This therapy represents a paradigm shift from palliative to rehabilitative treatment in CLBP.

☑ Integration into multidisciplinary care pathways enhances effectiveness, offering hope for patients with limited options.

Additional recommended reading:

1. Gilligan C, Volschenk W, Russo M, et al. Five-year longitudinal follow-up of restorative neurostimulation shows durability of effectiveness in patients with refractory chronic low back pain associated with multifidus muscle dysfunction. *Neuromodulation.* 2024;27:930-943.

2. Deckers K, De Smedt K, van Buyten JP, et al. Restorative neurostimulation for chronic low back pain: Clinical results from prospective trials. *Neuromodulation.* 2015;18(6):478-486.

3. Russo M, Deckers K, Eldabe S, et al. Optimizing patient selection for spinal neurostimulation in low back pain. *Pain Pract.* 2018;18(7):825-834.

4. Carayannopoulos A, Johnson D, Lee D, et al. Precision Rehabilitation After Neurostimulation Implantation for Multifidus Dysfunction in Nociceptive Mechanical Chronic Low Back Pain. *Arch Rehabil Res Clin Transl.* 2024;6(2):100333. Published 2024 Mar 21.

5. Tieppo Francio V, Westerhaus BD, Carayannopoulos AG, Sayed D. Multifidus dysfunction and restorative neurostimulation: a scoping review. *Pain Med.* 2023;24(12):1341-1354.

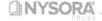

Regenerative Medicine

Regenerative medicine treatments for chronic pain

86

Why this topic is important

Chronic pain significantly impairs quality of life, with traditional treatments often failing to address the underlying pathology. Regenerative medicine, including platelet-rich plasma (PRP), mesenchymal stem cells (MSCs), and bone marrow aspirate concentrate (BMAC), offers a novel approach to managing pain through tissue repair and anti-inflammatory mechanisms. While promising, inconsistent evidence and a lack of standardized protocols have limited widespread adoption. This comprehensive consensus report by D'Souza et al. (2024) outlines current best practices and areas for further research, offering clinicians guidance in applying these innovative therapies.

Objectives of this update

- Summarize evidence-based guidelines for regenerative medicine in pain management.

- Discuss the efficacy of injectable biologics for specific chronic pain conditions.

- Highlight safety considerations and gaps in knowledge.

What is new

- **Consensus guidelines**: Developed by a multidisciplinary panel, these guidelines provide recommendations on using PRP, MSCs, and other biologics for conditions like osteoarthritis, tendinopathies, and neuropathic pain.

- **Condition-specific evidence**: PRP offers long-term benefits for lateral epicondylitis, while MSCs show potential in intervertebral disc disease and knee osteoarthritis.

- **Peri-procedural practices**: New protocols recommend holding NSAIDs before procedures to enhance biologic efficacy and using leukocyte-rich or leukocyte-poor PRP formulations based on pathology.

- **Safety and regulatory insights**: Injectable biologics are generally safe, but strict adherence to FDA guidelines for minimally manipulated products is essential.

Key findings

Evidence for specific conditions

- **Osteoarthritis (OA)**

  - PRP injections provide superior long-term pain relief and functional improvement compared to corticosteroids and hyaluronic acid for knee OA.

  - MSCs show mixed results for knee OA, with some studies demonstrating significant improvements in pain and function while others do not.

- **Tendinopathies**

  - PRP is effective for lateral epicondylitis, with better long-term outcomes than corticosteroid injections.

  - Evidence for PRP in Achilles tendinopathy and rotator cuff injuries remains inconsistent, with ongoing research needed.

- **Neuropathic pain**

  - Early evidence suggests PRP and MSCs may alleviate pain from discogenic back pain and diabetic neuropathy, but data are limited.

Mechanisms of action

- Injectable biologics release growth factors, cytokines, and extracellular vesicles that promote anti-inflammatory and regenerative processes.

- MSCs offer additional benefits by responding to the microenvironment and modulating immune responses.

Safety and tolerability

- Regenerative therapies have favorable safety profiles, with minor side effects such as transient swelling and discomfort.

- Rare complications, such as infection or inflammatory reactions, are reported with improper preparation or administration.

Challenges and limitations

- High variability in preparation methods (e.g., leukocyte-rich vs. leukocyte-poor PRP) complicates comparisons across studies.

- Regulatory constraints and lack of insurance coverage pose barriers to widespread adoption.

Clinical implications

- **Patient selection**

  - Regenerative medicine is most effective for patients with mild-to-moderate OA, refractory tendinopathies, or specific neuropathic pain conditions.

  - Pre-treatment counseling should emphasize the delayed onset of benefits compared to traditional therapies.

- **Standardization of protocols**

  - Clinicians should adhere to guidelines for PRP preparation (e.g., leukocyte-rich for tendinopathies, leukocyte-poor for joints) and administration timing.

  - Avoid peri-procedural NSAIDs and consider multimodal approaches, such as combining biologics with physical therapy.

- **Safety monitoring**

  - Use FDA-compliant products and sterile techniques to minimize risks.

  - Monitor patients for rare adverse events and educate them on expected post-procedure symptoms.

Key takeaways

☑ Regenerative medicine offers a promising, minimally invasive approach to managing chronic pain, particularly in osteoarthritis and certain tendinopathies.

☑ PRP provides long-term benefits with a strong safety profile, while MSCs show emerging potential for more complex conditions like intervertebral disc disease.

☑ Standardized protocols and adherence to regulatory guidelines are critical for optimizing outcomes and ensuring patient safety.

☑ Further high-quality research is needed to establish the various biologics' dosing, preparation, and comparative efficacy.

Additional recommended reading:

1. D'Souza RS, Her YF, Hussain N, et al. Evidence-based clinical practice guidelines on regenerative medicine treatment for chronic pain: A consensus report. *J Pain Res.* 2024;17:2951-3001. doi:10.2147/JPR.S480559.

2. Mishra A, Skrepnik N, Edwards S, et al. Platelet-rich plasma significantly improves outcomes in patients with chronic tennis elbow: A double-blind, prospective, multicenter, randomized controlled trial. *Am J Sports Med.* 2014;42(2):463-471.

3. Bennell KL, Hunter DJ, Paterson KL. Platelet-rich plasma for the management of hip and knee osteoarthritis. *Curr Rheumatol Rep.* 2017;19(5):24.

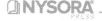

Cell transplantation and platelet-rich plasma for disc degeneration-related back and neck pain

87

Why this topic is important

Back and neck pain resulting from intervertebral disc degeneration are the leading causes of disability worldwide. Traditional treatments, including pain management and invasive surgeries like spinal fusion, fail to address the underlying degenerative processes and often result in suboptimal outcomes. Regenerative approaches, such as cell transplantation and platelet-rich plasma (PRP), offer novel therapeutic options targeting the root causes of discogenic pain. This systematic review by Schol et al. (2024) explores their efficacy, safety, and clinical significance, positioning these therapies as a potential shift in managing disc degeneration-related pain.

Objectives of this update

- Highlight the clinical significance of cell transplantation and PRP therapies for discogenic pain.

- Compare outcomes with standard interventions, such as spinal fusion.

- Evaluate the safety profiles of regenerative therapies in this context.

What is new

- **Long-term efficacy:** Both cell transplantation and PRP achieved clinically significant pain and disability reductions for up to two years, matching outcomes seen with spinal fusion.

- **Expanded patient outcomes:** PRP and cell-based treatments improved radiographic measures like disc height and hydration, suggesting a regenerative effect beyond symptom relief.

- **Favorable safety profile:** Serious adverse events were rare, with most side effects limited to transient post-injection pain or swelling.

- **Treatment comparability:** Pain and functional improvements with cell and PRP therapies were comparable, giving clinicians flexibility in treatment selection based on patient needs.

Key findings

Clinical outcomes

- **Pain relief:**
  - Cell therapy and PRP consistently reduced pain scores by an average of 3.8 points (63.8%) from baseline, meeting the minimal clinically important difference (MCID).
  - Improvements were sustained for up to 24 months in most trials.

- **Functional improvement:**
  - Disability scores (Oswestry Disability Index) decreased significantly in treated cohorts, with mean reductions aligning with MCID thresholds.

- **Radiographic changes:**
  - Treated discs exhibited better hydration and structural preservation, as indicated by improvements in magnetic resonance imaging (MRI) parameters like disc height and Pfirrmann grades.

Comparisons with spinal fusion

- Pain and disability outcomes were comparable between regenerative therapies and spinal fusion at two-year follow-up, but regenerative approaches avoided the risks of adjacent segment disease associated with surgery.

Safety

- Both PRP and cell therapies were well-tolerated, with no serious complications reported across trials.
- Mild side effects, such as injection site discomfort, resolved without intervention.

Discussion of findings

- **Mechanisms of action**
  - Cell transplantation rejuvenates degenerated discs by replenishing cell populations, promoting proteoglycan production, and modulating inflammatory pathways.

- PRP delivers growth factors and anti-inflammatory cytokines that stimulate disc repair and reduce pain sensitization.

- **Clinical implications**
  - These findings position regenerative therapies as less invasive, safer alternatives to surgery for disc degeneration, especially in patients with mild-to-moderate disease.

- **Heterogeneity in outcomes**
  - Variability in study designs, patient selection, and product preparation highlights the need for standardization in regenerative protocols.

- **Study limitations**
  - The high risk of bias in many studies and the limited number of randomized controlled trials necessitate further research to validate findings and optimize protocols.

Clinical implications

- **Patient selection**
  - Ideal candidates are those with mild-to-moderate disc degeneration confirmed by MRI and refractory to conventional therapies.

- **Procedure considerations**
  - PRP and cell transplantation require precise intradiscal injection techniques and adherence to sterile protocols.

- **Combination approaches**
  - Multimodal strategies combining regenerative therapies with physical rehabilitation may maximize long-term benefits.

- **Informed consent**
  - Patients should be counseled on the delayed onset of effects and the investigational nature of these therapies.

Key takeaways

☑ Cell transplantation and PRP significantly reduce pain and improve function in patients with discogenic back and neck pain, with sustained benefits for up to two years.

☑ Both treatments are safe, with no major adverse events reported.

☑ Outcomes rival those of spinal fusion without the associated risks and complications.

☑ Standardized protocols and additional high-quality research are needed to refine treatment approaches.

Additional recommended reading:

1. Schol J, Tamagawa S, Volleman TNE, et al. A comprehensive review of cell transplantation and platelet-rich plasma therapy for the treatment of disc degeneration-related back and neck pain. *JOR Spine*. 2024;7:e1348. doi:10.1002/jsp2.1348.

2. Wu J, Zheng Y, Wang Y, et al. The efficacy of mesenchymal stem cell therapy for intervertebral disc degeneration: A systematic review and meta-analysis. *Stem Cells Dev*. 2020;29(2):179-187.

3. Tuakli-Wosornu YA, Terry A, Boachie-Adjei K, et al. Lumbar intradiscal platelet-rich plasma (PRP) injections: A prospective, double-blind, randomized controlled study. *PM R*. 2016;8(1):1-10.

Orthobiologic injections for discogenic chronic low back pain

88

Why this topic is important

Chronic low back pain (LBP) is a leading cause of disability worldwide, often linked to degenerative disc disease (DDD). Conventional treatments, such as physical therapy, medications, and surgery, have limited success in addressing the underlying pathology, leading to ongoing patient suffering. Orthobiologic therapies, including platelet-rich plasma (PRP) and bone marrow concentrate (BMC), offer regenerative potential by targeting the biological processes of disc degeneration. Understanding the safety and efficacy of these innovative therapies is essential to advance non-surgical treatment options for LBP. Recent findings by Navani et al. (2024) provide evidence on this topic.

Objectives of this update

- Assess the safety and effectiveness of intradiscal PRP and BMC injections for discogenic LBP.

- Compare the outcomes of PRP and BMC with placebo treatments.

- Explore the clinical implications of orthobiologic therapies in managing chronic disc-related pain.

What is new

- **Superior outcomes for orthobiologic therapies**: Both PRP and BMC demonstrated significant improvements in pain (Numeric Rating Scale) and function (Oswestry Disability Index) compared to placebo, with benefits sustained over 12 months.

- **Safety confirmed**: PRP and BMC were well-tolerated, with no serious adverse events, hospitalizations, or surgical interventions reported.

- **Cross-over success**: All placebo-treated patients transitioned to PRP or BMC after 3 months due to insufficient pain relief, highlighting the efficacy of orthobiologics.

- **Comparable efficacy**: No significant differences were observed between PRP and BMC regarding pain and functional outcomes, indicating both are viable options for managing discogenic pain. treatment selection based on patient needs.

Study design

This multicenter, prospective, randomized, placebo-controlled crossover trial involved 43 patients with discogenic LBP. Participants were randomized to receive saline (placebo), PRP, or BMC injections into the affected discs, with follow-ups at 1, 3, 6, and 12 months. Placebo patients with < 50% pain relief crossed over to active treatment (PRP or BMC) after 3 months.

Outcomes

- **Primary outcomes**: Pain (Numeric Rating Scale [NRS]) and function (Oswestry Disability Index [ODI]).

- **Secondary outcomes**: Patient satisfaction (NASS questionnaire), incidence of hospitalizations, and need for surgical interventions.

Intervention protocols

- **PRP**: Leukocyte-poor PRP prepared and injected intradiscally (1-2 mL).

- **BMC**: Bone marrow-derived concentrate injected similarly into the affected discs.

Key findings

Pain and functional improvement

- **PRP and BMC efficacy**: Both treatments showed statistically significant improvements in NRS pain scores and ODI at all follow-up points compared to placebo.

  - PRP reduced NRS scores from 6.8 to 2.5 at 12 months.

  - BMC showed similar reductions, with no significant differences between the two groups.

- **Placebo limitations**: Placebo injections provided minimal short-term relief, leading to crossover in all placebo patients after 3 months.

Safety profile

- No adverse events, infections, or complications were reported in any treatment group.

- Transient low back pain at the injection site was the most commonly reported side effect, resolving within a few days.

Cross-over outcomes

- Patients crossing from placebo to active treatments experienced significant pain and functional improvements at 12 months, underscoring the efficacy of orthobiologics.

Discussion of findings

- **Comparable efficacy of PRP and BMC**

  - Both treatments were equally effective in reducing pain and disability, offering clinicians flexibility in choosing the most appropriate therapy based on availability and cost.

- **Biological mechanisms**

  - PRP promotes tissue regeneration by releasing growth factors and anti-inflammatory cytokines.

  - BMC enhances repair through mesenchymal stem cells (MSCs), which modulate immune responses and support extracellular matrix production.

- **Clinical implications**

  - These findings validate orthobiologics as a viable alternative to surgery, particularly for patients unresponsive to conservative treatments.

- **Study limitations**

  - The small sample size and single-dose protocol limit generalizability. Larger trials with extended follow-ups are needed to confirm long-term benefits.

Clinical implications

- **Indications for use**
  - Orthobiologic therapies are recommended for patients with chronic discogenic LBP who are unresponsive to standard treatments.

- **Patient education**
  - Explain the regenerative nature of these treatments, emphasizing their delayed but sustained benefits.

- **Procedure considerations**
  - Use sterile preparation techniques and adhere to evidence-based protocols for PRP and BMC administration.

- **Monitoring and follow-up**
  - Regularly assess pain, function, and patient satisfaction to ensure therapeutic efficacy and safety.

Key takeaways

☑ PRP and BMC significantly reduce pain and improve function in patients with chronic discogenic LBP, with sustained benefits over 12 months.

☑ Both treatments are safe and well-tolerated, with no reported complications.

☑ PRP and BMC show comparable efficacy, allowing clinicians to choose based on patient preferences and resource availability.

☑ Orthobiologic therapies provide a non-surgical alternative for managing degenerative disc disease, particularly in cases unresponsive to conservative care.

Additional recommended reading:

1. Navani A, Ambach M, Calodney A, et al. The safety and effectiveness of orthobiologic injections for discogenic chronic low back pain: A multicenter, prospective, randomized controlled trial. *Pain Physician.* 2024;27:E65-E77.

2. Tuakli-Wosornu YA, Terry A, Boachie-Adjei K, et al. Lumbar intradiscal platelet-rich plasma (PRP) injections: A prospective, double-blind, randomized controlled study. *PM R.* 2016;8(1):1-10.

3. Pettine KA, Suzuki RK, Sand TT, et al. Autologous bone marrow concentrate intradiscal injection for the treatment of degenerative disc disease with three-year follow-up. *Int Orthop.* 2017;41(10):2097-2103.

Subacromial injection of platelet-rich plasma or corticosteroids for rotator cuff tendinopathy

89

Why this topic is important

Rotator cuff tendinopathy, characterized by pain and functional impairment, is a common cause of shoulder-related outpatient visits. While corticosteroid injections remain widely used, their short-term effects and lack of regenerative potential limit their utility. Platelet-rich plasma (PRP), with its pro-regenerative growth factors, offers a promising alternative for long-term pain relief and functional recovery. This study by Rossi et al. (2024) compares the efficacy of PRP and corticosteroids in managing rotator cuff tendinopathy over a 12-month follow-up period.

Objectives of this update

- Assess the comparative effectiveness of PRP versus corticosteroids for pain relief and functional improvement.

- Evaluate long-term outcomes and failure rates associated with each treatment.

- Highlight the safety and tolerability of PRP in rotator cuff tendinopathy.

What is new

- **Sustained benefits of PRP**: PRP demonstrated superior pain relief and functional improvement at 12 months compared to corticosteroids, highlighting its regenerative potential for long-term outcomes.

- **Lower failure rates**: PRP was associated with significantly fewer treatment failures (12% vs. 30%), reducing the need for repeat interventions.

- **Improved sleep quality**: For the first time, PRP was shown to improve sleep disturbances associated with shoulder pain, offering a holistic benefit beyond pain and function.

- **Safety advantages**: PRP was well-tolerated with no adverse events, whereas corticosteroid injections were linked to mild allergic reactions in some patients.

Study design

This double-blind, randomized controlled trial included 100 patients aged 18-50 years diagnosed with supraspinatus tendinopathy refractory to conservative treatments. Patients received either a single subacromial injection of PRP (n = 50) or corticosteroids (n = 50). Assessments were conducted at baseline and 1, 3, 6, and 12 months post-treatment.

Interventions

- **PRP injection**: Prepared using a leukocyte-poor technique (80% platelets at 1.6× concentration).

- **Corticosteroid injection**: Included 40 mg/mL triamcinolone with lidocaine.

Outcome measures

- **Primary outcome**: Pain, measured by Visual Analog Scale (VAS).

- **Secondary outcomes** include functional scores (ASES and SANE), sleep quality (PSQI), and failure rates.

- **Failure definition**: Persistent pain (VAS > 6) requiring repeat injection by 3 months.

Key findings

Pain reduction

- **Short-term (1 month)**: Corticosteroids re-duced initial pain more than PRP (VAS 2.4 vs. 3.4).

- **Medium-term (3-6 months)**: No significant differences were observed between groups.

- **Long-term (12 months)**: PRP showed superior pain relief compared to corticosteroids (VAS 1.68 vs. 2.3).

Functional outcomes

- **ASES and SANE scores**: PRP-treated patients achieved significantly higher scores at 12 months:

  - ASES: 89.8 (PRP) vs. 78.0 (corticosteroids).

  - SANE: 89.2 (PRP) vs. 80.5 (corticosteroids).

- **PSQI**: PRP also improved sleep quality more effectively (PSQI 2.7 vs. 4.0).

Failure rates

- PRP had a significantly lower failure rate than corticosteroids (12% vs. 30%).

Safety

- No adverse events were reported in the PRP group. Three patients in the corticosteroid group experienced allergic reactions.

Discussion of findings

- **Long-term superiority of PRP**

  - PRP's ability to provide sustained pain relief and functional improvement aligns with its regenerative effects, addressing the underlying pathology rather than merely masking symptoms.

- **Corticosteroid limitations**

  - While corticosteroids offer rapid pain relief, their benefits are transient, and they cannot reverse tendon degeneration or inflammation.

- **Failure rates and treatment durability**

  - The higher failure rate in the corticosteroid group emphasizes the need for repeat interventions, increasing the cumulative treatment burden.

- **Clinical relevance**

  - These findings support PRP as a more effective long-term solution for managing rotator cuff tendinopathy, particularly in younger, active patients.

Clinical implications

- **Patient selection**

  - PRP is particularly suitable for patients with mild-to-moderate tendinopathy who prioritize long-term recovery over immediate symptom relief.

- **Treatment protocols**

  - Single subacromial PRP injections are sufficient for significant improvements, reducing the need for repeat procedures.

- **Safety profile**

  - The absence of adverse events with PRP highlights its safety, making it a favorable alternative to corticosteroids.

Key takeaways

☑ PRP improves pain, function, and sleep quality, outperforming corticosteroids at 12 months.

☑ Corticosteroids offer faster short-term relief but are associated with higher failure rates and diminished long-term efficacy.

☑ PRP's regenerative properties make it a valuable option for younger, active patients seeking durable outcomes in rotator cuff tendinopathy.

Additional recommended reading:

1. Rossi LA, Brandariz R, Gorodischer T, et al. Subacromial injection of platelet-rich plasma provides greater improvement in pain and functional outcomes compared to corticosteroids at 1-year follow-up: A double-blinded randomized controlled trial. *J Shoulder Elbow Surg.* 2024;33(12):2563-2571. doi:10.1016/j.jse.2024.06.012.

2. Hurley ET, Hannon CP, Pauzenberger L, et al. Nonoperative treatment of rotator cuff disease with platelet-rich plasma: A systematic review of randomized controlled trials. *Arthroscopy.* 2019;35(6):1584-1591. doi:10.1016/j.arthro.2018.12.028.

3. Mohamadi A, Chan JJ, Claessen FM, et al. Corticosteroid injections give small and transient pain relief in rotator cuff tendinosis: A meta-analysis. *Clin Orthop Relat Res.* 2017;475(1):232-243. doi:10.1007/s11999-016-5002-1.

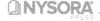

Platelet-rich plasma therapy for adhesive capsulitis

90

Why this topic is important

Adhesive capsulitis, commonly known as frozen shoulder, is a debilitating condition that impairs the functional range of motion and causes persistent pain. Affecting 2-5% of the general population, it can significantly diminish quality of life. While corticosteroid injections are a mainstay of treatment, concerns about their side effects, including tissue atrophy and cartilage damage, necessitate exploring safer, longer-lasting alternatives. Platelet-rich plasma (PRP) therapy, with its regenerative and anti-inflammatory properties, has emerged as a promising intervention. This update reviews evidence from a meta-analysis by Lin et al. (2023) comparing PRP with conventional treatments.

Objectives of this update

- Evaluate the efficacy of PRP therapy in improving range of motion, pain, and disability in adhesive capsulitis.

- Discuss the safety profile of PRP therapy.

- Provide clinical recommendations for integrating PRP into adhesive capsulitis management.

What is new

- **Sustained improvements in range of motion (ROM)**: PRP consistently outperformed corticosteroids in improving ROM, with significant gains in abduction, flexion, and external rotation at six and twelve months.

- **Long-term pain relief**: PRP achieved meaningful reductions in pain at 12 months, surpassing the minimum clinically important difference (MCID) and offering sustained benefits compared to corticosteroids.

- **Disability reduction**: PRP significantly improved disability scores, addressing functional limitations and quality of life more effectively than standard treatments.

- **Favorable safety profile**: PRP demonstrated excellent tolerability, with only minor transient side effects such as localized swelling and no serious adverse events reported.

Study design

A meta-analysis of 14 studies involving 1,139 patients assessed the effectiveness of PRP compared to corticosteroids and non-pharmacologic interventions. Outcomes were evaluated at short-term (1 month), medium-term (3 months), and long-term (6 months) follow-ups. Key measures included improvements in range of motion (ROM), pain (Visual Analog Scale [VAS]), and disability indices (e.g., Shoulder Pain and Disability Index).

- **Primary outcomes:** Changes in ROM (abduction, flexion, external rotation), pain, and disability.

- **Secondary outcomes:** Safety and adverse effects of PRP injections.

Key findings

Range of motion (ROM)

- **Short-term effects (1 month):**

  - PRP showed minimal improvements in passive ROM compared to corticosteroids.

  - No significant differences were observed between PRP and non-pharmacologic interventions like hydrodilation and ultrasound therapy.

- **Medium-term effects (3 months):**

  - PRP significantly improved passive abduction (+17.2 degrees), flexion (+17.7 degrees), and external rotation (+12.9 degrees) compared to corticosteroids.

  - Similar benefits were observed in comparison to non-pharmacologic therapies.

- **Long-term effects (6 months):**

  - Sustained gains in ROM were noted, with PRP outperforming corticosteroids and non-pharmacologic options.

Pain relief

- **Short-term:**

  - There were no significant differences in VAS scores between PRP and other interventions.

- **Medium-term:**

  - PRP reduced VAS pain scores by -8.4 points, surpassing corticosteroid and non-pharmacologic therapies, though changes were below the minimum clinically important difference (MCID) of 15.

- **Long-term:**

  - PRP achieved meaningful pain relief (VAS -19 points), exceeding the MCID and significantly outperforming other interventions.

Disability

- **Short-term:**

  - Small improvements in disability indices were observed with PRP compared to corticosteroids.

- **Medium-term:**

  - PRP showed a large effect size (standardized mean difference [SMD] -1.02) in reducing disability, significantly better than both corticosteroid and non-pharmacologic interventions.

Long-term:

  - Disability scores continued to improve, with PRP achieving a medium effect size (SMD -2.01) compared to other treatments.

Safety

- PRP was well-tolerated, with no significant adverse effects reported in the included studies.

- Minor side effects like transient pain and swelling were rare and self-limiting.

Discussion of findings

- **Advantages over corticosteroids:**

  - While corticosteroids provide short-term symptom relief, PRP offers sustained benefits in ROM, pain, and disability without the risk of tissue damage.

- **Mechanistic insights:**

  - PRP promotes tissue healing by delivering high concentrations of growth factors, reducing pro-inflammatory cytokines, and enhancing synovial repair.

- **Consistency across studies:**

  - Medium- and long-term improvements in PRP outcomes were consistent across diverse patient populations and intervention protocols, reinforcing its potential as a standard treatment for adhesive capsulitis.

- **Limitations:**

  - High heterogeneity in PRP preparation methods and injection protocols limits generalizability.

  - Few studies reported outcomes beyond 6 months, warranting further investigation into long-term efficacy.

Clinical implications

- **Indications for PRP therapy:**

  - PRP is recommended for patients with adhesive capsulitis seeking non-surgical interventions with sustained efficacy.

  - It is particularly suitable for those contraindicated for corticosteroids, such as individuals with diabetes or osteoporosis.

- **Integration into practice:**

  - Standardizing PRP preparation and injection protocols can improve the reproducibility of outcomes.

  - Combining PRP with physical therapy may further enhance functional recovery.

- **Patient counseling:**

  - Educate patients about the delayed onset of PRP benefits compared to corticosteroids, emphasizing long-term advantages.

Key takeaways

- ☑ PRP therapy offers significant medium- and long-term improvements in ROM, pain, and disability in adhesive capsulitis.

- ☑ Its safety profile makes it a viable alternative to corticosteroids, especially for patients with contraindications.

- ☑ Further research is needed to establish standardized PRP protocols and evaluate long-term outcomes beyond six months.

Additional recommended reading:

1. Lin HW, Tam KW, Liou TH, et al. Efficacy of platelet-rich plasma injection on range of motion, pain, and disability in patients with adhesive capsulitis: A systematic review and meta-analysis. *Arch Phys Med Rehabil.* 2023;104(11):2109-2122. doi:10.1016/j.apmr.2023.03.032.

2. Chang KV, Hung CY, Aliwarga F, et al. Comparative effectiveness of injection therapies in rotator cuff tendinopathy: A systematic review and meta-analysis. *Arch Phys Med Rehabil.* 2019;100(3):336-349. doi:10.1016/j.apmr.2018.03.012.

3. Hohmann E, Tetsworth K, Glatt V. Platelet-rich plasma versus corticosteroids for the treatment of plantar fasciitis: A systematic review and meta-analysis. *Am J Sports Med.* 2021;49(5):1381-1393. doi:10.1177/0363546521999155.

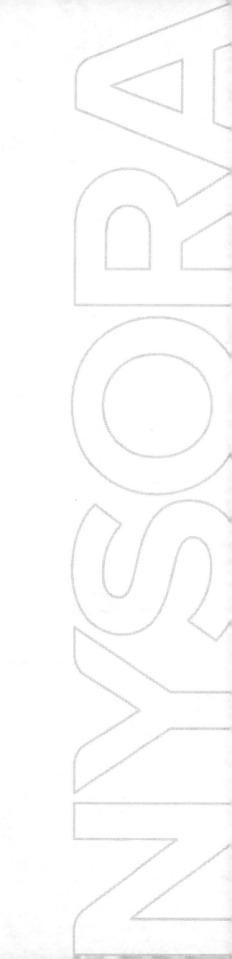

Platelet-rich plasma or corticosteroids for lateral epicondylitis

91

Why this topic is important

Lateral epicondylitis (LE), commonly referred to as tennis elbow, is a chronic overuse injury affecting the extensor tendons of the forearm. Characterized by persistent pain and functional limitations, it significantly impacts the quality of life and occupational performance. Traditional treatments, such as corticosteroid injections, provide rapid but short-lived relief and are associated with risks like tissue atrophy and tendon degeneration. Platelet-rich plasma (PRP), with its regenerative and anti-inflammatory properties, has emerged as a promising alternative for long-term pain relief and functional improvement. This review by Xu et al. (2024) compared PRP to corticosteroids for treating lateral epicondylitis.

Objectives of this update

- Compare the efficacy of PRP and corticosteroids for managing LE.

- Evaluate short- and long-term outcomes of pain, function, and safety.

- Provide clinical recommendations for integrating PRP into LE treatment protocols.

What is new

Recent evidence from a systematic review and meta-analysis by Xu et al. (2024) highlights the comparative benefits of PRP over corticosteroids for LE:

- **Long-term advantages:** PRP significantly outperformed corticosteroids in reducing pain and improving function at six months or longer, as evidenced by better VAS, DASH, and Mayo Elbow Performance scores.

- **Short-term limitations:** Corticosteroids provided better pain relief and functional improvement within the first two months, suggesting an early advantage for acute symptom management.

- **Sustained outcomes:** PRP demonstrated clinically meaningful and statistically significant benefits in long-term follow-up, with reduced failure rates and no reported tendon damage.

- **Safety profile:** Both treatments were well-tolerated, but PRP's regenerative properties avoid the tissue atrophy risks associated with corticosteroid use.

Study design

This systematic review and meta-analysis included 14 randomized controlled trials (RCTs) involving 1,020 patients with chronic LE. Participants received either PRP or corticosteroid injections, with follow-up durations ranging from 1 to 24 months. Outcomes included pain (VAS), functional scores (DASH, Mayo Elbow Performance), and adverse events.

Interventions

- **PRP injections**: Administered in varying concentrations, PRP was injected into the extensor tendon origin, typically prepared using leukocyte-rich protocols.
- **Corticosteroids**: Standard triamcinolone or methylprednisolone doses were often combined with a local anesthetic.

Outcomes

- **Primary outcomes**: Pain reduction (VAS) and functional improvement (DASH, Mayo Elbow Performance Score).
- **Secondary outcomes**: Adverse events and patient-reported treatment satisfaction.

Key findings

Pain reduction

- **Short-term (1-2 months)**: Corticosteroids were more effective, achieving a mean VAS reduction of 2.3 points compared to PRP's 1.5 points.
- **Long-term (6-12 months)**: PRP outperformed corticosteroids with sustained pain relief (mean VAS reduction of 3.8 vs. 1.2 points).

Functional improvement

- PRP significantly improved DASH and Mayo Elbow Performance scores at six months or longer, with mean score differences favoring PRP by over 10 points.
- Corticosteroids showed better functional improvement in the first two months but lacked durability, with many patients experiencing symptom recurrence by six months.

Safety

- PRP demonstrated an excellent safety profile, with minor, self-limiting side effects such as localized swelling and discomfort.
- Corticosteroids were associated with higher risks of tendon degeneration and skin atrophy.

Clinical implications

- **PRP is the preferred long-term option**
  - PRP offers durable pain relief and functional improvement, making it the ideal choice for patients seeking sustained recovery from LE.

- **Corticosteroids for acute symptoms**
  - Corticosteroids remain a valuable option for immediate relief in patients with severe, acute symptoms but should be used cautiously due to their short-lived benefits and potential adverse effects.

- **Tailored treatment strategies**
  - Combining PRP with rehabilitation protocols, such as physical therapy or eccentric exercises, may enhance long-term outcomes.

- **Patient education**
  - Patients should be informed about the delayed onset of PRP's benefits compared to corticosteroids, emphasizing its regenerative potential and long-term efficacy.

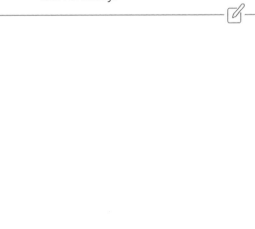

Key takeaways

☑ PRP provides superior long-term pain relief and functional improvement compared to corticosteroids for lateral epicondylitis, with sustained benefits at six months or longer.

☑ Corticosteroids offer faster symptom relief but have higher risks of adverse effects and symptom recurrence.

☑ PRP's regenerative properties and favorable safety profile position it as the treatment of choice for chronic LE.

☑ Combining PRP with physical therapy may further enhance outcomes, supporting a multimodal pproach to LE management.

Additional recommended reading:

1. Xu Y, Liang H, Wang W, et al. Platelet-rich plasma has better results for long-term functional improvement and pain relief for lateral epicondylitis compared with corticosteroids: A systematic review and meta-analysis. *Am J Sports Med.* 2024;52(1):10-21. doi:10.1177/03635465231234567.

2. Hurley ET, Lim Fat D, Moran CJ, et al. The efficacy of platelet-rich plasma for lateral epicondylitis: A systematic review and meta-analysis of randomized controlled trials. *Arthroscopy.* 2019;35(5):1461-1468. doi:10.1016/j.arthro.2018.12.011.

3. Krogh TP, Fredberg U, Stengaard-Pedersen K, et al. Corticosteroid injection therapy for lateral epicondylitis: A systematic review of randomized controlled trials. *Br J Sports Med.* 2013;47(17):1063-1070. doi:10.1136/bjsports-2012-091571.

Platelet-rich plasma injections for knee osteoarthritis

92

Why this topic is important

Knee osteoarthritis (OA) is a prevalent degenerative condition causing chronic pain, reduced mobility, and diminished quality of life. Conventional treatments such as corticosteroids or hyaluronic acid (HA) injections provide temporary symptom relief without addressing underlying degeneration. Platelet-rich plasma (PRP) therapy, leveraging biologically active growth factors to promote cartilage repair, has gained popularity as a regenerative treatment. Despite growing evidence supporting PRP, its application in knee OA remains inconsistent due to variable patient responses and a lack of standardized guidelines. This update is based on findings from the ESSKA-ICRS consensus paper (Kon et al., 2024), which evaluated over 200 clinical scenarios to develop recommendations for the appropriate use of PRP in knee OA.

Objectives of this update

- Summarize evidence-based recommendations for PRP in knee OA from the ESSKA-ICRS consensus.

- Identify patient populations most likely to benefit from PRP therapy.

- Address the appropriateness of PRP in various clinical scenarios.

What is new

- **Consensus clarity on appropriateness**: PRP is appropriate for patients aged ≤ 80 years with mild to moderate knee OA (Kellgren-Lawrence [KL] grades 0-III) after the failure of conservative or injective treatments. It is not recommended as the first treatment or for severe OA (KL grade IV).

- **Tailored recommendations**: Factors influencing PRP appropriateness include patient age, OA severity, joint effusion, and previous treatments, providing clinicians with a structured decision-making framework.

- **Treatment after failed injective approaches:** PRP showed the highest consensus (62.5%) for use after failure of corticosteroid or HA injections, underscoring its role in cases unresponsive to traditional therapies.

- **Patient-specific scenarios**: Over 200 clinical scenarios were rated, offering nuanced guidance for integrating PRP into practice.

Consensus on PRP indications

- **Appropriate use:**
  - PRP is suitable for mild-to-moderate OA (KL 0-III) after failed conservative (e.g., exercise, weight management) or injective (e.g., corticosteroid or HA) treatments.
  - Age ≤ 80 years with tibiofemoral involvement or patellofemoral OA without major effusion increases appropriateness.
- **Inappropriate use:**
  - PRP is not recommended as the first-line treatment before trying conservative measures or in patients with severe OA (KL IV).
  - Major effusion or advanced age (> 80 years) reduces the likelihood of PRP efficacy.
- **Uncertain scenarios:**
  - Scenarios involving KL IV OA, major effusion, or patellofemoral joint involvement are the most uncertain and require individualized clinical judgment.

Clinical scenarios examined

- Out of 216 scenarios, 84 (38.9%) were rated appropriate, 9 (4.2%) inappropriate, and 123 (56.9%) uncertain.
- Scenarios for mild-to-moderate OA after failed injective treatments reached the highest agreement.

Mechanisms of PRP in OA

PRP supports cartilage repair and inflammation modulation by delivering growth factors like platelet-derived growth factor (PDGF) and transforming growth factor-beta (TGF-β). These promote extracellular matrix production, reduce pro-inflammatory cytokines, and enhance joint homeostasis.

Factors influencing PRP efficacy

- **OA severity**: Mild and moderate OA (KL 0-III) respond better to PRP than advanced disease (KL IV).
- **Joint effusion**: Minor-to-mild effusion does not preclude PRP, but major effusion may dilute the injectate, reducing efficacy. Aspiration before PRP injection is recommended in such cases.
- **Patient age**: Outcomes decline in patients over 80 years, though PRP remains an option for individuals unsuitable for surgery.
- **PRP formulations**: Current evidence does not favor leukocyte-rich or leukocyte-poor PRP, but further studies are needed to refine preparation protocols.

Safety and tolerability

- PRP injections are well-tolerated, with most adverse events limited to transient pain or swelling at the injection site.
- No serious complications or infections were reported.

Clinical implications

- **PRP as a second-line therapy**
  - PRP is an effective option for patients unresponsive to HA or corticosteroids.
- **Avoidance in first-line treatment**
  - PRP should not replace conventional conservative approaches like physical therapy or weight management.

Procedure optimization
  - Joint aspiration for major effusion and sterile preparation of PRP are critical for optimizing outcomes.

- **Patient counseling**
  - Discuss delayed onset of symptom relief with patients, emphasizing the long-term benefits of PRP over symptomatic treatments.

Key takeaways

☑ PRP is appropriate for mild-to-moderate knee OA after conservative or injective treatment failure, particularly in patients aged ≤ 80 years.

☑ It is not recommended for first-line treatment or severe OA cases (KL IV).

☑ Individualized decisions are essential for uncertain scenarios, such as those involving major effusion or advanced age.

☑ PRP is a safe, effective option for managing knee OA within appropriate clinical contexts.

Additional recommended reading:

1. Kon E, de Girolamo L, Laver L, et al. Platelet-rich plasma injections for the management of knee osteoarthritis: The ESSKA-ICRS consensus. *Knee Surg Sports Traumatol Arthrosc.* 2024;32:2938-2949. doi:10.1002/ksa.12320.

2. Hurley ET, Lim Fat D, Moran CJ, et al. The efficacy of PRP for knee OA: A systematic review and meta-analysis. *Arthroscopy.* 2019;35(5):1461-1468.

3. Filardo G, Kon E, Di Matteo B, et al. PRP intra-articular knee injections for cartilage degeneration: Single vs. double spinning. *Knee Surg Sports Traumatol Arthrosc.* 2012;20:2082-2091.

Three doses or one dose of platelet-rich plasma in knee osteoarthritis

93

Why this topic is important

Knee osteoarthritis (KOA) is a progressive degenerative joint disease affecting millions worldwide. Non-surgical interventions, including intra-articular platelet-rich plasma (PRP) injections, are increasingly employed to alleviate pain and improve joint function. While PRP is known for its regenerative and anti-inflammatory properties, the optimal dosing frequency for maximum efficacy remains unclear. This systematic review and meta-analysis by Tao et al. (2023) explores whether multiple PRP injections provide superior outcomes compared to a single injection, offering evidence-based guidance for clinicians managing KOA.

Objectives of this update

- Compare the efficacy of single versus multiple PRP injections in alleviating pain and improving function in KOA patients.

- Evaluate the safety profile of multiple PRP doses.

- Discuss the clinical implications of multiple PRP injections for long-term KOA management.

What is new

- **Enhanced long-term pain relief**: Patients receiving three PRP doses reported significantly greater reductions in pain scores at 12 months compared to those receiving a single dose.

- **Improved functional outcomes**: Triple-dose therapy led to superior improvements in mobility and daily activities, as measured by WOMAC scores, sustaining benefits over a year.

- **Sustained symptom control**: Unlike single-dose PRP, three doses provided prolonged symptom relief, reducing the need for additional interventions.

- **Comparable safety profile**: Multiple PRP injections were as safe as a single dose, with only mild and transient adverse effects like injection site discomfort.

Study design

The systematic review included seven randomized controlled trials (RCTs) with 575 patients aged 20-80 treated for KOA. Patients received one, two, or three intra-articular PRP injections, with six to twelve months follow-ups. Primary outcomes included pain scores (measured via Visual Analog Scale [VAS]) and functional outcomes (Western Ontario and McMaster Universities Osteoarthritis Index [WOMAC]). Safety was assessed by analyzing adverse events (AEs).

Key findings

Pain relief

- **Triple-dose PRP:**

  - Patients receiving three PRP doses reported significantly better VAS pain scores at 12 months compared to single-dose recipients (mean improvement: -2.3 points).

  - Triple-dose therapy demonstrated sustained pain relief over the follow-up period, suggesting prolonged benefits.

- **Double-dose PRP:**

  - At the final follow-up, no significant differences were observed between the double- and single-dose groups, indicating that two doses may offer only transient benefits.

Functional outcomes

- Triple-dose PRP yielded superior improvements in WOMAC scores, with notable gains in mobility and daily activities. However, high heterogeneity across studies limited meta-analytic conclusions regarding functional outcomes.

Safety

- AEs were mild and included transient pain, swelling, and erythema at the injection site.

- No significant differences in safety profiles were observed between single, double, and triple-dose groups.

- Serious AEs, such as infections, were absent across all studies.

Mechanisms of action

PRP contains growth factors (e.g., platelet-derived growth factor, transforming growth factor-beta) that promote cartilage regeneration and reduce inflammation in KOA. Multiple doses may enhance these effects by providing sustained stimulation of cartilage repair and suppressing inflammatory mediators over a longer duration.

Discussion of findings

- **Efficacy of multiple doses:**

  - Triple-dose therapy consistently out-performed single-dose PRP in pain reduction, highlighting its potential for prolonged symptom relief.

  - The lack of significant differences between double- and single-dose groups suggests that therapeutic benefits plateau after a certain threshold of PRP administration.

- **Safety considerations:**

  - Multiple doses did not increase the risk of adverse effects, supporting their feasibility in clinical practice.

- **Study limitations:**

  - High variability in PRP preparation methods, injection intervals, and patient populations contributed to outcome heterogeneity.

  - Small sample sizes and limited long-term data restrict the generalizability of findings.

Clinical implications

- **Patient selection:**

  - Triple-dose PRP therapy may be especially beneficial for patients with moderate-to-severe KOA seeking non-surgical pain relief.

  - Individual factors, such as baseline pain intensity and activity levels, should guide treatment decisions.

- **Optimizing PRP administration:**

  - Standardizing PRP preparation protocols and dosing intervals can enhance consistency in clinical outcomes.

- **Long-term benefits:**

  - Sustained pain relief with triple-dose PRP highlights its potential to delay surgical interventions like total knee arthroplasty.

Key takeaways

☑ Triple-dose PRP therapy significantly reduces pain and improves function compared to a single dose, with sustained benefits up to 12 months.

☑ Double-dose PRP provides limited additional benefits over a single injection.

☑ Multiple PRP injections have a comparable safety profile to single-dose therapy, with only mild, transient adverse effects reported.

☑ Standardized protocols and larger RCTs are needed to refine PRP dosing strategies for KOA management.

Additional recommended reading:

1. Tao X, Aw AAL, Leeu JJ, Razak HRBA. Three doses of platelet-rich plasma therapy are more effective than one dose of platelet-rich plasma in the treatment of knee osteoarthritis: A systematic review and meta-analysis. *Arthroscopy.* 2023;39(12):2568-2576. doi:10.1016/j.arthro.2023.05.018.

2. Gormeli C, Gormeli G, Ataoglu B, et al. Multiple PRP injections are more effective than single injections and hyaluronic acid in knees with early osteoarthritis: A randomized, double-blind trial. *Knee Surg Sports Traumatol Arthrosc.* 2015;25(3):958-965. doi:10.1007/s00167-015-3737-7.

3. Filardo G, Kon E, Di Martino A, et al. Platelet-rich plasma vs hyaluronic acid to treat knee degenerative pathology: Study design and preliminary results of a randomized controlled trial. *BMC Musculoskelet Disord.* 2012;13:229. doi:10.1186/1471-2474-13-229.

Platelet-rich plasma in foot and ankle pathologies

94

Why this topic is important

Foot and ankle disorders, such as plantar fasciitis, Achilles tendinopathy, and ankle osteoarthritis, significantly impair mobility and quality of life. Platelet-rich plasma (PRP) therapy, leveraging autologous growth factors to promote healing, has gained traction in orthopedics. While PRP's regenerative potential is widely recognized, its efficacy across different foot and ankle conditions remains debated. This comprehensive review by Bagheri et al. (2023) synthesizes findings from recent studies to clarify the role of PRP in managing these pathologies.

Objectives of this update

- Assess the clinical efficacy of PRP in common foot and ankle conditions.

- Compare PRP with conventional treatments such as corticosteroids and surgery.

- Highlight challenges and recommendations for clinical application.

What is new

- **Long-term efficacy for plantar fasciitis**: PRP offers sustained pain relief and functional improvements over corticosteroids at six and twelve months, positioning it as a preferred treatment for chronic cases.

- **Variable outcomes in tendinopathies**: PRP demonstrates inconsistent benefits in Achilles tendinopathy, with midportion tendinopathy showing limited efficacy compared to eccentric exercises or shockwave therapy.

- **Enhanced outcomes for osteochondral lesions**: Combining PRP with microfracture surgery significantly improves pain and function compared to surgery alone, although evidence for isolated PRP use remains inconclusive.

- **Safety across conditions**: PRP maintains a strong safety profile, with no serious adverse events reported in studies, making it a low-risk alternative for various foot and ankle pathologies.

PRP preparation and mechanisms

PRP is derived from a patient's blood and contains platelets concentrated 2-5 times above baseline levels. It delivers growth factors, such as platelet-derived growth factor (PDGF) and vascular endothelial growth factor (VEGF), that modulate inflammation, stimulate angiogenesis, and support tissue repair. Variability in PRP preparation-leukocyte-rich (LR-PRP) versus leukocyte-poor (LP-PRP-influences its efficacy, with each variant better suited to specific conditions.

Key findings

Plantar fasciitis

- **Comparison with corticosteroids:**

  - PRP demonstrates superior long-term pain relief and functional improvement.

  - A systematic review of nine RCTs highlighted PRP's greater efficacy in reducing pain (Visual Analog Scale [VAS]) at six and twelve months compared to corticosteroids.

  - Corticosteroids carry risks like plantar fascia rupture and fat pad atrophy, making PRP a safer option for many patients.

- **Functional outcomes:**

  - PRP improved scores on the American Orthopedic Foot and Ankle Society (AOFAS) scale at six and twelve months, surpassing corticosteroids.

Achilles tendinopathy

- **Limited evidence for efficacy:**

  - Systematic reviews indicate PRP injections provide no consistent advantage over placebo or eccentric loading exercises for midportion tendinopathy.

  - VISA-A scores (Victorian Institute of Sport Assessment - Achilles) show comparable improvements with PRP and sham injections.

- **Insertional tendinopathy:**

  - PRP outcomes rival extracorporeal shock-wave therapy (ESWT), but the evidence is insufficient to recommend PRP as a primary treatment.

Achilles tendon ruptures

- Randomized controlled trials report no significant improvement in pain, function, or healing rates with PRP compared to placebo.

- PRP does not appear to enhance outcomes in nonsurgical or surgical management of acute ruptures.

Osteochondral lesions of the talus (OLT)

1. **Supplemental role:**

   - PRP combined with microfracture surgery improves function and reduces pain compared to microfracture alone.

   - Long-term benefits remain uncertain, with mixed findings on chondral regeneration observed in imaging studies.

2. **Conservative management:**

   - Intra-articular PRP injections yield modest short-term pain relief but lack robust evidence for routine use.

Hallux rigidus

- A case series suggests that PRP-enhanced arthroplasty improves pain, function, and range of motion (ROM).

- However, the lack of control groups and limited studies necessitate caution in adopting PRP for this condition.

Ankle osteoarthritis

- The only RCT comparing PRP to saline injections reported no significant differences in AOFAS scores or pain relief.

- Further studies are required to validate PRP's role in this pathology.

Clinical implications

- **Condition-specific recommendations**

  - **Strong evidence**: PRP is recommended for plantar fasciitis, especially in patients with corticosteroid contraindications.

  - **Weak evidence**: Due to inconsistent outcomes, PRP should be used cautiously for Achilles tendinopathy, tendon ruptures, and OLTs.

- **Selection of PRP type**

  - LP-PRP is preferable for inflammatory conditions like plantar fasciitis.

  - LR-PRP may be more effective for tendon disorders due to its higher inflammatory modulation capacity.

- **Integration into multimodal care**

  - Combining PRP with physical therapy or minimally invasive procedures like microfracture surgery may enhance outcomes.

- **Need for standardization**

  - Variability in PRP preparation and application techniques underscores the need for standardized protocols to optimize efficacy and comparability.

Key takeaways

☑ PRP offers significant benefits for plantar fasciitis, with superior long-term efficacy compared to corticosteroids.

☑ Evidence for PRP in Achilles tendinopathy, tendon ruptures, and OLTs is inconsistent, warranting cautious application.

☑ PRP preparation methods and dosing protocols need standardization to reduce variability in outcomes.

☑ Further high-quality trials are necessary to clarify PRP's role across various foot and ankle pathologies.

Additional recommended reading:

1. Bagheri K, Krez A, Anastasio AT, et al. The use of platelet-rich plasma in pathologies of the foot and ankle: A comprehensive review of the recent literature. *Foot Ankle Surg.* 2023;29(6):551-559. doi:10.1016/j.fas.2023.07.010.

2. Hurley ET, Hannon CP, Pauzenberger L, et al. Nonoperative treatment of rotator cuff disease with platelet-rich plasma: A systematic review of randomized controlled trials. *Arthroscopy.* 2019;35(6):1584-1591. doi:10.1016/j.arthro.2018.12.028.

3. Elghawy AS, Yausep OE, Paget DA. Platelet-rich plasma for cartilage restoration: Focus on osteochondral lesions of the talus. *J Orthop Res.* 2022;40(3):711-721.

The impact of platelet dose on the efficacy of platelet-rich plasma therapy for musculoskeletal conditions

95

Why this topic is important

Platelet-rich plasma (PRP) therapy has gained significant attention as a regenerative treatment for musculoskeletal conditions, including osteoarthritis (OA) and tendinopathies. The procedure involves injecting a concentrated solution of platelets and growth factors to stimulate healing and tissue repair. Despite its popularity, there remains substantial variability in PRP preparation methods, dosing protocols, and clinical outcomes. Identifying the optimal platelet dosage is crucial for standardizing treatment and maximizing therapeutic benefits while minimizing costs. This review by Barrigan et al. (2024) provides evidence on the effects of platelet dose on the efficacy of PRP therapy for musculoskeletal conditions.

Objectives of this update

- Evaluate the influence of platelet dosage on pain relief, functional improvement, and chondroprotection in musculoskeletal conditions.

- Examine specific dose-response relationships across conditions such as knee osteoarthritis and tendinopathies.

- Provide clinical recommendations for determining effective PRP doses in practice.

What is new

- **Dose-dependent efficacy**: High-dose PRP (> 10 billion platelets) demonstrated superior pain relief and functional improvements, particularly in knee osteoarthritis, compared to low- and medium-dose PRP.

- **Condition-specific responses**: Higher platelet doses were more effective for tendon conditions like lateral epicondylopathy, but the benefits varied for other tendinopathies, suggesting localized factors influence efficacy.

- **Sustained long-term benefits**: High-dose PRP improved pain and function for up to two years, outperforming lower doses in durability.

- **Safety across doses**: All platelet dose levels had favorable safety profiles, with no increase in adverse events, even at higher doses. alternative for various foot and ankle pathologies.

Study design

This systematic review and meta-analysis assessed 66 clinical studies investigating PRP for knee OA, hip OA, and tendinopathies. Platelet doses were categorized into three groups: low (< 5 billion), medium (5-10 billion), and high (> 10 billion). Outcomes were measured at 6 months, 1 year, and 2 years post-treatment, focusing on pain (VAS), function (WOMAC, IKDC), and patient-reported outcomes.

Inclusion criteria

- Randomized controlled trials (RCTs) and prospective cohort studies with at least 20 patients.

- Studies reporting platelet counts, injection volumes, and follow-up data.

- Excluded animal studies, meta-analyses, and studies with less than six months follow-up.

Key findings

Platelet dose and efficacy in osteoarthritis (OA)

- **Low-dose PRP (< 5 billion platelets):**

  - Showed modest improvements in WOMAC scores compared to control groups at 6 months (MD 6.93).

  - Minimal differences in VAS pain scores.

- **Medium-dose PRP (5-10 billion platelets):**

  - Significant improvements in pain (VAS MD 0.31) and function at 6 months, though benefits plateaued at 1 year.

- **High-dose PRP (> 10 billion platelets):**

  - Most effective for improving WOMAC (MD 14.8) and VAS scores (MD 1.32).

  - A consistent dose-response relationship was observed, with greater efficacy in reducing symptoms and enhancing function over time.

Tendinopathy outcomes

- Tendinopathy studies showed variable responses depending on the anatomical site and platelet dose.

- For lateral epicondylopathy, higher platelet doses (> 7 billion) correlated with superior pain relief and functional outcomes at 6 months.

- No significant improvements were noted in patellar tendinopathy when platelet doses were below 3 billion.

Safety and tolerability

- PRP was well-tolerated across studies, with transient side effects such as mild swelling, erythema, and injection site pain.

- No significant increase in adverse events was associated with higher platelet doses, underscoring the safety of dose escalation.

Discussion of findings

- **Dose-dependent efficacy**

  - High-dose PRP consistently outperformed low- and medium-dose regimens in OA, demonstrating significant pain reduction and functional improvement.

  - For tendinopathies, the benefits of higher doses varied by condition, suggesting localized factors influence PRP's efficacy.

- **Long-term benefits**

  - High-dose PRP achieved sustained symptom relief and chondroprotection for up to 2 years, particularly in knee OA.

  - Medium-dose PRP showed diminishing returns beyond 1 year, indicating that optimal dosing is critical for prolonged outcomes.

- **Clinical relevance**

  - Standardizing PRP doses is essential to reduce outcome variability and improve practice reproducibility.

Clinical implications

- **Optimizing dose selection**
  - Doses exceeding 10 billion platelets per injection provide the most reliable benefits in pain and function for knee OA.
  - Medium doses (5-10 billion) may suffice for mild cases or cost-sensitive patients.

- **Tailoring PRP therapy**
  - Consider condition-specific responses: higher doses are more effective for OA, while tendon conditions may require site-specific adjustments.

- **Implementation challenges**
  - Variability in PRP preparation and reporting underscores the need for adopting standardized protocols, such as those outlined in the Minimum Information for Biologics in Orthopedics (MIBO) guidelines.

Key takeaways

☑ High-dose PRP (>10 billion platelets) consistently provides superior pain relief and function outcomes, particularly for knee osteoarthritis.

☑ Medium-dose PRP offers moderate benefits but may not sustain long-term improvements.

☑ PRP is well-tolerated across all dose ranges, with a favorable safety profile.

☑ Standardized dosing protocols are essential to enhance clinical outcomes and comparability.

Additional recommended reading:

1. Berrigan W, Tao F, Kopcow J, et al. The effect of platelet dose on outcomes after platelet-rich plasma injections for musculoskeletal conditions: A systematic review and meta-analysis. *Curr Rev Musculoskelet Med.* 2024. doi:10.1007/s12178-024-09922-x.

2. Filardo G, Di Matteo B, Kon E, et al. Platelet-rich plasma in tendon-related disorders: Results and indications for use. Curr Pharm Biotechnol. 2012;13(7):1186-1192.

3. Andia I, Maffulli N. Platelet-rich plasma for managing pain and inflammation in osteoarthritis. *Nat Rev Rheumatol.* 2013;9(12):721-730.

Psychology, Psychiatry & Neuroscience

Psychologically based interventions for adults with chronic neuropathic pain

96

Why this topic is important

Neuropathic pain, resulting from lesions or diseases of the somatosensory nervous system, is notoriously challenging to treat with pharmacotherapy alone. Chronic neuropathic pain can lead to significant disability and emotional distress, often requiring a multidisciplinary approach. Psychologically based interventions (PBIs) such as cognitive-behavioral therapy (CBT) and mindfulness are well-established for general chronic pain but remain underexplored in neuropathic pain populations. This scoping review by Oguchi et al. (2024) identifies and synthesizes available evidence on PBIs for neuropathic pain, highlighting their potential efficacy and the need for further research.

Objectives of this update

- Summarize evidence on the types and efficacy of PBIs in chronic neuropathic pain.

- Highlight the specific outcomes targeted by these interventions.

- Assess whether current evidence supports a systematic review.

What is new

- **Broad therapeutic diversity:** The review categorized PBIs into four major approaches-CBT, mindfulness/meditation, trauma-focused therapy, and hypnosis-with CBT being the most extensively studied.

- **Positive outcomes:** Almost 50-66% of studies reported significant improvements in pain, disability, or distress following PBI.

- **Randomized controlled trails (RCT):** Thirteen RTCs were identified, but only nine had sufficient sample sizes (≥20 participants per arm), indicating room for higher-quality studies.

- **Systematic review potential:** The evidence base has grown sufficiently to justify a new systematic review.

Study design

A scoping review methodology was applied, covering 33 eligible studies published up to February 2023. Studies included adults with neuropathic pain persisting for at least three months and interventions rooted in psychological frameworks. Key outcomes were pain intensity, pain-related disability, and emotional distress.

Psychological interventions identified

- **Cognitive-behavioral approaches (48%):**
  - Standard CBT, acceptance and commitment therapy (ACT), and exposure-based therapy.
  - Delivered in individual or group settings, facilitated by trained professionals.

- **Mindfulness/meditation (30%):**
  - Standalone mindfulness, mindfulness-based stress reduction (MBSR), or mindfulness-based cognitive therapy (MBCT).
  - Often supplemented with home practice.

- **Trauma-focused therapy (12%):**
  - Eye movement desensitization and reprocessing (EMDR) and accelerated resolution therapy.

- **Hypnosis (9%):**
  - Including self-hypnosis and hypnotic cog-nitive therapy.

Neuropathic pain conditions included

- Diabetic neuropathy, spinal cord injury, phantom limb pain, postherpetic neuralgia, and peripheral neuropathies.

Key findings

Pain outcomes

- Significant reductions in pain intensity were reported in nearly half of the studies.
- CBT and mindfulness were particularly effective, with reductions sustained over three to six months.

Disability and distress outcomes

- Improvements in disability (e.g., functional limitations) were observed in most CBT-based and mindfulness interventions.
- Emotional distress (anxiety and depression) decreased significantly in trauma-focused therapies and mindfulness programs.

Delivery formats and follow-up

- Group interventions showed similar efficacy to individual formats, often delivered by interdisciplinary teams.
- Follow-up durations varied but rarely extended beyond six months, highlighting a gap in long-term data.

Safety and feasibility

- PBIs demonstrated excellent safety profiles, with high adherence and low attrition rates across studies.

Clinical implications

- **Expanding treatment options**
  - PBIs should be considered as part of multidisciplinary pain management strategies, particularly when pharmacotherapy is insufficient.

- **Tailored interventions**
  - Patient characteristics, including pain type and psychological comorbidities, should guide the selection of interventions.
  - CBT remains the most versatile approach, while mindfulness and trauma-focused therapies may suit specific conditions like phantom limb pain.

- **Integration into practice**
  - Training healthcare providers in psychological techniques can expand access to these therapies.
  - Digital platforms may offer scalable delivery methods, especially for mindfulness and CBT.

Key takeaways

☑ PBIs such as CBT and mindfulness significantly reduce pain, disability, and emotional distress in chronic neuropathic pain populations.

☑ Trauma-focused therapies and hypnosis show promise but require further validation.

☑ Current evidence justifies a systematic review to refine clinical guidelines and identify knowledge gaps.

☑ Incorporating PBIs into routine care offers a safe, effective alternative to pharmacotherapy, especially for patients with complex pain presentations.

Additional recommended reading:

1. Oguchi M, Nicholas MK, Asghari A, et al. Psychologically based interventions for adults with chronic neuropathic pain: A scoping review. *Pain Med.* 2024;25(6):400-414. doi:10.1093/pm/pnae006.

2. Eccleston C, Fisher E, Vervoort T, et al. Psychological therapies for the management of chronic neuropathic pain: An updated review. *Pain.* 2020;161(9):1918-1928.

3. McCracken LM, Vowles KE. Acceptance and commitment therapy and mindfulness for chronic pain: Model, process, and progress. *Am Psychol.* 2014;69(2):178-187.

Emotion regulation and pain catastrophizing in patients with chronic pain

97

Why this topic is important

Chronic pain affects an estimated 50 million individuals in the United States, leading to diminished quality of life, restricted daily functioning, and substantial healthcare costs. Psychological factors, particularly emotion regulation and pain catastrophizing, play pivotal roles in modulating the experience of pain. Pain catastrophizing, defined as magnifying, ruminating on, or feeling helpless about pain, has been identified as a key predictor of adverse pain outcomes. This update, based on Yuan et al. (2024), explores the dynamic relationship between emotion regulation difficulties and pain catastrophizing, emphasizing their combined impact on pain severity and interference in patients with chronic pain.

Objectives of this update

- Explore how emotion regulation difficulties contribute to pain catastrophizing and exacerbate chronic pain.

- Highlight the mediating role of pain catastrophizing in the relationship between emotion regulation and pain outcomes.

- Provide insights for developing psychosocial interventions targeting these factors.

What is new

- **The mediating role of pain catastrophizing**: The study found that pain catastrophizing fully mediates the relationship between emotion regulation difficulties and pain outcomes, with stronger effects on pain interference than severity.

- **Specific emotion regulation deficits**: Non-acceptance of negative emotions and lack of emotional awareness are key components driving pain catastrophizing.

- **Clinical prioritization**: Addressing catastrophizing alongside improving emotional regulation may benefit chronic pain management strategies significantly.

Study design

The study employed a cross-sectional design involving 120 patients with chronic non-cancer pain taking opioid medications. Participants completed self-reported measures assessing emotion regulation difficulties, pain catastrophizing, pain severity, and interference, with structural equation modeling (SEM) used to evaluate direct and indirect effects.

Measures

- **Emotion regulation**: Assessed with the Difficulties in Emotion Regulation Scale (DERS-18), which evaluates six dimensions, including emotional awareness, accep-tance, and impulsivity.

- **Pain catastrophizing**: Measured using the Pain Catastrophizing Scale (PCS), focusing on helplessness, rumination, and magnification.

- **Pain outcomes**: The Brief Pain Inventory (BPI) captured pain severity and its interference with daily activities.

Key findings

Pain catastrophizing as a mediator

- Pain catastrophizing fully mediated the relationship between emotion regulation and both pain severity and interference.

  - **Pain interference**: Indirect effects through catastrophizing explained 25% of the variance.

  - **Pain severity**: Indirect effects accounted for 14% of the variance.

Emotion regulation deficits driving catastrophizing

- Non-acceptance of negative emotions and a lack of emotional awareness were strongly associated with higher levels of catastrophizing.

- Poor emotional coping strategies were linked to a greater sense of helplessness and magnification of the pain experience.

Differential impact on pain outcomes

- Emotion regulation and catastrophizing had stronger effects on pain interference than pain severity, emphasizing their role in functional impairments and quality of life.

Mechanisms linking emotion regulation and catastrophizing

- **Emotional avoidance**: The inability to accept or manage negative emotions fosters catastrophizing, which in turn amplifies pain-related distress.

- **Cognitive focus**: Rumination of pain arises from poor emotional coping strategies, perpetuating a cycle of magnification and helplessness.

Clinical implications

- **Screening and assessment**

  - Evaluate patients for emotion regulation deficits using tools like the DERS-18 to identify at-risk individuals.

  - Include assessments for pain catastro-phizing to tailor interventions more effectively.

- **Targeted interventions**

  - Develop interventions focused on enhancing emotional awareness and acceptance.

  - Introduce cognitive-behavioral techniques to reduce rumination and helplessness.

- **Integrated care models**

  - Collaborate across disciplines to combine psychological and medical treatments, addressing pain's emotional and physical components.

Key takeaways

☑ Emotion regulation deficits, particularly non-acceptance and lack of awareness, significantly exacerbate pain through increased catastrophizing.

☑ Pain catastrophizing mediates the effects of emotion regulation on pain severity and interference, offering a clear target for intervention.

☑ Integrating emotional and cognitive strategies into chronic pain management can improve functional outcomes and reduce distress.

Additional recommended reading:

1. Yuan Y, Schreiber K, Flowers KM, et al. The relationship between emotion regulation and pain catastrophizing in patients with chronic pain. *Pain Med.* 2024;25(7):468-477. doi:10.1093/pm/pnae009.

2. Sullivan MJL, Bishop SR, Pivik J. The Pain Catastrophizing Scale: Development and validation. *Psychol Assess.* 1995;7(4):524-532.

3. McCracken LM, Vowles KE. Acceptance and Commitment Therapy and mindfulness for chronic pain: Model, process, and progress. *Am Psychol.* 2014;69(2):178-187.

The role of chronic pain acceptance in moderating suicidal cognitions

98

Why this topic is important

Chronic pain affects millions worldwide, often leading to severe psychological burdens, including heightened suicide risk. Pain severity is closely linked to perceived burdensomeness-the feeling that one is a liability to others-which is a known contributor to suicidal ideation. Despite these risks, not all individuals with chronic pain develop suicidal thoughts, highlighting the importance of identifying protective factors. This update is based on findings by Hale et al. (2023), which demonstrated that chronic pain acceptance-a psychological construct emphasizing adaptive living despite pain-could buffer the effects of pain severity on perceived burdensomeness and suicidal cognitions.

Objectives of this update

- Explore the relationships between pain severity, perceived burdensomeness, and suicidal cognitions.

- Highlight the moderating role of chronic pain acceptance in mitigating suicide risk.

- Provide actionable insights for integrating pain acceptance strategies into clinical practice.

What is new

- **Conditional indirect effects**: Chronic pain acceptance significantly moderates the pathway from pain severity to suicidal cognitions through perceived burdensomeness, reducing the impact of these relationships.

- **Attainable treatment target**: A pain acceptance score of just 0.38 standard deviations above the mean effectively buffers the association between pain severity and perceived burdensomeness, suggesting a practical intervention goal.

- **Broad clinical applicability**: Findings emphasize that even modest improvements in pain acceptance can reduce suicide risk, offering a scalable therapeutic focus.

Study design

The study included 207 participants with chronic pain (mean duration 3.8 years) recruited from military clinics. Participants completed validated self-report measures of pain severity, perceived burdensomeness, suicidal cognitions, and chronic pain acceptance. Conditional process modeling was used to test the mediated relationship between pain severity and suicidal cognitions via perceived burdensomeness, with chronic pain acceptance as a moderator.

Measures

- **Pain severity**: Assessed using the West Haven-Yale Multidimensional Pain Inventory.

- **Perceived burdensomeness**: Measured via the Interpersonal Needs Questionnaire.

- **Suicidal cognitions**: Evaluated using the Suicide Cognitions Scale, which reliably predicts suicidal behaviors.

- **Pain acceptance**: Measured with the Chronic Pain Acceptance Questionnaire.

Key findings

Indirect effects and moderation

- **Mediation pathway**: Perceived burdensomeness fully mediated the relationship between pain severity and suicidal cognitions, accounting for 89% of the total effect.

- **Moderation by pain acceptance**: Chronic pain acceptance moderated both key pathways:

  ◦ **Pain severity → Perceived burdensomeness**: The relationship weakened as pain acceptance increased and became nonsignificant at higher acceptance levels.

  ◦ **Perceived burdensomeness → Suicidal cognitions**: High pain acceptance buffered this association, reducing the impact of burdensomeness on suicidal thoughts.

Clinical significance of pain acceptance

- **Tipping point**: An acceptance score of 0.38 standard deviations above the mean mitigated the mediated relationship.

- **Incremental benefits**: Even small increases in pain acceptance significantly reduced suicide risk, underscoring the clinical value of targeting acceptance in therapy.

Sample characteristics and context

- Participants primarily included active-duty military personnel, a group at elevated suicide risk, making these findings particularly relevant to high-risk populations.

Mechanisms of protection

- **Cognitive reframing**: Pain acceptance shifts focus from reducing pain to enhancing engagement in meaningful activities, reducing feelings of helplessness and burden.

- **Social connectivity**: Acceptance facilitates participation in social and occupational roles, reducing perceived burdensomeness and thwarted belongingness, both central to suicide risk.

Implications for treatment

- **Therapeutic interventions**: Acceptance and Commitment Therapy (ACT) directly targets pain acceptance, making it a powerful tool for reducing suicidal cognitions in chronic pain patients.

- **Military and veteran care**: Given the high prevalence of chronic pain and suicide risk in military populations, integrating pain acceptance strategies into standard care is particularly critical.

Clinical implications

- **Screening and assessment**
  - Use validated measures like the Chronic Pain Acceptance Questionnaire to identify patients with low acceptance scores who may be at higher suicide risk.

- **Targeted interventions**
  - Incorporate Acceptance and Commitment Therapy or similar interventions to bolster pain acceptance.
  - Emphasize goal-setting and activity engagement as part of pain management plans.

- **Multidisciplinary approach**
  - Integrate psychological and physical therapies to address the multifaceted nature of chronic pain and its psychological sequelae.

- **Outcome monitoring**
  - Regularly evaluate changes in pain acceptance, perceived burdensomeness, and suicidal cognitions to gauge treatment effectiveness and adjust strategies as needed.

Key takeaways

☑ Perceived burdensomeness mediates the relationship between pain severity and suicidal cognitions, but chronic pain acceptance significantly buffers these effects.

☑ Even modest increases in pain acceptance can substantially reduce suicide risk, providing a practical and achievable target for intervention.

☑ Acceptance and Commitment Therapy is a highly effective approach for promoting pain acceptance and reducing psychological distress in chronic pain patients.

☑ Screening for pain acceptance and perceived burdensomeness should be integrated into suicide prevention efforts, particularly in high-risk populations like military personnel.

Additional recommended reading:

1. Hale W, Vacek S, Crabtree M, et al. The benefits of making peace with pain: Chronic pain acceptance moderates the indirect effect of perceived burdensomeness between pain severity and suicidal cognitions. *Pain Med.* 2023;24(8):993–1000. doi:10.1093/pm/pnad042.

2. McCracken LM, Vowles KE, Eccleston C. Acceptance of chronic pain: Component analysis and a revised assessment method. *Pain.* 2004;107(1-2):159-166. doi:10.1016/j.pain.2003.10.012.

3. Racine M. Chronic pain and suicide risk: A comprehensive review. *Prog Neuropsychopharmacol Biol Psychiatry.* 2018;87:269-280. doi:10.1016/j.pnpbp.2017.08.020.

Predicting quality of life in phantom limb pain using neuropsychiatric drugs and neurophysiological markers

99

Why this topic is important

Phantom limb pain (PLP) is a debilitating condition experienced by up to 80% of amputees, profoundly affecting physical, emotional, and social well-being. Managing PLP requires interventions that address not only pain but also the broader impacts on health-related quality of life (HR-QOL). While existing studies have explored predictors of HR-QOL in PLP, the role of neurophysiological metrics like intracortical facilitation (ICF) and the impact of pharmacological treatments such as gabapentin remain underexplored. This update, based on findings from Costa et al. (2024), investigates these factors to refine treatment approaches for improving HR-QOL in patients with PLP.

Objectives of this update

- Identify the impact of neurophysiological markers and medication use on HR-QOL in PLP patients.

- Discuss how findings can guide personalized treatment strategies for PLP.

- Highlight the implications of neuroplasticity in PLP management.

What is new

- **Neurophysiological marker as a predictor**: Intracortical facilitation (ICF) in the affected hemisphere was identified as a positive predictor of HR-QOL.

- **Gabapentin's paradoxical effect**: Despite its widespread use, gabapentin was associated with poorer HR-QOL, indicating the need for critical evaluation of its role in PLP management.

- **Domain-specific insights**: ICF positively influenced subdomains such as social functioning, bodily pain, and vitality, while gabapentin negatively impacted mental health, bodily pain, and vitality.

Study design

This cross-sectional analysis utilized baseline data from a previous clinical trial involving 92 lower-limb amputees with chronic PLP. Participants underwent neurophysiological evaluations using transcranial magnetic stimulation and completed HR-QOL assessments using the Short Form-36 (SF-36) questionnaire. Key predictors included ICF and medication usage, with multivariate regression analyses performed to adjust for confounders like age, sex, time since amputation, and amputation level.

Measures

- **Health-related quality of life (HR-QOL)**: Assessed via SF-36, covering eight subdomains (e.g., bodily pain, social functioning).

- **Neurophysiological data**: ICF and motor-evoked potential amplitudes measured cortical excitability.

- **Medication usage**: Focused on gabapentin, pregabalin, and antidepressants.

Key findings

HR-QOL predictors

- **Intracortical facilitation (ICF)**: Higher ICF in the affected hemisphere was associated with improved HR-QOL, with a 1-unit increase in ICF correlating to a 4.6-point rise in SF-36 scores.

- **Gabapentin use**: Linked to poorer HR-QOL, with users showing a 12.8-point decrease in SF-36 scores compared to non-users.

Subdomain-specific effects

- **ICF**: Positively influenced social functioning, bodily pain, and vitality.

- **Gabapentin**: Negatively impacted mental health, bodily pain, and vitality.

Multivariate models

- ICF improved the odds of better HR-QOL by over four times.

- Gabapentin use decreased the odds of higher HR-QOL by 76%, even after adjusting for pain severity.

Neuroplasticity and HR-QOL

- ICF reflects neuroplastic adaptation post-amputation, potentially indicating better motor control of the phantom limb and reduced cortical maladaptation.

- Interventions targeting cortical excitability, such as exercise, neuromodulation, and phantom limb control, may enhance HR-QOL by promoting favorable neuroplastic changes.

Gabapentin's paradoxical role

- While intended to manage neuropathic pain, gabapentin's potential interference with adaptive neuroplasticity may contribute to poorer HR-QOL.

- Its chronic use may blunt excitatory synaptic processes critical for recovery, underscoring the need for personalized pharmacological strategies.

Clinical implications

- **Screening and monitoring**

  - Use ICF as a potential marker to evaluate neuroplasticity and predict treatment outcomes.

  - Regularly assess the impact of medications like gabapentin on HR-QOL, considering alternatives if necessary.

- **Tailored treatments**

  - Combine neuromodulation techniques, physical therapies, and cognitive interventions to optimize ICF and reduce maladaptive cortical changes.

- **Informed prescribing practices**

  - Reassess the long-term use of gabapentin in PLP management, focusing on patient-reported outcomes and side effects.

- **Domain-specific interventions**

  - Integrate neurophysiological and psycho-logical insights by addressing vitality, social functioning, and pain perception with multimodal therapies.

Key takeaways

☑ Intracortical facilitation (ICF) is a promising neurophysiological predictor of HR-QOL in PLP patients, highlighting the importance of neuroplasticity in recovery.

☑ Gabapentin is associated with poorer HR-QOL, necessitating critical evaluation of its use in chronic PLP.

☑ Domain-specific approaches focusing on social functioning, vitality, and pain perception can improve targeted outcomes in PLP care.

☑ Combining neurophysiological markers and patient-centered therapies may refine treatment strategies, enhancing HR-QOL in PLP populations.

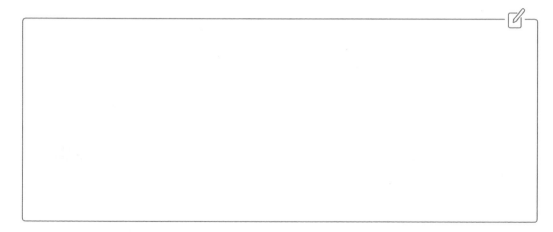

Additional recommended reading:

1. Costa V, Pacheco-Barrios K, Gianlorenço AC, et al. Neuropsychiatric drugs and a neurophysiological marker as predictors of health-related quality of life in patients with phantom limb pain. *Pain Med.* 2024;25(11):679-686. doi:10.1093/pm/pnae053.

2. Pacheco-Barrios K, Pinto CB, Saleh Velez FG, et al. Understanding intracortical excitability in phantom limb pain: A multivariate analysis. *Neurophysiol Clin.* 2021;51(2):161-173.

3. Nikolajsen L, Finnerup NB, Kramp S, et al. A randomized study of the effects of gabapentin on post-amputation pain. *Anesthesiology.* 2006;105(5):1008-1015.

Psychological factors influencing pain medication use in adolescents with chronic pain

100

Why this topic is important

Chronic pain affects up to 25% of adolescents, significantly impairing their physical, emotional, and social functioning. Pain management in this population often involves medications despite limited evidence supporting their efficacy for chronic conditions. Psychological factors, such as anxiety, depression, and pain catastrophizing, may influence medication use independently of pain intensity, potentially leading to misguided reliance on pharmacological treatments. Understanding these associations is crucial for developing interventions that target maladaptive pain coping strategies and reduce inappropriate medication use. This update is based on findings from Roman-Juan et al. (2024), which examined the role of psychological factors in predicting pain medication use among adolescents with chronic pain.

Objectives of this update

- Investigate the associations between psychological factors (anxiety, depression, and pain catastrophizing) and pain medication use in adolescents.

- Determine whether these associations persist after accounting for demographic and pain-related variables.

- Provide insights into targeted interventions for reducing medication dependence in this population.

What is new

- **Independent role of pain catastrophizing**: Pain catastrophizing emerged as the only significant predictor of pain medication use after controlling for age, sex, pain intensity, and pain interference.

- **No moderating effect of sex**: Contrary to prior studies in adults, sex did not moderate the relationship between psychological factors and medication use in adolescents.

- **High prevalence of medication use**: Over 78% of adolescents with chronic pain reported using pain medications, with nonsteroidal anti-inflammatory drugs (NSAIDs) being the most common.

Study design

This cross-sectional study included 320 adolescents aged 12-18 years with chronic pain lasting at least three months. Participants completed validated measures assessing pain characteristics, psychological factors, and medication use. Hierarchical logistic regression was used to determine the influence of anxiety, depression, and pain catastrophizing on medication use, adjusting for demographic and pain-related variables.

Measures

- **Pain severity and interference**: Assessed using the Pediatric PROMIS Pain Interference scale and a numerical rating scale for pain intensity.

- **Psychological variables**: Anxiety and depression were measured using the PROMIS Pediatric Profile Form; pain catastrophizing was assessed via the Pain Catastrophizing Scale for Children.

- **Medication use**: Adolescents reported whether they used medications such as NSAIDs, paracetamol, or others for pain management in the previous three months.

Key findings

Prevalence and types of medication use

- **High usage rates**: 78% of adolescents used pain medications, with 89% reporting NSAID use and 52% using non-opioid analgesics like paracetamol.

- **Association with pain characteristics**: Pain interference, but not pain intensity, was significantly associated with higher medication use.

Role of psychological factors

1. **Univariate analyses**: Anxiety, depression, and pain catastrophizing were significantly associated with medication use.

2. **Multivariate analyses:**

   - After adjusting for sex, age, pain intensity, and interference, only pain catastrophizing remained a significant predictor.

   - For every unit increase in pain catastrophizing score, the odds of medication use increased by 10%.

No sex moderation

- Unlike studies in adults, sex did not influence the associations between psychological factors and medication use, suggesting similar effects across male and female adolescents.

Discussion

- **Mechanisms linking catastrophizing to medication use**

   - Pain catastrophizing amplifies perceived threat and helplessness, increasing reliance on external solutions like medications.

   - Adolescents with high catastrophizing may seek medication as a coping mechanism, even when pain intensity does not warrant its use.

- **Implications for intervention**

   - Targeting pain catastrophizing through cognitive-behavioral strategies can reduce medication dependence by fostering adaptive coping skills.

   - School-based programs promoting pain education and resilience could prevent maladaptive behaviors in adolescents with chronic pain.

- **Clinical context**

   - High rates of NSAID use highlight the need for monitoring potential side effects, especially given the limited long-term safety data for adolescents.

Clinical implications

- **Screening and assessment**
  - Incorporate routine screening for pain catastrophizing in adolescents with chronic pain to identify those at risk for inappropriate medication use.
- **Non-pharmacological interventions**
  - Introduce psychological therapies, such as Cognitive Behavioral Therapy or Acceptance and Commitment Therapy, focusing on reducing catastrophizing and enhancing pain management skills.

- **Education and awareness**
  - Educate families and adolescents about the risks of over-relying on medications and the benefits of non-pharmacological strategies.

- **Multidisciplinary approach**
  - Collaborate with psychologists, physiotherapists, and educators to deliver comprehensive pain management plans.

Key takeaways

☑ Pain catastrophizing significantly predicts pain medication use in adolescents, independent of pain intensity or interference.

☑ Psychological interventions targeting catastrophizing can reduce inappropriate reliance on medications.

☑ Screening and addressing psychological factors should be integral to chronic pain management in adolescents.

☑ High rates of medication use in this population warrant close monitoring and emphasis on non-pharmacological strategies.

Additional recommended reading:

1. Roman-Juan J, Sánchez-Rodríguez E, Solé E, et al. Psychological factors and pain medication use in adolescents with chronic pain. *Pain Med.* 2024;24(10):1183-1188. doi:10.1093/pm/pnad075.

2. Fisher E, Law E, Dudeney J, et al. Psychological therapies for the management of chronic and recurrent pain in children and adolescents. *Cochrane Database Syst Rev.* 2018;(9):CD003968.

3. Eccleston C, Fisher E, Cooper TE, et al. Pharmacological interventions for chronic pain in children: An overview of systematic reviews. *Pain.* 2019;160(8):1698-1707.